OXFORD MEDICAL PUBLICATIONS

Cunningham's Manual of Practical Anatomy

Cunningham's Manual of Practical Anatomy

Fifteenth edition

G. J. ROMANES C.B.E.,
B.A., Ph.D., M.B., Ch.B., F.R.C.S.Ed., F.R.S.E., Hon. D.Sc.
Emeritus Professor of Anatomy in the University of Edinburgh

Volume One
Upper and lower limbs

Oxford New York Tokyo
OXFORD UNIVERSITY PRESS

OXFORD
UNIVERSITY PRESS

Oxford University Press is a department of the University of Oxford.
It furthers the University's objective of excellence in research, scholarship,
and education by publishing worldwide. Oxford is a registered trade mark of
Oxford University Press in the UK and in certain other countries

Published in India by
Oxford University Press
YMCA Library Building, 1 Jai Singh Road, New Delhi 110001, India

First Edition published in 1893
Fifteenth Edition 1986
Reprinted 1987 (with corrections), 1989, 1992, 1993
1996, 1997, 1998, 1999, 2000 (three times), 2001, 2002 (twice), 2003 (twice), 2004 (five times),
2005 (twice), 2006, 2007, 2009 (twice), 2010
Reprinted 2011, 2012, 2013, 2014, 2015, 2016

ISBN 978-0-19-922909-3

Printed in India by Thomson Press (India) Ltd.

Contents

Preface to the Fifteenth Edition

This edition has been extensively revised with a view to reducing the length of the text as far as possible commensurate with retaining the type of information which is necessary for an understanding of the structure of the human body at least sufficient to permit the intelligent examination of patients. In spite of this the length of the volumes has been increased principally by the introduction of many new figures which should assist the student without increasing the amount of reading matter. In addition and because shorter courses in anatomy make it increasingly difficult for the student to encompass several books, the introduction (Volume 1) has been expanded to cover a number of important items and there is a brief introduction to development in Volume 2 together with additional sections on the embryology of some of the parts of the trunk where a knowledge of development helps to clarify and is of importance to an understanding of the anatomy and of the clinically important anomalies which may arise. These sections are extensively illustrated with new diagrams intended to help the student to gain an appreciation of a complex subject with the minimal amount of extra reading matter. For the same reason and because of its importance for an appreciation of the new imaging techniques, an atlas of transverse sectional anatomy has been included together with similar scans produced by computerized tomography. These increase the sectional illustrations which have always been a feature of the book and are of particular importance to clinical work because they show the close packing of organs in a manner which is difficult to appreciate by dissection alone. Examples are also given of ultrasound and nuclear magnetic resonance scans so that the student may be aware of the type of information which modern imaging techniques can supply and which make a knowledge of sectional anatomy of increasing importance to clinical work.

The number of more conventional radiographs has also been increased to show the detail which more recent techniques (e.g. double contrast) can demonstrate and which permit the visualization of early pathological changes, e.g. in the mucosa of the gastro-intestinal tract.

The author is particularly indebted to Professor Emeritus Eric Samuel, C.B.E., for supplying most of the new radiographs and CT scans and to the Department of Medical Radiology of the University of Edinburgh for the CT scans of the head and the NMR scan of the author's cranium.

It is hoped that these many additions will increase the usefulness of the *Manuals* and help to make them a more complete text for the overburdened medical and dental students as well as serving the purposes of many of the students in the professions allied to medicine.

Edinburgh G. J. R.
January 1986

General introduction

For descriptive purposes the human body is divided into head, neck, trunk, and limbs. The trunk is subdivided into chest or thorax and belly or abdomen. The abdomen is further subdivided into abdomen proper and the pelvis. The student acquires first-hand knowledge of the relative positions of the various structures in the body by dissecting it region by region. He requires an anatomical vocabulary which must be adequate to define precisely the relevant positions of these structures, and he should have an elementary knowledge of the kinds of structures he will encounter—this is the purpose of the following introduction.

Terms of position

The body, or any detached part of it, usually lies horizontally on a table during dissection, but the dissector must remember that terms descriptive of position are always used as though the body was standing upright with the upper limbs hanging by the sides and the palms of the hands directed forwards. This is the **anatomical position. Superior** or **cephalic** (towards the head) therefore refers to the position of a part that is nearer the head of a supposedly upright body, while **inferior** means nearer the feet. **Caudal** (towards the tail) can replace inferior in the trunk.

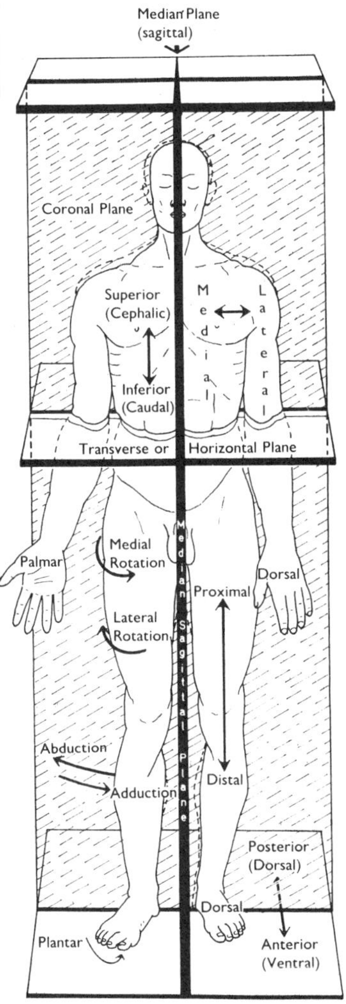

Fig. 1. A diagram illustrating the use of some anatomical terms referring to position and movement.

Anterior means nearer the front of the body and **posterior** means nearer the back. **Ventral** and **dorsal** may be used instead of anterior and posterior in the trunk and have the advantage of being appropriate also for four-legged animals (*venter*=belly; *dorsum*=back). In the hand, **dorsal** commonly replaces posterior, and **palmar** replaces anterior. In the foot, the corresponding surfaces are superior and inferior in the anatomical position, but these terms are usually replaced by **dorsal** (**dorsum** of the foot) and **plantar** (*planta*=the sole).

Median means in the middle. Thus the **median plane** is an imaginary plane that divides the body into two apparently equal halves, right and left. The **anterior** and **posterior median lines** are the edges of that plane on the front and back of the body. A structure is usually said to be median when it is bisected by the median plane. **Medial** means nearer the median plane, and **lateral** means further away from that plane. The presence of two bones, one lateral and the other medial, in the forearm (radius and ulna) and leg (fibula and tibia) allows the use of the adjectival forms of the names of these bones as synonyms of medial and lateral, i.e. **ulnar** or **radial** side in the forearm, and **tibial** or **fibular** side in the leg. The words outer and inner, or their equivalents **external** and **internal** are used only in the sense of nearer the surface or further away from it in any direction; they are not synonymous with medial and lateral. **Superficial**, meaning nearer the skin, and **deep**, meaning further from it, are the terms most usually used when direction is of no importance.

A **sagittal plane** may pass through any part of the body parallel to the median plane. A **coronal plane** is a vertical plane at right angles to the median plane.

Proximal (nearer to) and **distal** (further from) indicate the relative distances of structures from the root of that structure, e.g. the root of the limb.

Middle, or its Latin equivalent *medius*, is the usual adjective indicating a position between superior and inferior or between anterior and posterior, but **intermediate** is commonly used for a position between lateral and medial.

The terms **superolateral** and **inferomedial**, or **antero-inferior** and **postero-superior**, or any other combination of the standard terms may be used to show intermediate positions in much the same way as the points of the compass are described.

Terms of movement

All movements take place at joints and may occur in any plane, but are usually described in the sagittal and coronal planes. *Movements of the trunk in the sagittal plane* are known as **flexion** (bending anteriorly) and **extension** (straightening or bending posteriorly). *In the limbs*, flexion is applied to the movement which carries the limb anteriorly and folds it; extension to the movement which carries it posteriorly and straightens it. At the ankle, confusion is avoided by the use of the terms **plantar flexion** (movement towards the sole) and **dorsiflexion** (movement towards the dorsum). *Movements of the trunk in the coronal plane* are known as **lateral flexion**, while in the limb they are called **abduction** (movement away from the median plane) and **adduction** (movement towards the median plane). *At the wrist* abduction (**radial deviation**) refers to movement of the hand towards the radial (thumb) side and adduction (**ulnar deviation**) to the movement towards the ulnar (little finger) side. *In the fingers and toes*, abduction means the spreading apart and adduction the drawing together of the digits in the plane of the finger or toe nails. In the hand this movement is away from or towards the line of the middle finger, in the foot it is away from or towards the line of the second toe. The *thumb* lies in a plane at right angles to that of the fingers. Hence abduction and adduction, respectively, carry the thumb anteriorly and posteriorly.

Rotation is the term applied to the movement in which a part of the body is turned around its own longitudinal axis. In the limbs, lateral and medial rotation refer to the direction of movement of the anterior surface. A special movement in the forearm which appears to be rotation is the rotation of the radius only on the stationary ulna. The hand moves with the radius and is turned so that the palm faces posteriorly (**pronation**). The opposite movement (**supination**) returns the hand to the anatomical position. Because these movements can be summated to shoulder joint rotation, their range is always tested with the elbow flexed.

Structures met in dissection

The **skin** consists of a superficial layer of avascular, stratified squamous epithelium, the **epidermis**, and a deeper, vascular, dense fibrous tissue, the **dermis**, which sends small peg-like protrusions into the epidermis. These protrusions form the minute bleeding points which appear when a thin layer is cut from the surface of the skin and they help to bind the epidermis to the dermis by increasing the area of contact between them. The skin is separated from the deeper structures (muscles and bones) by two layers of fibrous tissue, the superficial and deep fasciae.

The superficial fascia

This fibrous mesh, filled with fat, connects the dermis to the underlying sheet of deep fascia, and is particularly dense in the scalp, the back of the neck, the palms of the hands, and the soles of the feet, thus binding the skin firmly to the deep fascia in these situations. In other parts of the body its looseness and elasticity allow the skin to be moved freely yet return it to its original position.

The thickness of the superficial fascia varies with the amount of fat in its meshes. It is thinnest in the eyelids, the nipples and areolae of the breasts, and in some parts of the external genital organs where there is no fat. In a well-nourished body, the **fat** in the superficial fascia rounds off the contours, but its distribution and amount varies in the sexes. The smoother outline of a woman's figure, due to the greater amount of subcutaneous fat, is a secondary sex-character. The fat is an insulating layer and accounts for the increased resistance of the female to cold in comparison with the male. This insulation is partly overcome in hot conditions by the passage of much venous blood through the large veins of the superficial fascia—veins which are contracted in cold conditions forcing the venous blood to return through the veins deep to the deep fascia. The superficial fascia also contains small arteries, lymph vessels, and nerves of the skin; a few lymph nodes are embedded in it.

Vessels

The **blood vessels** consist of **arteries, capillaries**, and **veins.**

Blood vessels

Arteries

These are tubes which convey blood from the heart to the tissues at high pressure. The largest artery in the body is the elastic aorta which begins at the heart and is approximately 2.5 cm in diameter. It gives rise to a number of branches which vary in size with the volume of tissue each has to supply.

These branch and re-branch, often unequally, and, becoming successively narrower, have progressively more muscle and less elastic tissue in their walls. The smallest arteries (<0.1 mm in diameter) are known as **arterioles.** They transmit blood into the capillaries and are entirely muscular.

The large **elastic arteries** resist a high internal pressure and their elastic recoil smooths out the intermittent pumping action of the heart to produce a continuous flow of blood. The contraction and dilatation of the **muscular arteries**, controlled by the sympathetic nervous system, determines the volume of blood distributed through each. This is essential for directing blood to the active tissues and for maintaining the blood pressure in a system which has a potential capacity greatly in excess of the circulating blood volume.

In many tissues the smaller arteries unite with one another, forming tubular loops called **anastomoses.** Such anastomoses occur especially around the joints of the limbs, in the gastrointestinal tract, at the base of the brain, and elsewhere. They are of importance in maintaining the circulation when one of the arteries to the tissue is blocked. In these circumstances the remaining arteries enlarge gradually to produce a **collateral circulation.** In some tissues the degree of anastomosis between adjacent arteries may be so slight that blockage of one cannot be compensated for by its neighbours. As a result, the piece of tissue supplied by the blocked artery dies. Such **end-arteries** are particularly important in the eye, the brain, the lungs, the kidneys, and the spleen.

Blood capillaries

These microscopic tubes form a network through which the arterioles discharge blood into the smallest tributaries of the veins. The capillary walls consist of a single layer of flattened **endothelial cells** through which substances are exchanged between the blood and the tissues. The amount of blood flowing through the capillaries (and its pressure) is determined by the degree of contraction of the arterioles, and this is related to the activity of the tissue which they supply. The capillaries may be short-circuited by **arteriovenous anastomoses.** These contractile vessels form direct communications between the smaller arteries and veins. When they open, they permit a considerable blood flow to occur without involving the capillaries. Such anastomoses occur in many parts of the body, especially in exposed parts of the skin and the walls of some organs. The increased flow which they permit produces greater heat transfer without a consequent rise in the metabolic rate of the tissue which they would supply through the capillaries. Thus they are used to promote heat loss from the skin and to warm air which is being drawn into the lungs through the cavities of the nose.

Veins

The pumping action of the heart forces the blood through the arteries and capillaries, but is mostly spent by the time the blood reaches the veins from the capillaries. The more sluggish flow of blood in the veins is aided (1) by compression from the contracting muscles surrounding them, and (2) by the fall in pressure in the thorax with each inspiration which draws venous blood into the thorax as well as air. Because of the low pressure of the veins, the flow of blood is easily retarded in them, even by light compression, though this is usually overcome because there are multiple venous pathways. The presence of **valves** in the veins prevents any tendency to backward flow of the blood. The positions of the valves in the superficial veins of the forearm can be seen as localized swellings when the veins arc distended with blood by being compressed at the elbow.

It was the demonstration of valves in the veins by Fabricius that led William Harvey (1578–1657) to discover the circulation of the blood. Whenever possible, the student should slit open the veins in the different parts of the body to see the position and structure of the valves.

Veins in the superficial fascia are dilated when heat loss is necessary. The deep veins accompany arteries as **venae comitantes**—an arrangement for heating the venous blood as it returns to the heart from cold extremities and for allowing surrounding muscles to act as venous pumps. Communications between superficial and deep veins permit the superficial veins to drain their blood into deep veins emptied by muscular contraction [Fig. 124].

Lymph vessels

These are fine tubes that contain a clear fluid called lymph. They are much more numerous in tissues adjacent to epithelial surfaces (skin and alimentary and respiratory tracts) than elsewhere and are absent from the central nervous system. **Lymph** passes into the tissues through the walls of the blood capillaries. It permeates all the tissues of the body and provides the mechanism for exchange of substances between the tissues and the blood. Lymph is drained by the lymph vessels and by absorption into the venous ends of the blood capillaries. More lymph is produced in active tissues and in inflamed tissues where the blood capillary endothelium becomes excessively permeable. This excess is usually removed by the lymph vessels but its accumulation in inflammation is one of the causes of swelling. Thus there is a continuous flow of lymph from the alimentary canal, some part of which is nearly always active, but the flow is intermittent from parts which are sometimes at rest, e.g. the limbs.

Lymph is collected from the tissues by a closed network of fine **lymph capillaries** which have a similar structure to blood capillaries but are wider and less regular in shape. They are more permeable to particulate matter and cells than blood capillaries. Small lymph vessels drain this capillary plexus. These unite to form larger lymph vessels many of which converge on each primary lymph node. The lymph passes through this node and leaves it in a vessel which usually converges on a secondary and, through it, on a tertiary lymph node as one of many similar vessels. Thus the lymph drains through a number of lymph nodes and is gathered into larger and larger lymph vessels before returning to the blood stream by entering the great veins at the root of the neck. The vessels which carry lymph to a node are called **afferent vessels;** those that carry it away from a node are **efferent lymph vessels** (*ad*=to; *ex*=from; *fero*=carry).

Lymph nodes are firm, gland-like structures which act as filters for lymph and phagocytes carried in it. Nodes vary in size from a pin-head to a large bean and are one of the two main sources of the lymphocytes of the blood (the other is the bone marrow). They tend to decrease in size with age unless enlarged by inflammation or tumour growth, but they normally are difficult to distinguish from the fat in which they lie unless coloured by particles of foreign material which are carried to them through the lymph vessels in scavenger cells (**phagocytes**), e.g. carbon in the lymph nodes of the lung. In the limbs, the lymph nodes are largest and most numerous in the **armpit** (axilla) and groin. They are usually found in groups which are linked to each other by lymph vessels.

The flow of lymph through the lymph vessels depends on the movements of the body aided by the low pressure in the great veins at the root of the neck and the presence of multiple **valves** in the lymph vessels though not in the capillary plexuses. These valves are so closely set that a distended lymph vessel has a beaded appearance.

The lymph vessels in the superficial fascia drain the capillary plexuses of the skin. They converge directly on the important groups of lymph nodes situated mainly in the axilla [Fig. 42], the groin [Fig 179], and the neck. Most lymph nodes are situated close to the deep veins along which the deep lymph vessels run.

Only the largest lymph vessels can be demonstrated by dissection, *but the great importance of this system in the reaction to infection and in the spread of disease—either bacterial infection or cancerous tumours—makes it necessary for the student to know the main routes of lymph drainage and particularly the positions of the primary lymph nodes which drain lymph from the various parts of the body.* This information makes it possible for the clinician to determine the position in the body of a pathological condition which is causing enlargement of a particular group of primary lymph nodes and to gauge the extent of the spread of the disease by the involvement of secondary or tertiary lymph nodes.

Nerves

These are whitish cords consisting of large numbers of exceedingly fine filaments (**nerve fibres**) of variable diameter, bound together in bundles by fibrous tissue. Nerves have considerable tensile strength and are capable of being stretched to a moderate degree without damage. The fibrous tissue which confers this strength forms a delicate sheath (**endoneurium**) around each nerve fibre, encloses the individual bundles of nerve fibres in a cellular and fibrous sheath (**perineurium**), and binds the bundles together with a dense fibrous layer (**epineurium**).

Each nerve fibre consists of the process of a nerve cell enclosed in a series of **sheath cells** arranged end to end. Each of these sheath cells, which surrounds a nerve cell process of larger diameter, forms one segment of a discontinuous, laminated, fatty sheath, the **myelin sheath.** Such fibres are white in colour and are called **myelinated nerve fibres.** The thinner nerve cell processes, simply enclosed in the sheath cells, are grey in colour, and are called **non-myelinated nerve fibres.**

Nerve fibres transmit messages (**nerve impulses**) either from the central nervous system to the various structures of the body or from these structures to the central nervous system. The fibres which carry impulses from the central nervous system are called **efferent.** Many of these pass to the muscles to make them contract and are therefore often called **motor nerve fibres.** Those which carry impulses to the central nervous system are known as **afferent** fibres. The information which they transmit from the skin and deeper tissues often evokes subjective sensations within the central nervous system, hence they are often called **sensory nerve fibres.** In addition to the impulses which they carry, nerve fibres also transmit substances in both directions in the nerve cell process. Thus there is a flow of materials to and from the nerve cells which give rise to these processes.

Nerves may branch or unite with one another, usually at acute angles. When they do so there is usually no division and *never* any fusion of individual nerve fibres, but only the passage of some of the nerve fibres into a separate bundle or the entry of two or more bundles into a single sheath. A similar process of rearrangement of fibres between the bundles occurs throughout the length of all nerves. Nerve fibres frequently branch extensively near their termination, though they may give off such branches (**collaterals**) at any point between adjacent sheath cells and their segments of myelin in myelinated nerve fibres. The gaps between the segments of myelin are known as **nodes.**

Nerves may be classified as: (1) **cranial nerves** which are attached to the brain and emerge from the skull or cranium; (2) **spinal nerves** which are attached to the spinal medulla and escape from the vertebral column through the intervertebral foramina.

Spinal nerves

There are 31 pairs of these, named after the groups of vertebrae between which they emerge—8 cervical, 12 thoracic, 5 lumbar, 5 sacral, and 1 coccygeal. All these nerves emerge caudal to the corresponding vertebrae except the cervical. The first seven cervical emerge cranial to the corresponding vertebrae while the eighth emerges between the seventh cervical and first thoracic vertebrae.

Spinal nerves are attached to the spinal medulla by two roots—ventral and dorsal [Fig. 2].

The **ventral root** consists of bundles of efferent fibres which arise from nerve cells in the spinal medulla. The **dorsal roots** consist of bundles of afferent fibres. These arise from a cluster of nerve cells which forms a swelling (the **spinal ganglion**) on each dorsal root. Each of these ganglion cells sends one process into the spinal nerve and another into the spinal medulla through the dorsal root.

The two roots unite at the ganglion in the intervertebral foramen to form the trunk of the spinal nerve. This short trunk, which thus consists of a mixture of efferent and afferent fibres, divides into a **ventral ramus** and a **dorsal ramus** as it emerges from the intervertebral foramen. *Do not confuse the rami (branches) into which the nerve divides with the roots by which it is formed*, for every ramus contains both efferent and afferent fibres.

The small **dorsal ramus** passes backwards into the muscle on the back of the vertebral column (erector spinae). Here it divides into lateral and medial branches which supply that muscle, and one of them sends a branch to the overlying skin. These cutaneous branches of the dorsal rami form a row of nerves on each side of the midline of the back [Fig. 28].

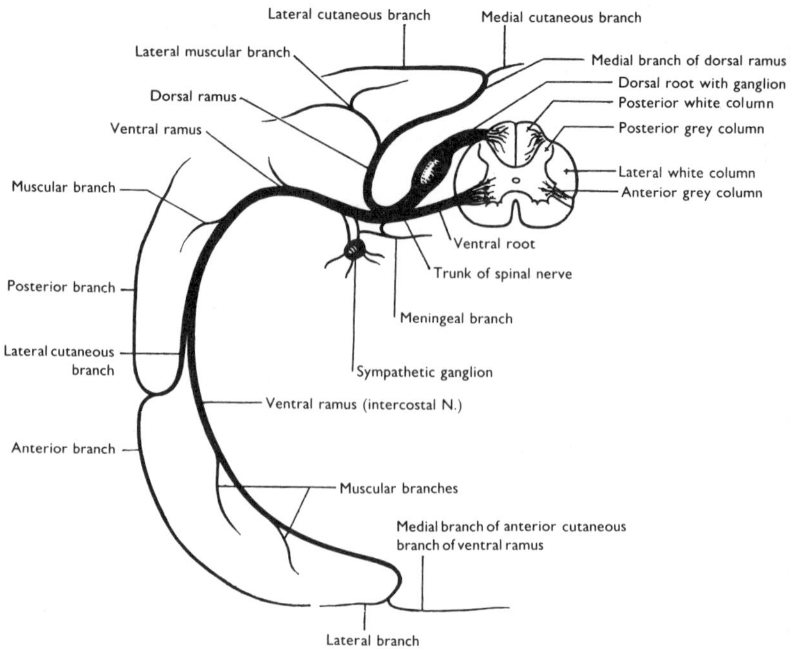

Fig. 2. Diagram of a typical spinal nerve. Note that the medial branch of the dorsal ramus is represented as distributed to skin, whilst the lateral branch terminates at a deeper level in muscle. Both branches, however, supply muscles; and in the lower half of the body it is the lateral branch that supplies skin.

The large **ventral rami** run laterally. The *thoracic* ventral rami run along the lower border of the corresponding ribs. They form the intercostal (upper eleven) and subcostal (twelfth) nerves (*costa*=a rib). Each of these ventral rami supplies the strip of muscle in which it lies and gives off lateral and anterior cutaneous branches. These, together with the cutaneous branch of the dorsal ramus, supply a strip of skin from the posterior median line to the anterior median line. This strip of skin supplied by a single spinal nerve is known as a **dermatome**, though no area of skin is supplied solely by a single spinal nerve because adjacent dermatomes overlap. The total mass of muscle supplied by a single spinal nerve is a **myotome.** Muscles receive afferent as well as efferent nerve fibres.

The ventral rami of the *cervical, lumbar, sacral*, and *coccygeal nerves* are more or less plaited together to form **nerve plexuses.** The cervical (with part of the first thoracic) form the cervical and brachial plexuses, the latter supplying most of the nerves to the upper limb. The lumbar, sacral, and coccygeal ventral rami co-operate to form plexuses of the same name. The first two are mainly concerned with the nerve supply of the lower limb.

Soon after its formation, each ventral ramus receives a slender bundle of non-myelinated nerve fibres (the **grey ramus communicans**) from the corresponding ganglion of the **sympathetic trunk.** This trunk is formed by a row of ganglia (groups of nerve cells) united by nerve fibres. It extends from the base of the skull to the coccyx, one on each side of the vertebral column. The nerve fibres in each grey ramus arise from the cells in a sympathetic trunk ganglion. The fibres which enter each ventral ramus are distributed through all its branches. They also enter every branch of each dorsal ramus by coursing back in the corresponding ventral ramus to enter the dorsal ramus. These **sympathetic nerve fibres** supply the muscles of the blood vessels and of the hairs (arrectores pilorum) and the sweat glands. Thus each spinal nerve carries efferent fibres to these involuntary structures in addition to those which it transmits from the ventral root to the muscles which are under the control of the will (voluntary).

The thoracic and upper two or three lumbar ventral roots and rami contain an additional group of fine, myelinated fibres. These leave the ventral ramus as a slender branch (**white ramus communicans**) which enters the sympathetic trunk. Within the trunk, the fibres of the white ramus communicans run longitudinally. They end on the nerve cells in the ganglia throughout the length of the sympathetic trunk. Through these nerve fibres the central nervous system controls the activity of all the nerve cells in the sympathetic trunk. Thus it can alter the secretion of sweat, the amount of blood flowing

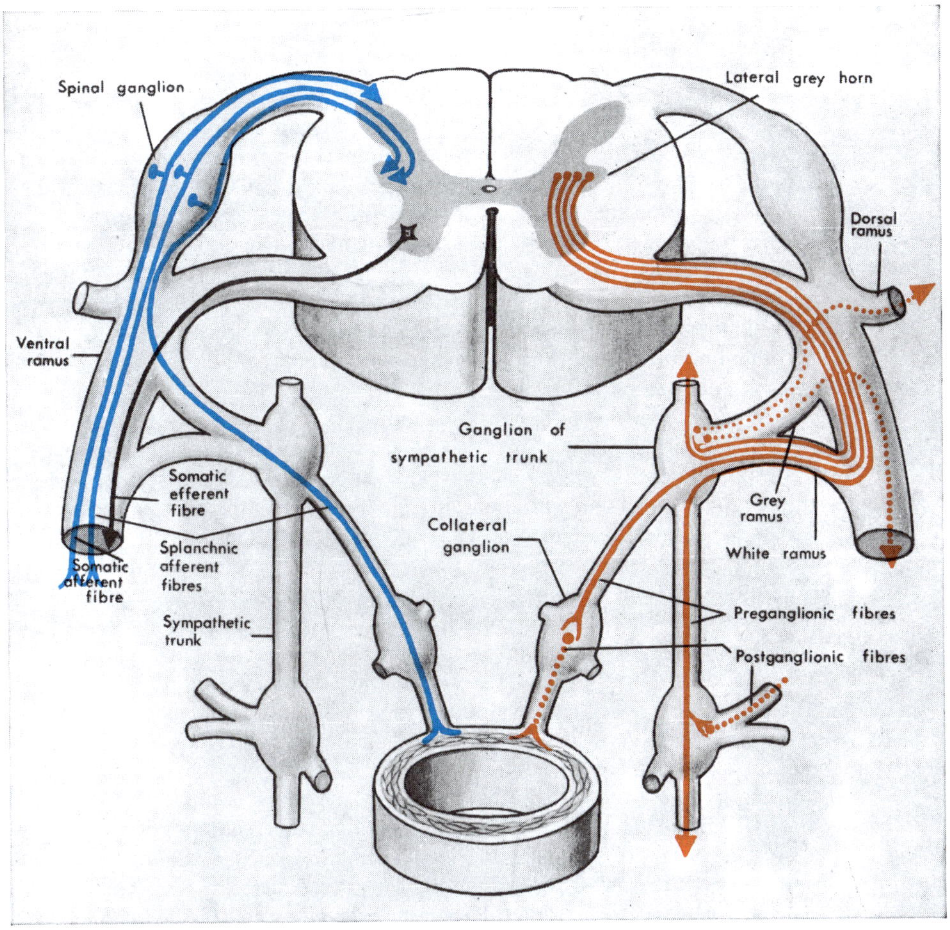

Fig. 3. Scheme showing relation of sympathetic system to spinal nerves and spinal medulla.

Sympathetic efferent fibres (pre- and postganglionic, red) are shown on the right side; a somatic efferent fibre (black) and somatic and visceral afferent fibres (blue) on the left.

through the various tissues, and the erection of hairs (goose-flesh) throughout the body by way of the processes of the sympathetic nerve cells that are distributed through the spinal (and cranial) nerves. It is important to note that the nerve fibres which connect the central nervous system to the sympathetic nervous system run only in the first thoracic to second or third lumbar spinal nerves. If all these nerves or the white rami communicantes arising from them were cut, the sympathetic nervous system would be separated from the control of the central nervous system. This would result in the loss of a number of responses which arise from afferent impulses discharging directly into the central nervous system over the dorsal roots, e.g. the sweating and dilatation of skin vessels on exposure to heat and the contraction of skin vessels with goose-flesh in response to cold or fear.

Since fibres of the white rami communicantes end in the ganglia of the sympathetic trunk, they are known as **preganglionic nerve fibres**, while those of the grey rami communicantes are known as **postganglionic nerve fibres** because they arise from the cells of the ganglia. Postganglionic fibres are present in every branch of all the nerves [see also Vol. 2, p. 165].

From the information given above, it should be clear that branches of nerves to skin (cutaneous branches) are not entirely sensory but also contain sympathetic efferents. Similarly, branches to muscles are not entirely efferent but also contain sensory fibres and sympathetic fibres. Thus the signs of nerve injury are not simply paralysis of muscle and loss of sensation, but also loss of sweating, blood-vessel control, and goose-flesh.

In addition to its grey rami communicantes to the spinal nerves and equivalent branches to the cranial nerves, the sympathetic trunk distributes postganglionic fibres through branches which pass on to the arteries of the body wall, limbs, head, and neck. Hence there is a dual route via nerves and arteries to these structures from the sympathetic trunk ganglion cells. The internal organs (viscera), including the gut tube from mouth to anus, also receive postganglionic sympathetic nerve fibres. These arise from separate sympathetic ganglia closely associated with the arteries which supply these organs and pass to these organs along the arteries as **periarterial plexuses** of nerve fibres. These visceral or **splanchnic ganglia** are brought under the control of the central nervous system through preganglionic nerve fibres which emerge in the white rami communicantes, enter the sympathetic trunk, and pass through it to the splanchnic ganglia as **splanchnic nerves.** They appear as branches of the sympathetic trunk but merely pass through it, emerging at every level to run to the splanchnic ganglia which lie at that level in early development. Subsequently, the developing viscera and their splanchnic ganglia move caudally relative to the vertebral column and to the sympathetic trunks and the nerves to which they are attached by rami communicantes so that the splanchnic nerves come to run caudally from the sympathetic trunk in the adult.

Many **afferent nerve fibres** which innervate sensory nerve endings in the viscera travel with the sympathetic nerve fibres (in rami communicantes, sympathetic trunk, splanchnic nerves, and periarterial plexuses) but have no functional connection with them, merely transmitting their sensory information directly to the central nervous system through the dorsal roots of the spinal nerves. They are, therefore, part of the general sensory system and not of the sympathetic nervous system which can be defined as *a peripheral efferent system* in that the nerve cells which innervate the effector organs, e.g. smooth muscles or glands, lie completely outside the central nervous system.

The viscera and the eye also receive an additional efferent innervation from the **parasympathetic nervous system** which is not found in other parts of the body. This consists of peripheral ganglion (nerve) cells in small groups (ganglia) or scattered in or near the viscera which they innervate and not primarily associated with the arterial supply. These parasympathetic ganglion cells usually affect the structures which they innervate, e.g. glands and smooth muscle of the gut tube, by the release of acetyl choline from the terminals of their short postganglionic fibres (**cholinergic nerve fibres**) while the sympathetic postganglionic fibres usually act by the release of noradrenaline (**adrenergic fibres**) although the sympathetic innervation of **sweat glands** is effected by the release of acetyl choline.

Like the sympathetic ganglion cells, parasympathetic ganglion cells are controlled by the central nervous system through preganglionic nerve fibres which arise from cells in the central nervous system and emerge from it in certain cranial nerves and the second, third, and fourth sacral nerves to pass to its ganglion cells. Because of this the parasympathetic nervous system is sometimes called the **craniosacral part** of the involuntary (autonomic) nervous system while the sympathetic nervous system, for the same reason, is the **thoracolumbar part** of the involuntary nervous system. These two parts together form the **autonomic nervous system** and their balanced activities control the visceral structures of the body.

The routes taken by the parasympathetic nerve fibres (pre- and postganglionic) are also routes for the distribution of **afferent visceral nerve fibres** which have no peripheral functional connection with the parasympathetic system but discharge directly into the central nervous system through the appropriate cranial and spinal nerves.

It is important to appreciate that preganglionic fibres of the autonomic nervous system **synapse** with the cells of its ganglia. Hence drugs which act on synapses will affect the central nervous control over the autonomic nervous system but will have no effect on the transmission of afferent impulses through sensory ganglia where there are *no synapses*.

Deep fascia

Deep fascia is the dense, inelastic membrane which separates the superficial fascia from the underlying structures. It is continuous with the fibres of the superficial fascia, and sends wide partitions or **septa** between the muscles from its deep surface. Thus it ensheathes the muscles and the vessels and nerves which lie between them. These sheaths form a major part of the attachment of many muscles for they pass deeply to become continuous with the fascia which surrounds and is tightly adherent to the bones (**periosteum**). The sheaths also form tunnels within which the muscles slide independently of the adjacent muscles; hence such **intermuscular septa** are well developed between adjacent muscles of different function. Such tunnels are frequently thickened to form restraining bands or **retinacula** that hold the tendons in position and form pulleys within which the tendons slide where they change direction, e.g. at wrist and ankle. When muscles contract, they tighten within their sheaths and compress the veins within and between them. Thus they form effective pumps for the return of venous blood; the dense deep fascia and septa in the legs playing a major role in the return of blood from these dependent extremities. It follows that severe wasting of the muscles of the legs or extensive damage to the deep fascia which surrounds them leads to a poor venous return with the accumulation of blood and fluid in the legs (**oedema**).

Fascia reacts readily by laying down collagen fibres parallel to any forces applied to it. Thus it becomes thickened to form (1) glistening **aponeuroses** where muscles are attached to it; (2) **retinacula** where it is stretched by tendons curving round it; (3) **ligaments** where there are forces tending to separate bones which meet at a joint.

Ligaments are strong bands of inelastic, white, fibrous tissue which connect bones, more especially at joints. Their basic structure is the same as that of tendons, but their margins are usually less well defined since they are thickenings in the general mass of fascia and are not called upon to slide on adjacent tissues as tendons do.

Muscles

The muscles are the red flesh of the body and form nearly half of its weight. They produce movement for they can be shortened (contracted) at will so as to approximate the structures to which they are attached. Each muscle has at least two attachments, one at each end, and its actions can readily be predicted from a knowledge of these attachments. However, muscles are most often used in complex groupings, even in apparently simple movements, so that paralysis of a single muscle may scarcely be noted except for a degree of weakness of the movements in which it plays a part. Most muscles, nevertheless, play a key role in some movement and a knowledge of this is of considerable importance in the diagnosis of muscle paralysis—an essential element in determining the presence, site, and degree of injury to nerves.

Muscles are used in a number of different ways. They may shorten and thus produce a movement (**concentric action**). If the tension developed by a muscle is equal to the load against which it is acting, then it helps to fix a part of the body (**isometric contraction**) as in holding the arm outstretched. If the tension developed in a muscle is less than the load acting against it, the muscle will lengthen while active, thus paying out gradually (**excentric action**) to control the speed and force of a movement in the direction opposite to that normally produced by the muscle when it is shortening, e.g. in lowering the arm to the side or a heavy weight to the floor. To test this, place your left hand on the skin over your right deltoid muscle, i.e. on the lateral surface of the shoulder below its tip. Now abduct the arm till it is horizontal and feel the deltoid muscle hardening as it contracts (concentric action). Note that as long as you hold the arm in this position the deltoid remains contracted and hard (isometric contraction). Now slowly lower the arm towards the side and the note that the deltoid remains contracted throughout the action (excentric action) but at once becomes soft, i.e. stops contracting, if, the hand is pressed down against an obstruction while the arm is being lowered.

When a muscle shortens, either or both ends may move, but it is usual to consider one end (**the origin**) as fixed while the other (**the insertion**) moves. Which attachment moves is determined by other forces in action at the time and is not an intrinsic property of the individual muscle. Thus muscles passing from the leg into the foot will move the foot when it is off the ground, but will move the leg on the foot when the foot is on the ground. Similarly, muscles which are used to pull downwards on a rope can also be used to climb up it.

The fleshy part of a muscle (the **muscle belly**) is composed of bundles of **muscle fibres** held together by fibrous tissue within which they slide during contraction. The ends of the muscle fibres are attached through the medium of fibrous tissue but there may be so little of this that the belly appears to be attached directly to bone. More usually the fibrous tissue forms long, inelastic cords (tendons or sinews) or a thin, wide sheet (**aponeurosis:** *neuron* and *nervus* originally meant sinew) depending on the arrangement of the muscle fibres. **Tendons** usually extend over the surface or into the substance of the muscle and thus increase the surface area for its attachment. Tendons also enable a muscle (a) to act at a distance, e.g. muscles of the forearm that act on the fingers; and (b) to change the direction of its pull by passing round a fibrous or bony pulley, e.g. the tendons in a flexed finger. Tendons which are compressed against a bony surface, e.g. the ball of the big toe, are frequently protected by the development in their substance of a small, cartilage-covered, **sesamoid bone** which slides on (*articulates with*) that surface and prevents occlusion of the blood supply during compression.

Where two flat sheets of muscle meet each other they usually become tendinous and these fibres interlock (interdigitate) to form a linear tendinous strip (**raphe**) uniting the muscles. Such raphes, unlike tendons or ligaments, can be stretched along their length by the separation of their interdigitating fibres even though the muscles forming them cannot be pulled apart. Thus the flat muscles of the two sides of the abdominal wall meet in the anterior median plane forming the largest raphe in the body, the linea alba, which stretches freely in extension of the trunk but holds the muscles together so that they can compress the abdomen effectively.

The *power of a muscle* depends on the number and diameter of its fibres. The number may be increased by arranging the fibres obliquely to the line of the tendon and thus packing more but shorter fibres into the same space. Thus **bipennate muscles**, e.g. dorsal interossei of the hand [Fig. 100], have fibres which converge on a central tendon like barbs of a feather, and **multipennate muscles**, e.g. deltoid and subscapularis, have a series of such intramuscular tendinous sheets. The obliquity of the fibres reduces the power of each but not proportionately to the increase in number of fibres. The diameter and power of individual muscle fibres is increased by exercise because of an increase in the number of contractile elements (myofibrils) in each fibre.

Muscle fibres can only contract to 40 per cent of their fully stretched length. Thus the short fibres of pennate muscles are more suitable where power rather than range of contraction is required. This limitation in the *range of contraction* affects all muscles and those which act over several joints may be unable to shorten sufficiently to produce the full range of movement at all of them simultaneously (**active insufficiency:** e.g. the fingers cannot be fully flexed when the wrist is also flexed). Likewise, the opposing muscles may be unable to stretch sufficiently to allow such movement to take place (**passive insufficiency**). For both these reasons it is often essential to use other muscles (called fixators or **synergists** in this type of action) to fix certain of the joints so that the others can be moved effectively, e.g. fixation of the wrist during full flexion of the fingers in clenching the fist.

Most muscles are attached to the bones close to the joints on which they act. Thus they lose mechanical advantage over the fulcrum (joint) but gain in speed and range of movement through the levers (bones) on which they act. In many cases, muscles which are clustered round a joint are less concerned with the movement of that joint than with maintaining its stability in any position. Thus they act as ligaments (extensile) of variable length and tension in place of the usual ligaments which would inevitably restrict movement, e.g. at the shoulder joint.

The manner in which a muscle acts on a joint depends on its position relative to the joint. It should be remembered, however, that any muscle may act concentrically, isometrically, or excentrically [p. 9].

In addition to the main artery and nerve which enter most limb muscles at distinct **neurovascular hila**, numerous small arteries enter elsewhere. The vessels of muscles directly attached to bone anastomose with its vessels and are of importance in the repair of fractures at these sites.

Nerves which enter muscles carry impulses which cause the muscle to contract, but they also transmit sensory impulses from the muscle and tendon to the central nervous system whereby the tension and degree of contraction may be measured. Such nerves also transmit sympathetic nerve fibres to the blood vessels in the muscle. It is possible to stimulate contraction in individual muscles by the application of appropriate electrical impulses to the skin overlying the neurovascular hilus. Such 'motor points' may be used to diagnose the state of innervation of a muscle.

Muscles are often classified in groups by the principal action which they have on a particular joint, e.g. flexors, extensors, abductors, adductors, etc. [see p. 1]. This is not a satisfactory classification because the different parts of one muscle may have very different functions, e.g. the anterior fibres of deltoid [p. 59] are flexors of the shoulder while the posterior fibres are extensors) and a single muscle may be a flexor of one joint and an extensor of another, e.g. rectus femoris [p. 146]. Unfortunately, the terms flexor and extensor are also used to designate the groups of muscles in the limbs which develop respectively from the ventral and dorsal sheets of muscle irrespective of the actual functions of the individual muscles. These 'flexor' groups of muscles are supplied by the anterior divisions of the ventral rami of the spinal nerves entering the limb and are thus differentiated from the 'extensors' which are supplied by the posterior divisions.

Bursae and synovial sheaths

Where two structures slide freely over each other, e.g. muscle, tendon, or skin over bone or fascia, the friction between them is reduced by the presence of a **bursa**. This is a closed sac lined with a smooth synovial membrane which normally secretes a small amount of glutinous fluid into the sac. When there is irritation or infection of the bursa, the secretion is increased and the bursa becomes swollen, tight, and tender, as in a bunion. Similar **synovial sheaths** enclose tendons where the range of movement is considerable, e.g. the tendons sliding in the fingers [Fig. 77].

Joints

A joint is present where two bones come together whether there is movement between them or not. *Joints without movement* are those where

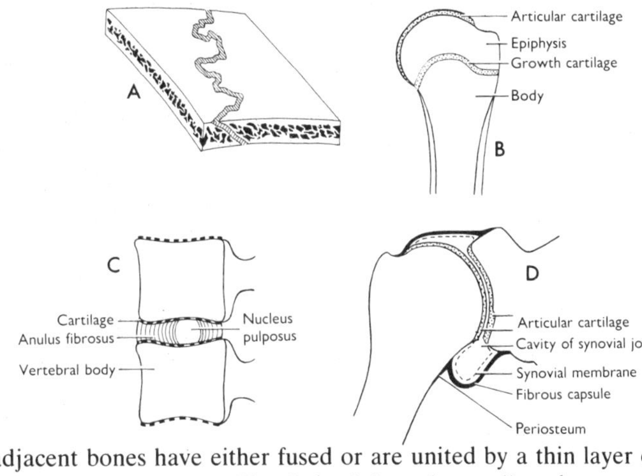

Fig. 4. Diagrams to show four types of joints.
A. A suture between two skull bones. In this the bones are firmly bound together by a thin layer of dense fibrous tissue which does not allow movement, but permits the addition of new bone to the adjacent surfaces, thus assisting in growth of the bones.
B. Section through the proximal end of the growing humerus; the two parts of the bone, epiphysis and body, are joined by a layer of firm, growing cartilage. No movement is possible, the joint is a temporary one concerned with the growth in length of the body, and is called a synchondrosis. When growth ceases this joint is replaced by bone, forming a synostosis, a fate which also overtakes sutures.
C. Section through an intervertebral disc joining two vertebral bodies. A thick laminated fibrous sheath (anulus fibrosus) of great strength encloses a pulpy central mass (nucleus pulposus). The flexibility of the disc allows limited movement between the vertebrae, the range increasing with the thickness of the disc.
D. Section through the shoulder joint to show the parts of a synovial joint. Such joints have a cavity which extends between the ends of the bones which are covered with slippery, hyaline cartilage, and the whole is enclosed in a fibrous sheath or capsule lined with synovial membrane. This type of joint allows the maximum freedom of movement which is limited only by the shape of the articular surfaces, and the length and strength of the fibrous capsule and ligaments.

the adjacent bones have either fused or are united by a thin layer of dense fibrous tissue or cartilage. The first of these is usually a late stage in the development of one of the other two [Fig. 4 (A), (B)]. *Joints with a small amount of movement* are those where the bones are held together with a thick layer of fibrous tissue or fibrocartilage, e.g. the discs between the bodies of the vertebrae. *Joints with the maximum amount of movement* are **synovial joints.** Here the bearing surfaces of the bones are covered with firm, slippery, **articular cartilage** and slide on each other in a narrow cavity containing lubricant **synovial fluid.** Outside the cavity, the bones are held together by a tubular sheath of fibrous tissue (the **fibrous capsule** or **fibrous membrane)** which is a continuation of the periosteum between the two bones and is sufficiently loose to permit movement. It may be strengthened in certain situations where it will not interfere with movement or where it is required to limit such movement. Such strengthenings form some of the **ligaments of the joint** and are usually named from their position, e.g. radial and ulnar collateral ligaments of the elbow joint. Thus, in the hinge-like elbow joint, the anterior and posterior parts of the capsule are lax, while the collateral ligaments lie approximately as radii of the arc of movement and thus remain tight in all positions, effectively holding the bones together.

All the structures which immediately surround the joint cavity, except the articular cartilage, are separated from that cavity by **synovial membrane.**

The bones which articulate at synovial joints are of many different shapes to permit particular movements while preventing others. Thus the surfaces of the bones may be flat (**plane joint**) permitting only slight gliding movements e.g. in some of the joints between the bones of the hand and foot) and giving some resilience to an otherwise rigid structure. More usually the surfaces of the articulating bones are curved. The greatest number of different movements is obtained from the **ball-and-socket** type of joint, e.g. shoulder and hip joints, in which the spheroidal end of one bone fits into a cup-shaped recess in the other. Where the cup is shallow, e.g. the shoulder joint, the range of each movement is great but the intrinsic strength and stability is decreased in comparison with joints having a deep cup, e.g. the hip joint. Three types of joints allow movements in only two directions at right angles to each other—usually flexion/extension and abduction/adduction—but permit little or no rotation: (1) **condyloid joints**, e.g. the joints of the knuckles where the fingers meet the hand, have a bony configuration similar to the ball-and-socket type of joint but rotation is limited by the ligaments; (2) the **ellipsoid joint**, e.g. the wrist joint, is also like a ball-and-socket joint, but the radius of curvature of the surfaces is long in one direction and short at right angles to this—like a sausage fitted into a curved trough; (3) in the **saddle** type of joint, e.g. the carpometacarpal joint at the base of the thumb, the articular suface of the bone is concave in one direction and convex at right angles to this—the convex surface of one bone fitting the concave surface of the other.

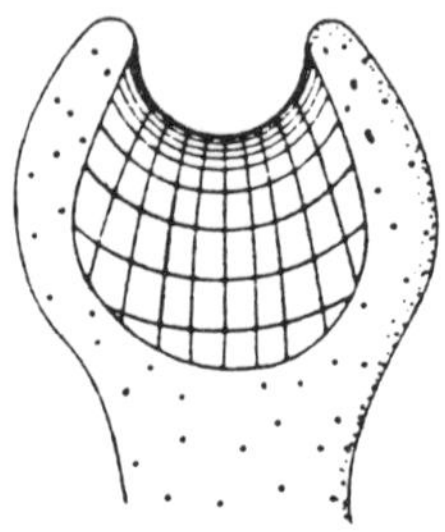

Fig. 5. A diagram to show the shape of the articular surface of a bone taking part in a saddle joint.

Two types of joints give movement around only one axis: (1) in **hinge joints**, e.g. the interphalangeal joints of the fingers and the ankle joint, the configuration of the bones and the arrangement of the ligaments prevent movements except those of flexion and extension; (2) in the **pivot joint**, e.g. the proximal radio-ulnar joint, a cylindrical bone lies in a ring formed by bone and ligament, the one element rotating on the other much as a door swings on the pin of a hinge. At such a joint only rotation is possible.

It should be remembered that many joints are used to achieve a single movement and that their combined actions are necessary for normal activity. It follows that damage to one joint may interfere with many movements.

In joints where considerable movement is required in many directions, e.g. the shoulder, the fibrous capsule is thin and lax throughout, being supported by muscles which closely surround the joint and are able to be stretched to the required degree, but can be tightened to support the joint in any position. Where extreme mobility in one direction is required, e.g. at the knuckles or knee, the appropriate part of the fibrous capsule is entirely replaced by the tendon of a muscle.

The stability and complexity of movement at a joint are sometimes increased by placing a **disc** of fibrous tissue between the bones. This may have different curvatures on its two surfaces and thus convert a single joint into two, each having a different type of movement. It may also act as a shock absorber within the joint, or assist with the spreading of the synovial fluid between the bearing surfaces of joints which are under considerable pressure, e.g. the knee joint.

Bones

Bone is a living, vascular form of connective tissue in which the intercellular substance consists of dense, white fibrous tissue embedded in a hard calcium phosphate complex. The fibrous tissue imparts resilience to the bone, while the calcium salts resist compression forces.

Bone occurs in two forms. (1) **Compact bone** is dense and forms the tubular bodies of the long bones filled with yellow (fatty) bone marrow. It consists of longitudinal, laminated tubules of bone (**Haversian systems**), each of which transmits a capillary to maintain the bone cells lying in spaces (**lacunae**) between the laminae. The tubules are bound together by interstitial lamellae (remnants of partially replaced Haversian systems) and the capillaries within them arise at intervals from transversely placed arterioles which pierce the bone mainly from the marrow cavity. When compact bone is broken, the capillaries are torn and blocked by clotting. Thus the bone on either side of the fracture dies back to the next undamaged transverse vessel even in a

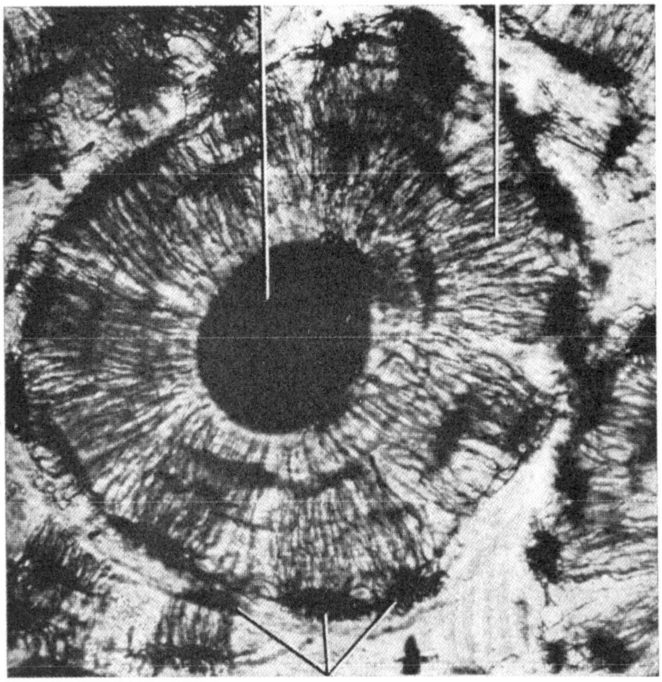

Fig. 6. Photograph of a ground section of bone showing a single Haversian system. The lacunae, canaliculi, and the central tubular cavity all appear black owing to their content of air. Note how the canaliculi stream towards the central cavity from which the blood supply of the osteocytes is derived.

clean break without damage to the main vessels in the marrow cavity most of which arise from a single, large **nutrient artery.** (2) **Cancellous bone** is a lattice of bone spicules. It occurs in the ends of long bones and fills the flat and irregular bones. The spaces between the spicules are filled with highly vascular bone marrow which is often of the red variety (blood-cell-forming).

The **periosteum** is a dense layer of fibrous tissue which covers the external surfaces of all bones, except where they articulate in synovial joints. It is continuous with muscles, tendons, ligaments, the fibrous capsules of joints, the deep fascia where a bone becomes subcutaneous and elsewhere through the intermuscular fibrous septa, and with the connective tissue (endosteum) of the marrow space through the substance of the bone.

Dried bones show a number of tell-tale marks which allow the student to learn much about the structures in contact with the bone. Bone is smooth (a) where it is covered in life by articular cartilage; (b) where it gives a fleshy attachment to muscles; and (c) where it is subcutaneous. It is often roughened where ligaments, aponeuroses, and tendons are attached, and has grooves lodging blood vessels, and holes (foramina) where arteries enter and veins leave the bone. Many of these features are more readily felt than seen, and they are of importance for they show the exact point of attachment of structures to the bone and so clarify their functions.

It is important for the student to determine the position of each bone in the body, to be able to identify the parts of the bones which are readily visible or palpable, and to check these findings by the use of radiographs.

Bones are usually classified according to their shape. (1) The **long bones** of the limbs vary in length from finger to thigh bones, but all tend to have enlarged, articular ends (composed of cancellous bone with a thin shell of compact bone) and a narrower, tubular **body** (shaft) of compact bone. Of the remainder (2) the **short bones**, e.g. of the wrist and the foot, (3) the **flat bones**, e.g. the sternum and vault of the skull, and (4) the **irregular bones**, e.g. the vertebral column, all consist of cancellous bone enclosed in compact bone of varying thickness, while (5) the **pneumatic bones** of the skull have the marrow cavity replaced by air spaces which are extensions of the nasal cavity and form resonating chambers.

Bones are formed during *development* in two ways.

1. The majority of bones are preformed in cartilage (**cartilage bone**) by the production of a cartilage model.

The cartilage model consists of cartilage cells buried in an apparently

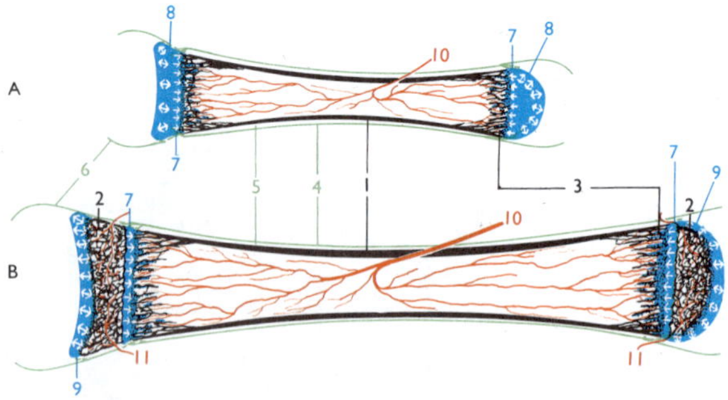

Fig. 7. Diagrams of two stages in the development of a long bone.
A. Before birth.
B. After birth.
Black, bone.
Blue, cartilage.
Blue with black dots, calcified cartilage.
Green, fibrous periosteum, perichondrium, and fibrous capsule of joints.
Red, arteries.
The white arrows indicate the direction of growth of the cartilage, that on the articular surfaces of the epiphyses being much less than in the growth cartilage. Note that there is no addition to the epiphyses from the growth cartilage, that cartilage grows interstitially and by addition from the perichondrium, and that the fibrous periosteum is attached only to the cartilaginous ends while the deeper, osteogenic layer is adding to the diameter of the bone. Hence the growth cartilage and the bone increase in width principally from periosteal and perichondrial additions. Note also the dual blood supply to the body and the epiphyses when these appear as secondary centres of ossification after birth. Short bones, e.g. carpus and tarsus, develop in the same manner as epiphyses and mostly appear after birth as do the epiphyses.
1. Body of bone (diaphysis).
2. Bone of epiphysis.
3. Zone of active ossification of calcified cartilage produced by growth cartilage and adding to the length of the bone (metaphysis).
4. Fibrous periosteum.
5. Osteogenic layer of periosteum.
6. Fibrous capsule of joint.
7. Growth cartilage.
8. Cartilaginous end before formation of epiphysis.
9. Cartilage which forms articular cartilage and adds to the articular surface of the epiphysis.
10. Nutrient artery (often single).
11. Epiphysial arteries (multiple) which arise from joint anastomosis.
The diagram does not show the arterial supply to the body of the bone from periosteal vessels which are responsible for approximately one-third of its thickness.

homogeneous matrix. This grows by the proliferation of its cells and the production of matrix by each of these. The model is then replaced by bone (ossification). This process begins in one of two ways.

A. In long bones, a supporting shell of bone is laid down by the periosteum on the external surface of the body of the model. The matrix of the cartilage internal to this calcifies and its contained cells die leaving spaces throughout the calcified cartilage. This is then invaded by phagocytic cells (**osteoclasts**) and blood vessels from the surrounding shell in such a manner that the spaces coalesce leaving spicules of calcified cartilage between them. These spicules, mainly longitudinal, are then strengthened by the action of bone-forming cells (**osteoblasts**) which lay down bone on the spicules to increase the strength of this temporary scaffolding. This process begins at the centre of the body and then spreads towards the ends which remain cartilaginous. Each cartilaginous end is continuous with the ossifying body through a zone of growing cartilage (**growth cartilage**) which adds new cartilage to the body at the same rate as the processes of calcification and ossification spread towards it. Thus the cartilaginous ends move away from the centre of the body, followed by a zone of active ossification (**metaphysis**) in calcified cartilage which produces cancellous bone. The external shell of bone increases in length at the same rate, so that its extremities always lie at the metaphysis. This process increases the length of the body of the bone, while its diameter is increased by the addition of bone to the external surface of the enclosing shell. This bone is produced by a highly cellular (osteogenic) layer which is characteristic of the **periosteum** of developing bones. As the shell increases in thickness, the need for the internal scaffolding of cancellous bone disappears and it is removed leaving a continuous marrow cavity. Thereafter, this cavity increases in transverse diameter at a slightly slower rate than bone is added to the external surface of the shell. These processes of bone removal are carried out by osteoclasts.

B. In short and irregular bones and in the ends of long bones, the same process occurs in the centre of the cartilage model without the production of an external shell of bone. Thus a centre of ossification begins and spreads outwards as the surrounding cartilage continues to grow until the adult size is reached. By this time, the ossification has replaced all of the cartilage except that which persists on the articular surfaces. At about the same time, the growth cartilages in the long bones stop growing and ossification from the body spreads into them. Thus fusion occurs between the ossification in the body and that in the cartilaginous ends. This brings growth in length to a halt. After this has happened in all the bones, there can be no further growth in length and the height of the individual is fixed.

The ossifications in the ends of the long bones (**epiphyses**) appear much later (at or after birth) than those in the bodies (**primary centres**, at approximately 8 weeks of intra-uterine life) and hence are often known as **secondary centres.** In short and irregular bones they form the primary centres, most of which do not appear till after birth. In all cases the ossification in cartilage forms cancellous bone, while that formed by the periosteum is compact bone, though cancellous bone can be turned into compact bone by continuation of the process of ossification.

Most long bones have epiphyses (secondary centres) at each end, but the growth in length occurs mainly at one end. At this **'growing end'** the epiphysis usually appears earlier and fuses with the body later than that at the non-growing end where fusion may occur considerably before growth ceases.

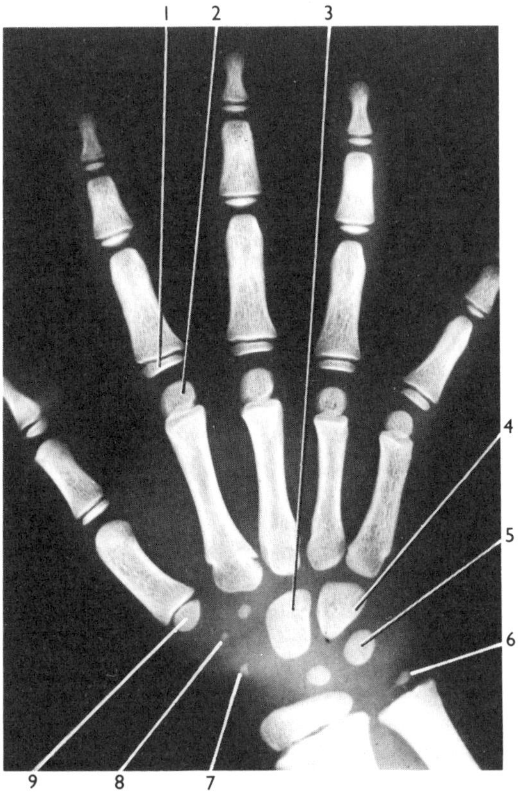

Fig. 8. Radiograph of the wrist and hand of a boy aged 7 years.
1. Phalangeal epiphysis.
2. Metacarpal epiphysis.
3. Capitate.
4. Hamate.
5. Triquetrum.
6. Distal epiphysis of ulna.
7. Scaphoid.
8. Trapezium.
9. Epiphysis of first metacarpal, normal position.

The presence of such 'growing ends' in long bones makes the injury to these ends in children much more serious than damage to the non-growing end. Since epiphyses are visible in radiographs and are separated from the body of the bone by a clear region of growing cartilage during growth, they have to be differentiated from fractures. It is useful, therefore, to know where epiphyses appear and when they are present. The student should not try to memorize all of these but should have a general indication of their times of appearance and fusion, realizing that there are marked individual variations. The growing ends in the upper limb are at shoulder and wrist, in the lower limb at the knee.

2. Bone may also be formed in connective tissue without the intervention of cartilage (**membranous ossification**). Here osteoblasts are produced which form many separate spicules of bone. These fuse to form a lattice around the capillaries of the connective tissue. This may persist as cancellous bone, or continued deposition of bone in the cavities of the lattice can turn it into compact bone. In either case, the formation of periosteum with a cellular, **osteogenic layer** on the external surfaces of a membrane bone permits the continued growth of the bone by deposition. Continuous periosteal deposition of the bone ceases at the end of growth. Then the cellular, osteogenic layer of the periosteum disappears, its outer, **fibrous layer** persisting and fusing with the surface of the bone. Osteogenesis from the periosteum can begin again when increased strength of a bone is required, e.g. when the weight or muscularity of the individual increases. It is also responsible for the surface irregularities of the bone where tendons and ligaments are attached and for much of the formation of new bone at the sites of fractures.

Absorption of unnecessary bone plays an important part in bone development. In addition to increasing the size of the marrow cavity and lightening the bone, it also maintains the normal external shape of the bone throughout its growth.

General instructions for dissection

The dissector requires one scalpel with a solid blade, two pairs of forceps, preferably with rounded points, a strong blunt hook or seeker, and a hand lens. The lens is especially useful as an aid to bridging the gap between gross and microscopic anatomy and can also help to throw light on the functions of many tissues.

Instruments

Deep to the skin, the body consists of a number of organs embedded in a matrix of fibrous connective tissue (**fascia**) which varies in density from a loose mesh to tough sheets or bundles of fibres. Dissection is the process of freeing the organs from this tissue and demonstrating the variations in its density. This can best be done by blunt dissection with a hook or forceps by pulling these through the loose layers of connective tissue. In this way it is possible to free organs without damaging blood vessels or nerves, the knife being reserved for cutting the skin and the dense layers of deep fascia which enclose many organs and partly conceal them.

Removal of the skin

One method is to remove the skin from the superficial fascia in a series of flaps which can be replaced to obviate drying of the part. It is probably better to cut through both skin and superficial fascia and remove both of them in one layer from the underlying deep fascia by blunt dissection. The blood vessels and nerves entering the superficial fascia through the deep fascia are easily found in this way and can be traced for some distance. The alternative of searching for their minute branches in the superficial fascia is a tedious and often unrewarding process. The student should be aware that the distribution of cutaneous nerves is of considerable clinical importance, but this is best learnt by reference to diagrams except in the case of the larger branches which are easily followed. In the superficial fascia, the nerves are almost always accompanied by a small artery and one or more minute veins. Larger veins are also found in the superficial fascia. They run a solitary course to pierce the deep fascia and drain into the deep veins. At such junctions, these superficial veins contain valves which prevent the reflux of blood from the deep veins.

Deep dissection

When the deep fascia has been uncovered and examined, proceed to remove it. This is made more difficult because it sends sheets between the various muscles enclosing each in a separate tunnel. Where a number of muscles arise together, the walls of these tunnels also give origin to muscle fibres and thus they form a tendinous sheet which appears to bind together adjacent muscles. Elsewhere it is relatively easy to strip the deep fascia from muscles for only delicate strands pass between the individual bundles of muscle fibres. *It is important to follow each muscle to its attachments and to define these accurately, for it is only in this way that the functions of a muscle can be determined.*

As each muscle is exposed and lifted from its bed, look for the neurovascular bundle entering its surface. Follow the structures in the neurovascular bundle back to the main nerve trunk and vessels from which they arise. Once these have been identified, it is relatively easy to follow them by blunt dissection and determine their other branches. In many situations it will be found that the arteries are accompanied by tributaries of the main vein which often obscure the artery and nerve. In these cases it is usually advisable to remove the veins so that a clearer view of the other structures can be obtained. In any case it will be found that there are usually multiple venous channels and that their arrangement is much less standard than that of the arteries. The arteries are less constant in their arrangement than the nerves.

Variation

It is obvious even to the casual observer that there are wide variations between persons. The same type of variation exists in the size, position, and shape of the various organs of the body in different individuals, just as the fingerprints and even the proteins of the body are unique to each individual. Therefore, no single account of the structure of the body exactly fits every individual, so the student must expect to find variations from the descriptions given in this book. For this reason, he should take every opportunity to look at the other bodies being dissected at the same time. Some of the variations are of considerable clinical importance, e.g. differences in the anastomotic arrangement between the arteries at the base of the brain, while others have no such significance, e.g. an extra belly to a particular muscle or the marked difference in the arrangement of the superficial veins even on the two sides of the body. One type of variation, not commonly seen in the dissecting room, is the **congenital abnormality** which arises from some defect in development. Many of these are so severe that they lead to death before or immediately after birth, while others, compatible with life outside the uterus, may cause considerable disability and early death, e.g. congenital defects of the heart. Other congenital defects may be present throughout life without any overt sign, and may only come to light at operation or as a result of investigation for some other condition, e.g. at X-ray examination. The student should understand, therefore, the main processes of development and the effects of its abnormalities on the structure and function of the various systems, even though there is insufficient space in this book to do more than draw attention to some of the major points.

Anatomy of the living body

It is unfortunate that the study of anatomy has to be carried out on the dead, preserved body in which the texture and appearance of the organs of the body has been altered. The student should remember that the purpose of such studies is to allow him to visualize the living body in action so that he can appreciate the effects of injury or disease, and can recognize an abnormality from his knowledge of the normal. To achieve this kind of information there is no substitute for the personal process of looking at the body by dissection while thinking of the functions of its various parts and checking these points by observation and palpation of the living body. Dissection is only a means to the end of a fuller understanding of function. It deals, for example, with simple concepts such as the arrangement of the valves in the veins and the more complex structure of the heart, without which the normal and abnormal circulation of the blood could not be understood properly. Similarly, a knowledge of the movements at joints, the muscles which move them, and the nerves which supply these structures is essential if the effects of injury or disease in any of these systems are to be understood and rational corrective measures undertaken. Moreover it forms the basis on which a patient can be advised that he will require to change his occupation and be retrained for some different activity which is compatible with a permanent disability.

As in any other study, dissection can become a meaningless chore unless the student approaches it with an enquiring mind and avoids the temptation of assuming that it is simply a method of learning a number of dead facts.

In this book there are paragraphs describing one method of dissection. These are only for the guidance of the student and need not be followed slavishly. Any method which the student may wish to follow to investigate the body in his own way will prove at least as effective for him.

Special techniques

X-ray

An increasing number of techniques are being established whereby the internal structure of the body can be assessed during life without surgical intervention. Of these the oldest is the use of X-rays. This technique depends on the differential absorption of X-rays by the various tissues of the body on their way through it to a sensitive film (or other recording apparatus) which is blackened by development in direct proportion to the amount of X-rays reaching it. Thus, if the exposure is correct, the film is deeply blackened outside the area shaded by the body and is completely clear where a tissue intervenes which absorbs all the penetrating X-rays. Compact bone and teeth are the most absorbent tissue while air, such as that contained in the lungs, windpipe, or intestine, is the least. Most other tissues, including fluid, have an equal, intermediate absorption per unit of thickness except fat which has a lower level of absorption though not as low as air.

Each point on the film (radiograph) has a density (blackness) which is directly proportional to the amount of X-rays reaching it and hence inversely to the sum of the absorptions of all the tissues which lie between the source of X-rays and that point on the radiograph. Hence in a postero-anterior radiograph of the chest [Fig. 1, Vol. 2] the lung fields are dark because the air they contain does not absorb X-rays as much as the vertebral column, breast bone (sternum), and the tissues lying between the two lungs (including the heart) and which overlap each other in the central white area. Also the absorption by the ribs, added to the absorption by the tissue in the lungs, etc., makes the ribs appear as lighter strips in the lung fields and the fuzzy, whiter areas in the medial parts of each lung are due to absorption by the larger blood vessels (fluid-filled) in these parts of the lungs.

In examining Fig. 1, Vol. 2, the following points should be noted.

1. The outlines of the heart and great vessels which arise from it are obvious on your right (left side of the patient) of the median white area because they project beyond the vertebral column and sternum into the lung fields and make a sharp contrast in absorption by comparison with that on your left where the vertebral column and sternum overlap the heart and vessels.

2. On each side the lower part of the lung field becomes lighter and this area has a sharp, curved inferior margin—absorption caused by the overlying breast in this female.

3. Air introduced into the abdominal (peritoneal) cavity makes the lower surface of the diaphragm (a thin partition between the thorax and abdomen) and the upper surfaces of the organs immediately below it obvious, though without that air only the upper surface of the diaphragm would have been seen because of its contrast with the lungs. The presence of the air in the upper part of the peritoneal cavity shows that this radiograph was taken with the patient in the erect position.

If the intensity of the X-rays or the length of exposure had been increased, the lung fields would have become darker and the breast and rib 'shadows' much less obvious though some detail of the vertebral column would have been visible. Conversely, it is possible to show minor differences in tissue absorption, e.g. fat versus tumour, most easily with low-intensity X-rays.

Thus radiographs show the outlines of structures where there is a change in X-ray absorption but cannot show the outline of two adjacent structures which have the same X-ray density. Clearly any hollow organ, e.g. blood vessel, gut tube, etc., which can be filled with a substance which absorbs X-rays more effectively than bone, e.g. heavy metals such as barium [Figs. 83,148,164, and 195; all in Vol. 2], or less effectively than the surrounding tissue, e.g. air, can make its outline obvious. The combination of both (double contrast) where a small amount of X-ray opaque material is introduced into a cavity followed by air allows the first to outline the internal surface so that irregularities are made visible by the contrast with the air [Fig. 203], while use of the X-ray opaque material alone merely produces a silhouette [Fig. 60].

Other special techniques

Three more recent techniques all produce pictures representing slices taken through the body at any desired level. All of these depend on special features of the tissues and all can be recorded in a digital form and reproduced in any desired manner which the information permits.

Computerized tomography

Computerized tomography is a technique which uses X-rays [Figs. 276A–290A, Vol. 2] and depends on the differences in absorption by different tissues—a feature which can be enhanced by the introduction of special materials. Once a series of transverse sections has been made and the results recorded in digital form it is possible to combine these in the computer and to construct images in a different plane if required.

Ultrasound

Ultrasound (sonar) can also be used to produce electronic pictures [Fig. 286B, Vol. 2] which represent the reflection of that ultrasound from surfaces where one tissue meets another. Unfortunately ultrasound cannot be used where there is air or bone because it is not transmitted through these, but it has the advantage that there is no evidence, unlike X-rays, of it having any damaging effects on even the most sensitive tissues. It is used, therefore, as a method of choice to scan the pelvis where there is the possibility of pregnancy and to determine gross abnormalities at an early stage. The method consists of passing an ultrasound transmitter and recorder over the skin and showing the computerized reflection on a cathode ray tube. The pictures produced are more difficult to read than computerized tomographs but represent sections taken through the body under the path of travel of the instrument. They are most useful when shown as a continuous recording (real time) which can take account of movements of tissues such as the heart valves.

Nuclear magnetic resonance

This is the latest technique. In this, protons can be made to resonate in a strong magnetic field when subjected to the appropriate radio wavelength. Such resonations are recorded, computed, and pictures produced electronically [Fig. 284, Vol. 3] which at the moment show densities representing the amount of water in the different tissues. This technique has very great potential for development and already shows much more detail than is possible with computerized tomography. When it is possible to use other elements in the tissues it should give much more information, including information about biochemical changes and the exact sites in which such changes are taking place.

The upper limb

Introduction

The parts of the upper limb are the shoulder, the arm or brachium, the forearm or antebrachium, and the hand.

The **shoulder** region includes the axilla or armpit, the scapular region or parts around the shoulder blade, and the pectoral or breast region on the front of the chest. The scapula or shoulder blade and the clavicle or collar bone [Figs. 11, 32, 49] are the bones of the upper limb girdle. They articulate with each other at the acromioclavicular joint, but their only articulation with the rest of the skeleton is where the clavicle articulates with the upper end of the sternum at the sternoclavicular joint. The mobile scapula is otherwise held in position entirely by muscles.

The **arm** is the part between the shoulder and the elbow or cubitus. Its bone is the humerus which articulates with the scapula at the shoulder joint.

The **forearm** extends from the elbow to the wrist. Its bones, the radius and ulna, articulate with the humerus at the elbow joint and with each other proximally and distally at the corresponding radioulnar joints. In the anatomical position (supine position of the forearm) the bones are parallel with the radius lateral to the ulna. When the palm of the hand faces posteriorly (prone position of the forearm) the distal end of the radius has rotated around the ulna so that the radius lies obliquely across the ulna. The movement producing this is called **pronation**, the reverse movement is **supination.**

The **hand** consists of the wrist or carpus, the hand proper or metacarpus, and the digits (thumb and fingers). The small wrist or carpal bones are in two rows (proximal and distal) each consisting of four bones. They articulate (a) with one another at the intercarpal joints, (b) proximally, with the radius at the radiocarpal joint, so that they move with the radius in pronation and supination, and (c) distally, with the metacarpal bones at the carpometacarpal joints. The small movements that occur at each of these joints summate to allow a considerable range of movement. Posteriorly the carpal bones are close to the skin, but anteriorly they are covered by muscles of the ball of the thumb (**thenar eminence**), the ball of the little finger (**hypothenar eminence**), and between these by the long tendons entering the hand from the forearm.

The hand proper has five metacarpal bones numbered 1 to 5, beginning with the thumb. Proximally their bases articulate with the distal row of carpal bones, and the 2nd to 5th articulate with each other (intermetacarpal joints) [Fig. 110]. Distally each articulates with the proximal phalanx of the corresponding digit.

The **digits** are: the thumb or pollex, the forefinger or index, the middle finger or digitus medius, the ring finger or annularis, and the little finger or minimus. Each finger has three phalanges though the thumb has only two, the proximal phalanx articulating with the corresponding metacarpal head at the metacarpophalangeal joint. The phalanges articulate with one another at the proximal and distal interphalangeal joints.

The pectoral region and axilla

In man the walls of the thorax form a conical structure which is flattened anteroposteriorly and has its apex truncated obliquely to form the **superior aperture of the thorax.** This is continuous above with the root of the neck and has as its margins the first thoracic vertebra, the first ribs, and the upper part of the sternum (manubrium). The upper limb is attached to the thorax by muscles and bones which diverge from the proximal part of the limb to the anterior and posterior surfaces of the thorax, thus leaving a three-sided pyramidal space (the **axilla**) between these two groups of muscles and bones and the lateral wall of the thorax. When the arm is by the side, the axilla is a narrow space. When the arm is abducted the volume of the axilla increases and its floor (base) rises, forming a definite 'armpit' and causing the muscular inferior margins of its anterior and posterior walls to stand out as the anterior and posterior **axillary folds.** The superior part of the axilla (apex) lies lateral to the first rib and is continuous over its superior surface with the superior aperture of the thorax below and the root of the neck above. This continuity permits blood vessels and nerves from the thorax and neck to enter the axilla on their way to the upper limb. They pass over the superior surface of the first rib behind the middle of the clavicle [Fig. 25].

The clavicle extends medially from its articulation with the scapula (acromioclavicular joint) on the superior surface of the shoulder to its articulation with the superolateral surface of the sternum (sternoclavicular joint)—the only articulation of an upper limb bone with a bone of the trunk. Thus the clavicle acts as a strut which transmits forces from the upper limb to the trunk and prevents the scapula, and hence the shoulder, from sagging downwards and medially under the weight of the limb as it does when the clavicle is broken. The scapula lies posterior to the axilla and is almost entirely covered with muscles. These either attach the scapula to the humerus or hold it to the thorax on which it can slide freely because of the absence of any bony articulation between it and the thoracic wall. Such movements of the scapula are limited only by its articulation with the clavicle and through it with the sternoclavicular joint around which these movements are forced to take place.

Surface anatomy

All points mentioned in this section should be confirmed on the living body and on specimens of the bones [Fig. 9].

The **clavicle** (collar bone) is palpable throughout its length. It follows a sinuous curve which is concave forwards in its lateral one-third but convex in its medial two-thirds to make room for the passage of vessels and nerves into the axilla. Draw a finger along your clavicle and note that its ends project above the acromion of the scapula laterally and the manubrium of the sternum medially. Thus the positions of these joints are easily identified, though the medial end of the clavicle is somewhat obscured by the attachment of the sternocleidomastoid muscle [Figs. 10, 26].

Between the medial ends of the clavicles is the **jugular notch** on the superior margin of the manubrium. Draw a finger downwards from this notch in the median plane till a blunt, transverse ridge is felt on the sternum. This **sternal angle** is the joint between the manubrium and the body of the sternum. It marks the articulation of the **cartilage of the second rib** with the side of the sternum. The second rib may be identified in this way even in obese subjects, for the sternal angle is always readily palpable. The other ribs are identified by counting downwards from the second. The anterior part of the first rib is hidden by the medial part of the clavicle. Immediately inferior to the lower end of the body of the sternum is a small, median depression, the **epigastric fossa** or 'pit of the stomach' which overlies the **xiphoid process**, the lowest piece of the sternum. The **cartilages of the seventh ribs** lie on either side of this fossa.

The **nipple** is very variable in position, even in the male, but usually lies over the fourth intercostal space, near the junction of the ribs with their cartilages. It is just medial to a vertical line passing through the middle of the clavicle (the **midclavicular line**).

The **infraclavicular fossa** [Fig. 15] is a depression inferior to the junction of the lateral and middle thirds of the clavicle. The pectoralis major muscle on the front of the chest and axilla lies medial to the fossa, while the deltoid muscle, which clasps the shoulder, is lateral to it. The **coracoid process** of the scapula can be felt just lateral to the fossa and under cover of the deltoid muscle, 2–3 cm below the clavicle.

Follow the clavicle laterally to its articulation with the **acromion**—a subcutaneous, flattened piece of the bone about 2.5 cm wide which lies in the top of the shoulder. The **acromioclavicular joint** can be felt as a slight dip, for

Fig. 9. Landmarks and incisions. For the bony landmarks of the upper limb, see illustrations of individual bones. Left forearm pronated, right supinated.

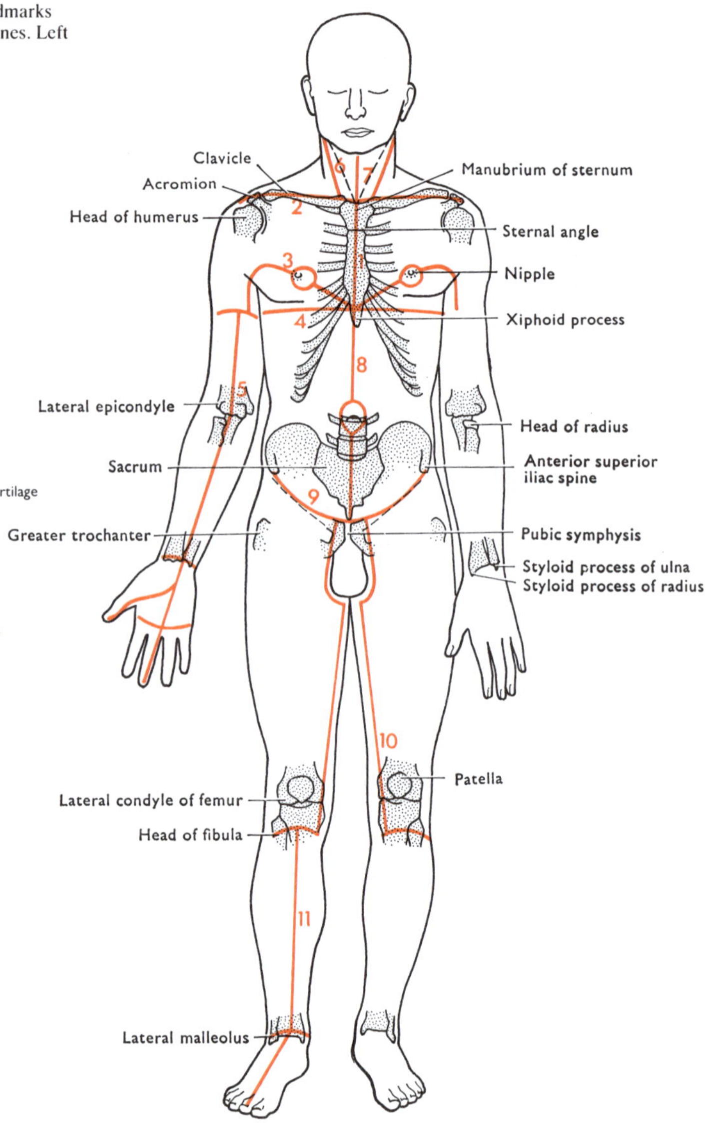

Fig. 10. Sternum (anterior view). The xiphoid process is missing.

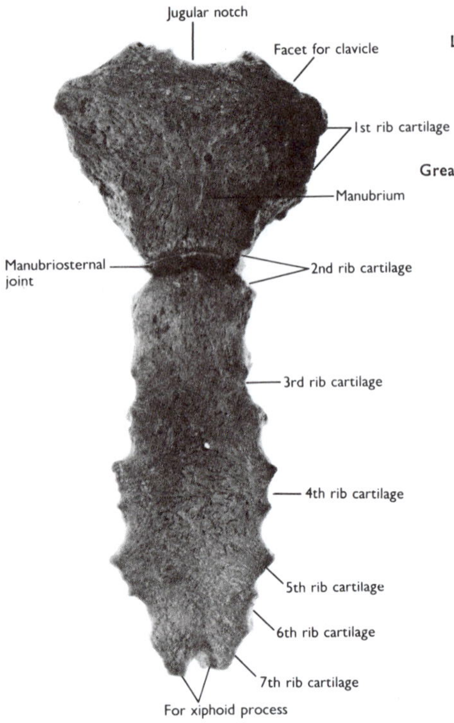

the clavicle projects slightly above the level of the acromion (*acron* = summit; *omos* = shoulder).

Raise the arm from the side, i.e. abduct it, to bring into view the hollow of the **axilla**, the anterior axillary fold (containing the pectoralis major muscle) and the posterior axillary fold (containing the latissimus dorsi and teres major muscles). The teres major is a thick, rounded muscle which connects the inferior angle of the scapula to the humerus and can be felt in the posterior axillary fold when the arm is raised above the head. The latissimus dorsi muscle extends from the lower part of the back to the humerus [Fig. 28]. It can be made to stand out by depressing the horizontal arm against resistance.

With the arm by the side, push the fingers into the axilla. The anterior and posterior walls are soft and fleshy, but the lateral margin of the scapula can be felt in the posterior wall. The medial wall is formed by the ribs covered by a sheet of muscle—the serratus anterior. In the lateral angle lie the biceps brachii and coracobrachialis muscles overlying and parallel to the humerus. Some of the large nerves in the axilla can be rolled between the fingers and the humerus, and the axillary artery can be felt pulsating. The head of the humerus laterally and the lateral border of the first rib medially can be felt by pushing the fingers up into the axilla.

Dissection

Make the skin incisions 1–4 shown in Fig. 9. Cut through the superficial fascia except in incision 2 where it is desirable to avoid cutting through the thin sheet of muscle (platysma) and the supraclavicular nerves [Fig. 13] which lie deep to it in that fascia. Carry incision 4 backwards as far as the posterior axillary fold.

Reflect the flaps of skin and superficial fascia laterally by blunt dissection, but do not detach them. Leave the nipple and surrounding skin in position as a landmark. Note the fibrous strands connecting the deep fascia to the skin, especially deep to the breast in the female, and the small neurovascular bundles passing from the anterior ends of the intercostal spaces into the skin. Follow the branches of one of these nerves medially and laterally as far as possible.

As the flap is separated from the skin of the neck along the clavicle, split the superficial fascia with a blunt instrument and try to find the branches of the supraclavicular nerves passing anterior to the clavicle to supply the skin of the upper part of the anterior thoracic wall and the shoulder.

When the reflexion of the lower flap reaches the anterior axillary fold, look for the lateral cutaneous branches of the intercostal nerves which pierce the chest wall just posterior to the fold. These will be found emerging through the deep fascia, one inferior to the other, in a vertical line. Follow the branches of one of them anteriorly and posteriorly as far as possible.

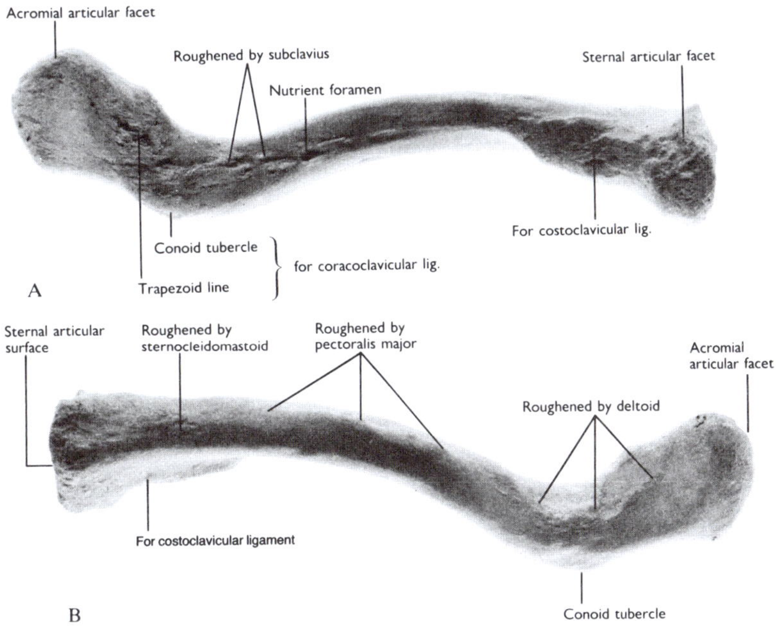

Fig. 11. (A) Right clavicle (inferior surface). (B) Right clavicle (superior surface).

Cutaneous nerves and vessels

On the anterior and lateral surfaces of the thoracic wall the cutaneous nerves are:

1. The supraclavicular nerves from the cervical plexus—principally the fourth cervical ventral ramus.

2. The anterior and lateral cutaneous branches of the ventral rami (intercostal nerves) of the thoracic nerves from the second inferiorly.

The **supraclavicular nerves** [Fig. 13] arise in the neck from the third and fourth cervical nerves. Diverging as they descend, the nerves pierce the deep fascia in the neck and cross the clavicle to supply the skin on the front of the chest and shoulder [Figs. 46, 47] down to a horizontal line at the level of the second costal cartilage. They are named, according to their positions, medial, intermediate, and lateral.

The **anterior cutaneous branches of the intercostal nerves** [Fig. 2] emerge from the intercostal spaces (except the first and occasionally the second) and pierce pectoralis major and the deep fascia to supply skin from the anterior median plane almost to a vertical line through the middle of the clavicle (midclavicular line). They are accompanied by branches of the internal thoracic artery which descends immediately deep to the costal cartilages. These perforating branches are enlarged in the second to fourth spaces to supply the mammary gland in the female. All have lymph vessels running with them from the skin of the anterior thoracic wall and medial part of the mammary gland to lymph nodes (**parasternal**) which lie beside the internal thoracic artery.

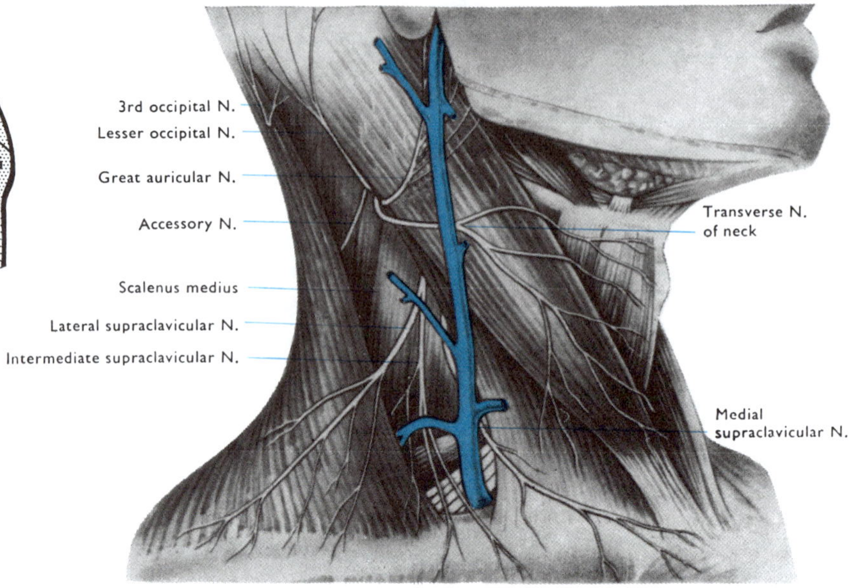

Fig. 13. Superficial branches of cervical plexus.

The **lateral cutaneous branches of the intercostal nerves** pierce the deep fascia as a vertical series a little posterior to the anterior axillary fold. Each enters the superficial fascia as anterior and posterior branches. They supply the remainder of the strip of skin innervated by that spinal nerve between the parts supplied by the anterior cutaneous branch and the dorsal ramus. See also page 6.

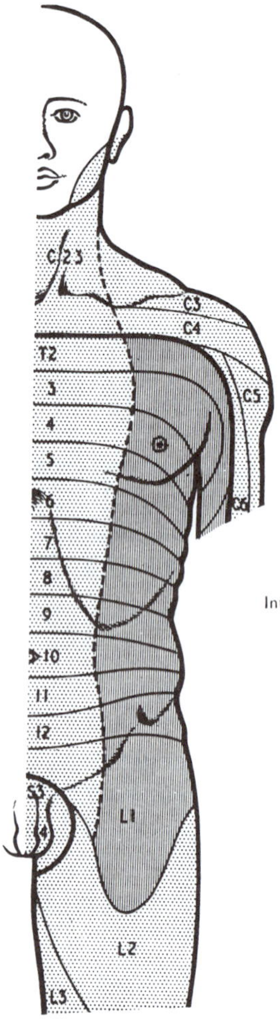

Fig. 12. Distribution of cutaneous nerves on the front of the trunk to illustrate the dermatomes.

The breast

The mamma or breast is made up of: (1) the mammary gland; (2) the fatty superficial fascia in which it is embedded; and (3) the overlying skin with the nipple and the surrounding zone of pigmented skin, the **areola.**

The mammary gland is rudimentary in the male, the nipple is small, and the areola is commonly surrounded by fine hairs. In the non-lactating female, the breast consists mainly of the fatty tissue of the superficial fascia in which are enclosed 15 to 20 lobes of rudimentary gland tissue radiating outwards from the nipple, thus giving the gland the shape of a flattened cone. Each lobe has a main **lactiferous duct** which is dilated to form a **lactiferous sinus** at the base of the nipple and, narrowing again, passes to open separately on its apex. The gland has no capsule but its lobes are separated by fibrous strands of the superficial fascia which pass from the skin to the deep fascia anchoring it to both.

The base of the gland extends from the margin of the sternum almost to the midaxillary line, and from the second to sixth ribs. It lies on the pectoralis major muscle except inferolaterally where it extends on to the origins of the serratus anterior and external oblique muscle of the abdomen from the ribs. The **'axillary tail'** passes superolaterally into the axilla to the level of the third rib, deep to pectoralis major [Fig. 14].

The apex of the gland, the **nipple**, lies a little below the mid-point of the gland and approximately over the fourth intercostal space unless the gland is pendulous. The nipple is free of fat but contains circular and longitudinal smooth muscle fibres which can erect or flatten it respectively. The skin of the nipple and areola contain modified sweat and sebaceous glands, particularly

Fig. 14. Dissection of the right mammary gland.

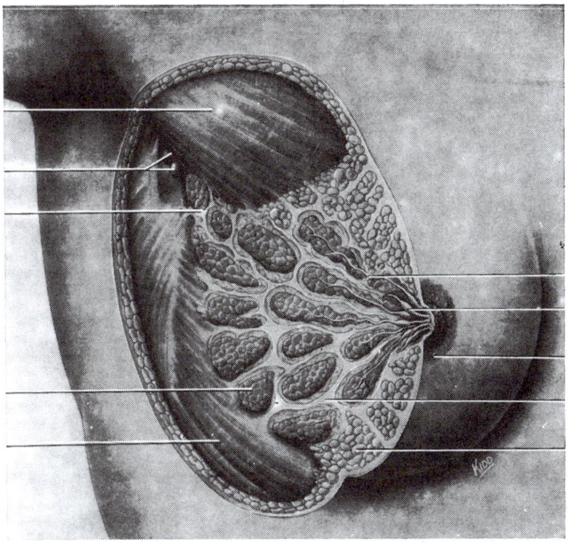

at the outer margin of the areola. The latter tend to enlarge in the early stages of pregnancy and shortly thereafter there is an increase in pigmentation in both nipple and areola which never return to their original colour. In the later stages of pregnancy, the greater part of the fat in the gland is replaced by the proliferation of its ducts and the growth of many secretory alveoli from their branching ends.

The gland receives its *blood supply* from perforating branches of the intercostal and internal thoracic arteries medially and from the lateral thoracic artery laterally.

Lymph vessels drain principally (A) to the axilla, (i) along the axillary tail to the **pectoral lymph nodes**, (ii) through the pectoralis major and clavipectoral fascia to the **apical axillary nodes** via the **infraclavicular nodes**, and (B) to the **parasternal nodes** on the internal thoracic artery by passing along the branches of that artery which supply the gland. Some also drain to the intercostal vessels and nodes, and, since there is communication of lymph vessels across the median plane, there may be drainage to the opposite side especially when some of the pathways are blocked by disease [Fig. 21].

Dissection

Attempt to pass a bristle through one of the ducts of the nipple and try to identify one of the lobes of the gland by blunt dissection. This is not usually very successful in the elderly female and should not be attempted in the male.

Deep fascia

The deep fascia covering the pectoralis major is continuous with the periosteum of the clavicle and sternum and passes over the infraclavicular fossa and deltopectoral groove (between pectoralis major and deltoid) to become continuous with fascia covering the deltoid. It curves over the inferolateral border of pectoralis major to become continuous with the fascia of the axillary floor (**axillary fascia**) which stretches between pectoralis major and latissimus dorsi and may contain muscle fibres from either. When the arm is abducted the axillary fascia rises into the axilla to form the armpit.

The **clavipectoral fascia** lies in the anterior wall of the axilla deep to pectoralis major. It extends from the clavicle to the axillary fascia and encloses the pectoralis minor muscle [Fig. 19].

Dissection

Divide the deep fascia in the deltopectoral groove to uncover the cephalic vein passing to the infraclavicular fossa. Occasional lymph nodes found beside the vein receive lymph from the adjacent superficial tissues and transmit it through the infraclavicular fossa to the apical nodes of the axilla [Figs. 21, 42].

Remove the fascia from the anterior parts of pectoralis major and deltoid and define their attachments.

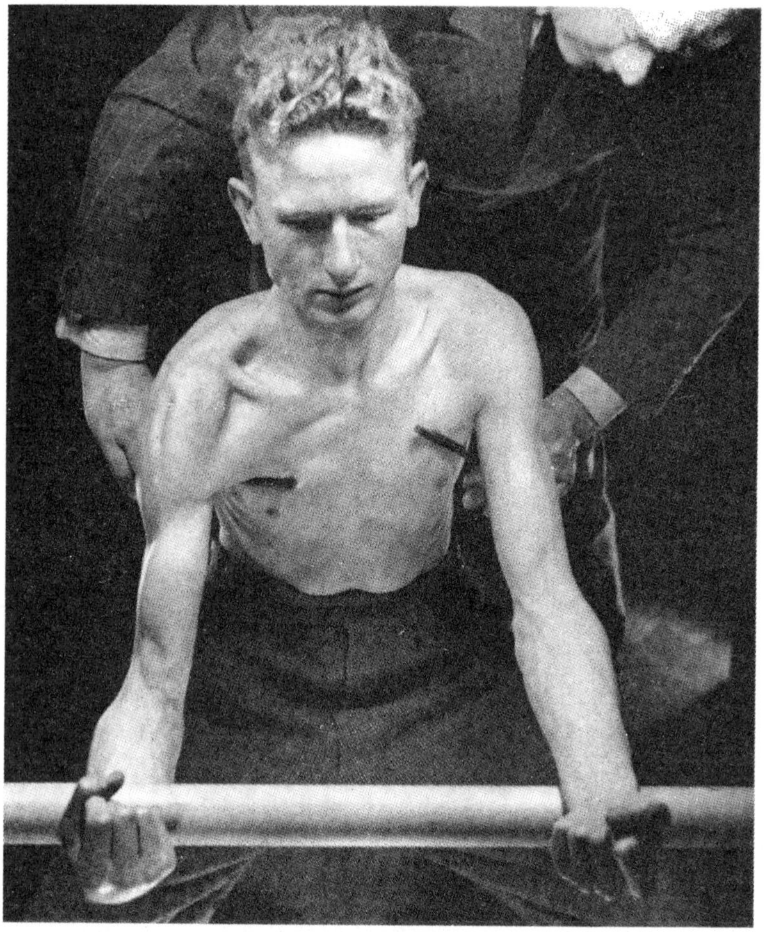

Fig. 15. Actions of pectoralis major. The subject's right arm is being raised and the left arm depressed against resistance. The clavicular part of the right muscle is active, the left is inactive, the reverse is the case with the sternocostal part. (From *Living anatomy* by R. D. Lockhart, 6th edn. Faber and Faber, London (1963).)

Pectoralis major

This powerful, fan-shaped muscle passes from the medial half of the front of the clavicle, the anterior surfaces of the sternum and upper six costal cartilages, and the aponeurosis of the external oblique muscle of the abdomen to the crest of the greater tubercle of the humerus [Fig. 53]. The abdominal part twists under the sternocostal part to form a U-shaped tendon with it at the insertion. The lowest, abdominal, fibres are inserted deep to the upper sternocostal fibres, while the intermediate fibres form the base of the U in the anterior axillary fold [Fig. 16].

The clavicular part passes inferolaterally, and fusing with the anterior layer of the U-shaped tendon, extends further inferiorly. The clavicular part lies at right angles to the abdominal and lower sternocostal fibres, hence these parts have different actions.

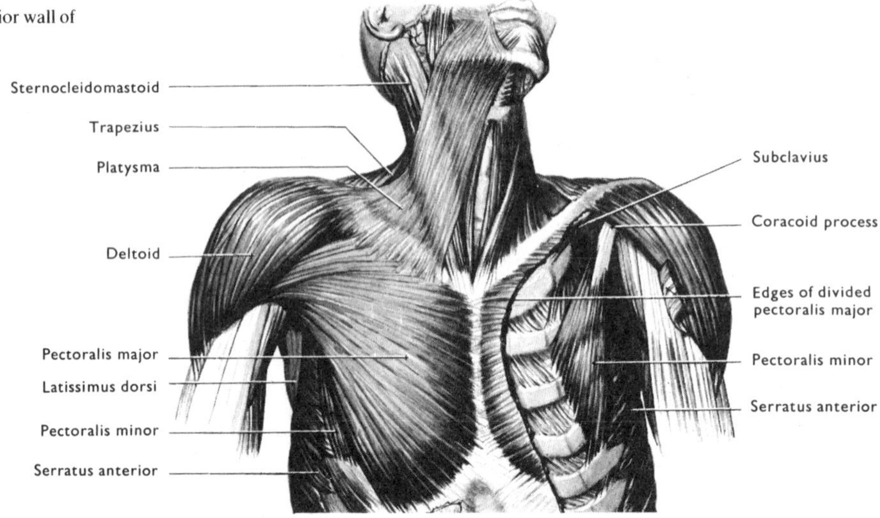

Fig. 16. Muscles of anterior wall of the trunk.

Actions. The pectoralis major is an adductor and medial rotator of the humerus. With the arm above the head, the lowest fibres act with latissimus dorsi to pull down the arm or raise the body as in climbing. The muscle can also return the extended humerus to the vertical position, then continue this flexion of the shoulder joint with its clavicular part which passes in front of the shoulder. **Nerve supply**: medial and lateral pectoral nerves.

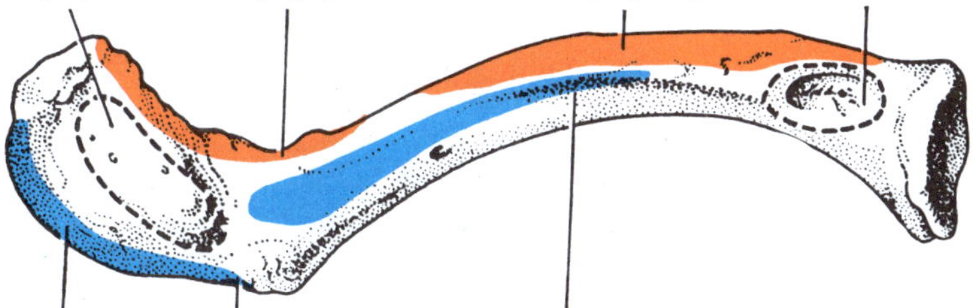

Fig. 17. Muscle attachments of inferior surface of right clavicle.

Axilla

Boundaries and contents

The anterior wall of the axilla extends from the clavicle to the **anterior axillary fold**. It consists of the two pectoral muscles, the subclavius muscle, and the fascia enclosing them [Fig. 19]. The posterior wall consists of: (1) superiorly, the lateral part of the costal surface of the scapula covered by subscapularis; (2) inferiorly, the **posterior axillary fold** formed by the teres major muscle with the latissimus dorsi winding round its lower border to reach its anterior surface [Fig. 22]. The convex medial wall is the lateral wall of the thorax (first five ribs and intercostal spaces) covered by serratus anterior. The humerus lies in the lateral angle covered by the upper parts of biceps and coracobrachialis muscles [Fig. 18].

The **apex** of the axilla (bounded by the clavicle, first rib, and upper border of the scapula) is continuous medially with the superior aperture of the thorax and the root of the neck. From them it receives the axillary vessels and

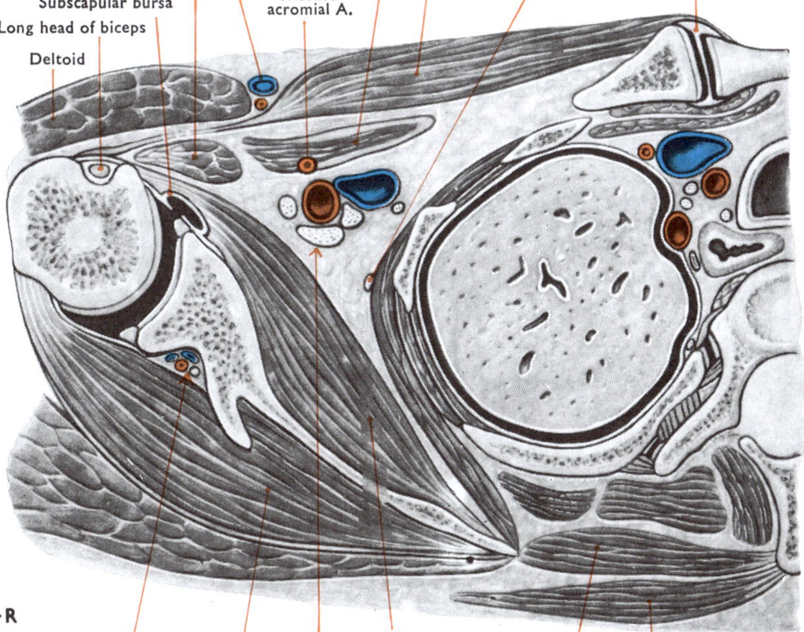

Fig. 18. Horizontal section at the level of shoulder joint (based on a section by Symington). The chief structures in the axilla and its walls are shown, and also the structures close to the left sternoclavicular joint.
A. Anterior.
P. Posterior.
L. Left.
R. Right.

the nerves of the brachial plexus. These descend through the lateral part of the axilla to the arm, and form the *contents of the axilla* together with the axillary lymph nodes and loose, fatty tissue.

Dissection

Cut across the clavicular head of pectoralis major below the clavicle and reflect it towards its insertion. The branches of the lateral pectoral nerve and thoraco-acromial artery pierce the clavipectoral fascia to enter it. Cut across the remainder of the pectoralis major about 5 cm from the sternum. Reflect its parts medially and laterally. A branch of the medial pectoral nerve pierces pectoralis minor to enter pectoralis major. Note the entire sheet of clavipectoral fascia, and then remove it from pectoralis minor, tracing that muscle to its attachments.

Follow the cephalic vein [Fig. 21] through the upper part of the clavipectoral fascia to the axillary vein, and the thoraco-acromial artery and the lateral pectoral nerve to their origins. Then expose the vessels and nerves in the axilla superior to pectoralis minor. Cut through the anterior layer of the clavipectoral fascia immediately inferior to and parallel with the clavicle to expose the subclavius muscle. Gently push a finger, inferior to that muscle, along the line of the axillary vessels. It will pass over the first rib, deep to the clavicle, into the root of the neck. If the finger is pressed medially between the axillary artery and vein, the firm resistance of the scalenus anterior muscle can be felt descending to the upper surface of the first rib between the artery and vein which are here called the subclavian vessels.

Pass a finger deep to the pectoralis minor through the lower part of the axilla. Lift it from the subjacent structures but preserve the medial pectoral nerve which enters its deep surface.

Fig. 19. Diagram of clavipectoral fascia as seen in an oblique section parallel to the axillary artery.

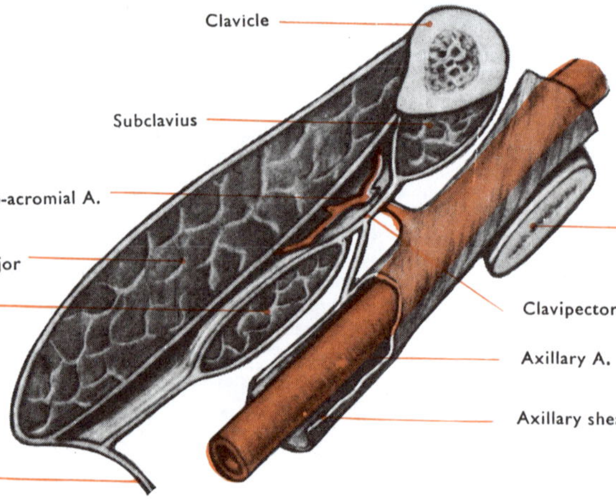

Pectoralis minor
[Figs. 20, 22]

This triangular muscle passes superolaterally from the third to fifth ribs, near their cartilages, to the upper surface of the coracoid process near its tip [Fig. 33]. **Action:** it pulls the scapula (and hence the shoulder) downwards and forwards. It raises the ribs in inspiration when the scapula is fixed. **Nerve supply:** medial pectoral nerve.

Dissection

Remove the loose connective tissue, fat, and lymph nodes from the axilla to expose its contents. Only a few of the large number of lymph nodes will be seen unless they are enlarged by disease, so it is not profitable to try to make a dissection of them, though they will be felt as slightly firmer structures amongst the fat. Lymph vessels will not be seen. Begin by exposing the coracobrachialis and short head of biceps muscles arising from the tip of the coracoid process. Then find the axillary artery and median nerve medial to these muscles and the **musculocutaneous nerve** entering the deep surface of coracobrachialis. Follow this nerve upwards and find its branch to the muscle.

Medial to the axillary artery is the axillary vein with the **medial cutaneous nerve of the forearm** between them and posterior to that the larger **ulnar nerve.** Find the **medial cutaneous nerve of the arm** medial to the vein. Trace it superiorly to a branch from the **intercostobrachial nerve** which usually joins it. Follow this branch upwards to the emergence of that nerve from the second intercostal space in the medial axillary wall, and trace that nerve downwards to the axillary floor and the medial side of the arm.

Inferior to the emergence of the intercostobrachial nerve (the lateral cutaneous branch of the second intercostal nerve) the equivalent branches of the lower intercostal nerves emerge in a vertical line posterior to pectoralis major and between the digitations (attachments) of the serratus anterior on each rib. Find the lateral thoracic artery and the long thoracic nerve descending on the lateral surface of the serratus anterior muscle which they supply [Fig. 20].

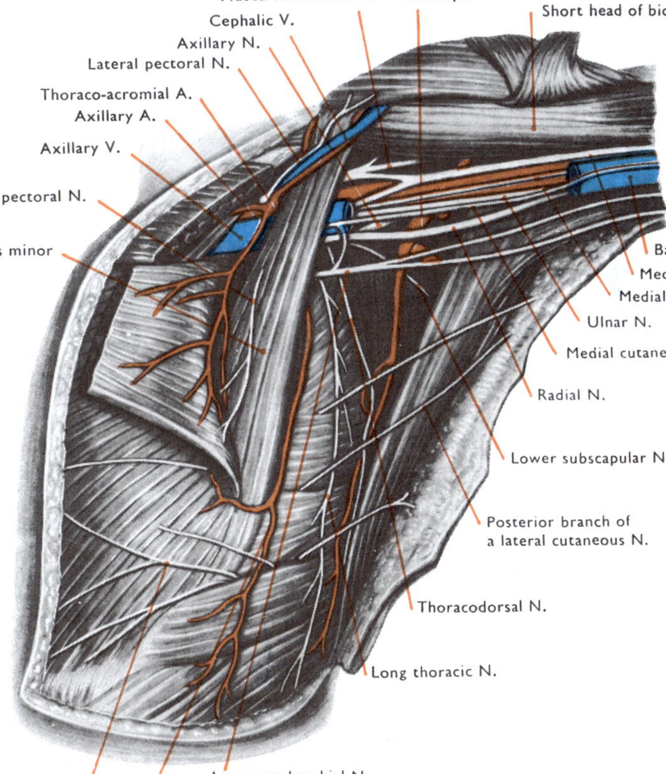

Fig. 20. Contents of axilla exposed by reflexion of pectoralis major and removal of fat, fascia, and lymph nodes. Part of axillary vein has been removed to display the medial cutaneous nerve of forearm and ulnar nerve.

Lateral cutaneous branches of the intercostal nerves

Each of these emerges from an intercostal space, and divides into anterior and posterior branches. They pierce, or pass between, the digitations of serratus anterior but play no part in supplying this muscle, the pectoral muscles, or latissimus dorsi over which their branches run. There is usually no lateral or anterior cutaneous branch from the first intercostal nerve. The lateral branch of the second (**intercostobrachial nerve**) emerges as a large, single branch and communicates with the medial cutaneous nerve of the arm and the lateral cutaneous branch of the third intercostal. Together these three nerves supply the skin of the medial side of the arm and the floor of the axilla.

Dissection

Expose the axillary artery and vein and the large nerves surrounding them. If necessary, remove the smaller tributaries of the vein in order to get a clear view of the nerves. Since the veins follow the corresponding branches of the artery, their loss is of no significance.

Identify and follow the **ulnar nerve.** It lies behind and between the artery and vein, while the **radial nerve** lies behind the artery. Trace the radial nerve upwards and, at the lower border of subscapularis [Fig. 22], find: (1) the **axillary nerve** passing backwards with the posterior humeral circumflex artery; (2) the posterior cutaneous nerve of the arm; (3) muscular branches to the long and medial heads of the triceps muscle.

Find the **subscapular artery** close to the axillary nerve. Trace it and its major branches, the circumflex scapular and thoracodorsal arteries. The latter runs to the chest wall parallel to the margin of latissimus dorsi together with the thoracodorsal nerve to that muscle. The **circumflex scapular artery** lies close to the nerve (lower subscapular) entering the teres major.

Cut across the pectoralis minor and follow the axillary vessels to the outer border of the first rib. Note that the medial, lateral, and posterior **cords of the brachial plexus** are disposed around the artery posterior to pectoralis minor, while all lie posterior to the artery at the level of the clavicle. Expose the anterior surface of subscapularis and identify the **upper subscapular nerve(s)** entering it. Follow the **upper** and **lower subscapular** and **thoracodorsal nerves** to their origin from the posterior cord of the brachial plexus [Figs. 20, 24].

Fig. 21. Lymph nodes and lymph vessels of axilla and mamma.

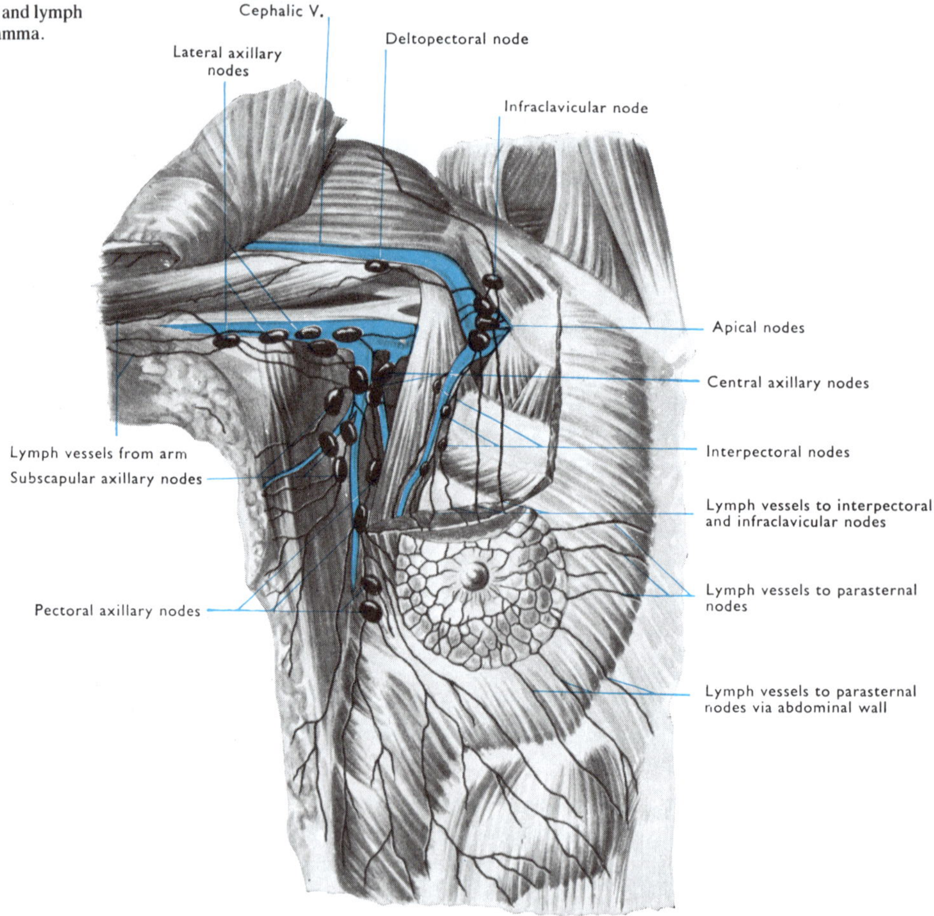

Axillary lymph nodes

These lymph nodes drain the lymph vessels of the upper limb and the superficial vessels of the trunk from the level of the clavicle to that of the umbilicus. The nodes are scattered throughout the fascia of the axilla and most transmit lymph towards the nodes at its apex (**apical nodes**). For descriptive purposes they are divided into groups, each of which lies in one angle of the axillary pyramid and drains a specific territory, though all communicate with those more centrally placed (**central nodes**). Thus the **lateral nodes** lie along the axillary vessels and drain the greater part of the upper limb. The **pectoral group** lie in the anteromedial angle, deep to pectoralis major, and drain the superficial tissues of the anterior and lateral parts of the thoracic and upper abdominal walls. The **subscapular group** lie along the subscapular vessels and drain lymph from the corresponding region on the back. The efferents [p. 4] of all these nodes pass to the apical group [Fig. 21] which also receives vessels from nodes on the cephalic vein and in the infraclavicular fossa. The efferents of the apical nodes form the **subclavian lymph trunk** which usually enters the subclavian vein.

Axillary artery

This is the main artery of the upper limb. It extends from the subclavian artery at the outer border of the first rib through the apex and lateral part of the axilla to become the brachial artery at the lower border of teres major, close to the humerus. For the purposes of description it is divided into three parts which lie respectively superior, posterior, and inferior to pectoralis minor. The cords of the brachial plexus lie posterior to the first part; are arranged around the second part according to their names; while the main nerves arising from the cords surround the third part.

The axillary artery supplies the structures in and surrounding the axilla by branches [Fig. 22]: (A) to the anterior axillary wall, including the clavicle, acromion, and anterior part of deltoid (**thoraco-acromial artery**); (B) to the medial axillary wall, including the lateral part of the mammary gland and surrounding structures (**superior** and **lateral thoracic arteries**); (C) to the posterior axillary wall (**subscapular artery**) including the scapula and muscles covering its posterior aspect through anastomoses of the branches of the artery (**circumflex scapular** and **thoracodorsal**) with branches from the subclavian artery (suprascapular and transverse cervical [Fig. 61]); (D) to the proximal part of the humerus, the muscles covering it, and the shoulder joint (anterior and posterior **circumflex humeral arteries** [Figs. 59, 61]).

Fig. 22. Dissection of axillary artery and its branches.

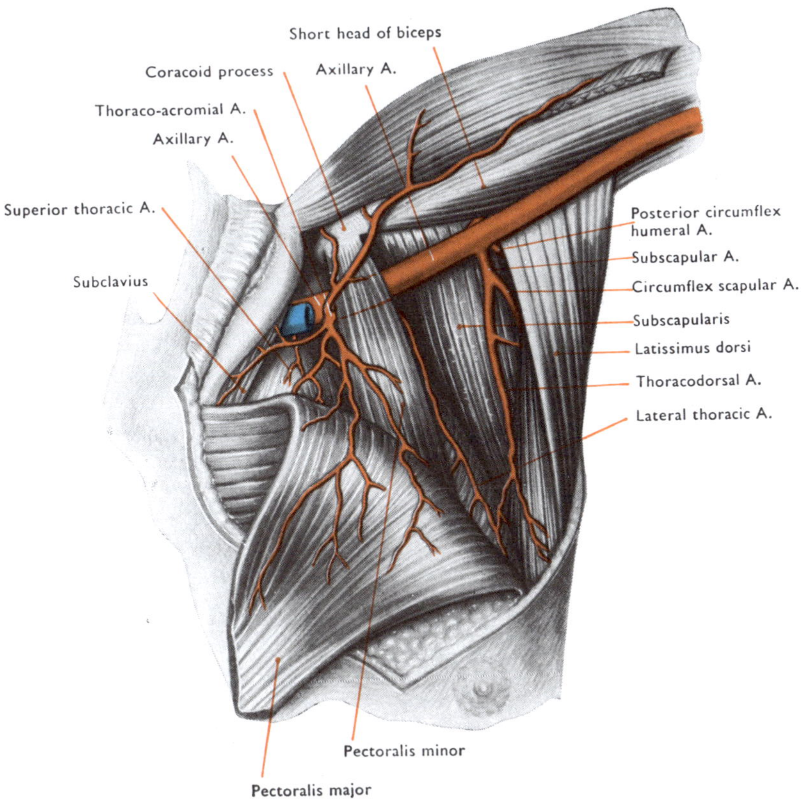

Axillary vein

This lies on the anteromedial aspect of the axillary artery and has the same extent. It is the continuation of the basilic vein and it receives tributaries corresponding to the branches of the axillary artery and also the **brachial veins,** inferiorly, and the cephalic vein, superiorly. It becomes the subclavian vein at the outer border of the first rib.

Subclavius

This small muscle arises from the adjacent parts of the upper surfaces of the first costal cartilage and rib and, passing parallel to the clavicle, is inserted into the groove on its inferior surface [Fig. 17]. **Action:** it holds the medial end of the clavicle against the articular disc of the sternoclavicular joint during movements of the shoulder girdle, thus preventing the clavicle from hammering against the disc in to-and-fro movements of the upper limb. **Nerve supply**: from the fifth and sixth cervical ventral rami [p. 5].

Dissection

Separate the subclavius from its costal attachment and turn it laterally to expose the strong costoclavicular ligament. Expose the anterior and superior surfaces of the articular capsule of the sternoclavicular joint as far as possible. Remove the anterior part of the articular capsule and identify the articular disc between the clavicle and the sternum, but leave the clavicle in position.

Sternoclavicular joint [Fig. 23]

This synovial joint is between the shallow notch at the superolateral angle of the manubrium of the sternum and the larger, medial end of the clavicle. A complete articular disc intervenes. The joint also extends on to the superior surface of the first costal cartilage and is the only point of articulation of the upper limb bones with the axial skeleton. Thus the clavicle forms a strut which maintains the scapula in position and transmits to the trunk forces applied to the upper limb, e.g. in falling on the outstretched hand. Functionally the joint behaves like a ball and socket with a wide range of movements since it has to move with each change in scapular position. It carries heavy loadings but the bony surfaces give little intrinsic stability. Consequently it is strengthened by powerful ligaments which are designed to prevent dislocation of the medial end of the clavicle from the shallow fossa on the sternum. The **articular capsule** is attached close to the articular margins of the bones. It is thickened anteriorly and posteriorly to form the anterior and posterior **sternoclavicular ligaments**.

The **articular disc** is a nearly circular plate of fibrocartilage attached at its margins to the articular capsule and dividing the joint into two separate synovial cavities. Its strongest attachments are to the upper surface of the medial end of the clavicle and to the sternum and first costal cartilage at their junction. It assists the costoclavicular ligament in preventing the upward displacement of the medial end of the clavicle, and acts as a shock-absorber of compression forces applied from the upper limb.

The **costoclavicular ligament** is a powerful band which passes upwards and

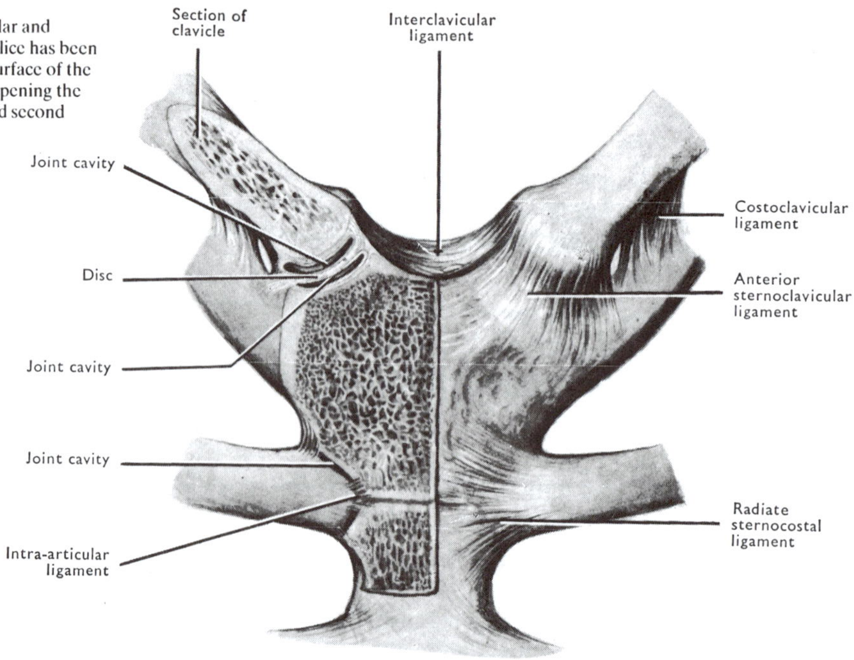

Fig. 23. Sternoclavicular and sternocostal joints. A slice has been cut from the anterior surface of the sternum and clavicle, opening the left sternoclavicular and second chondrosternal joints.

laterally from the junction of the first rib and its cartilage to a rough area on the inferior surface of the clavicle near its medial end [Fig. 11].

The **interclavicular ligament** passes between the medial ends of the two clavicles and is fused with the articular capsules and the jugular notch of the sternum.

The brachial plexus

The **roots** of this important plexus which supplies the upper limb are the ventral rami of the lower four cervical nerves, the greater part of the ventral ramus of the first thoracic nerve, and a small twig each from the ventral rami of the fourth cervical and second thoracic nerves.

The ventral rami of the fifth and sixth cervical nerves unite to form the **superior trunk** [Fig. 24]; the seventh cervical remains single and continues as the **middle trunk,** while the eighth cervical and first thoracic unite to form the **inferior trunk**. A short distance above the clavicle, each of these trunks splits into an anterior and a posterior division. The three **posterior divisions,** *which supply the extensor muscles and skin on the back of the limb,* unite to form the **posterior cord** of the plexus—the lowest posterior division being the smallest. Of the three **anterior divisions,** *which supply the flexor muscles and skin on the front of the limb,* the upper two unite to form the **lateral cord** of the plexus, and the lower passes distally as the **medial cord**. The plexus begins in the lower part of the neck (**supraclavicular part:** ventral rami and trunks), and passes as divisions behind the middle third of the clavicle into the apex of the axilla. Here (**infraclavicular part**) the cords lie posterior to the axillary artery (first part) but, descending posterior to pectoralis minor, they pass into positions relative to the artery (second part) which correspond to their names. The plexus ends at the lower border of pectoralis minor by dividing into a number of nerves.

The plexus is so arranged that each cord and the nerves which arise from it contain nerve fibres from more than one spinal (segmental) nerve. Thus the lateral cord contains nerve fibres from the cervical (C) nerves 5–7 [Fig. 24], the medial cord from C. 8 and thoracic (T.) 1 (and 2), and the posterior cord from C. 5–8 (and T. 1). *A knowledge of these 'segmental values' is of importance in the diagnosis of injuries to the spinal nerves or to the spinal medulla from which they arise.*

Branches of the brachial plexus

1. Arising in the neck but distributed to the upper limb.

The **dorsal scapular nerve** (C. 5), to the rhomboid muscles and levator scapulae, passes postero-inferiorly a little superior to the brachial plexus. It

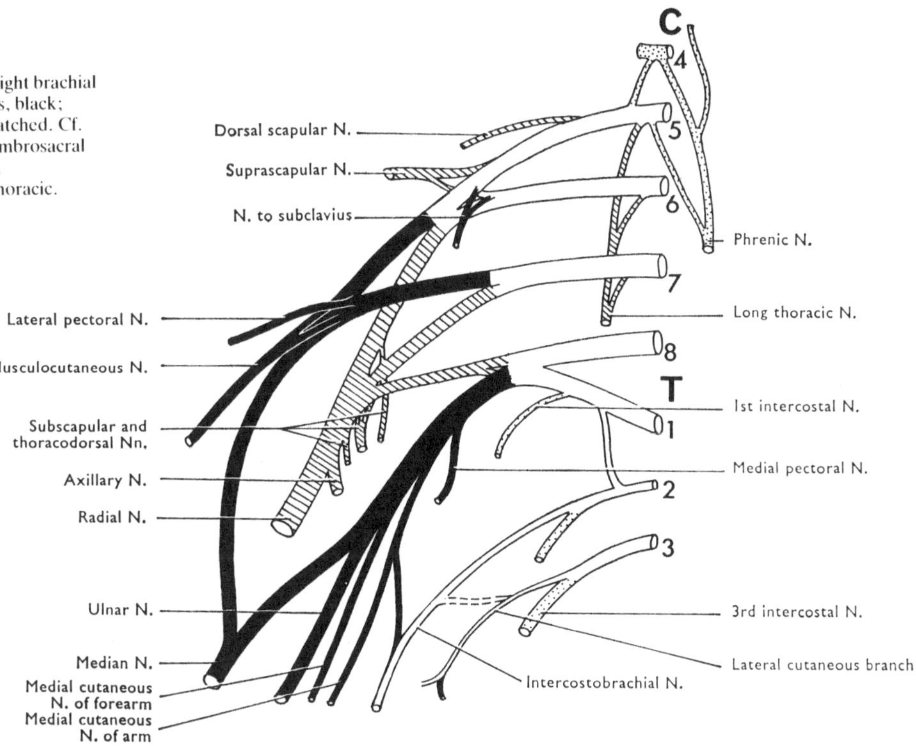

Fig. 24. Diagram of right brachial plexus. Ventral offsets, black; dorsal offsets, cross hatched. Cf. arrangement of the lumbrosacral plexus, Figs. 126, 145.
C = cervical, T = thoracic.

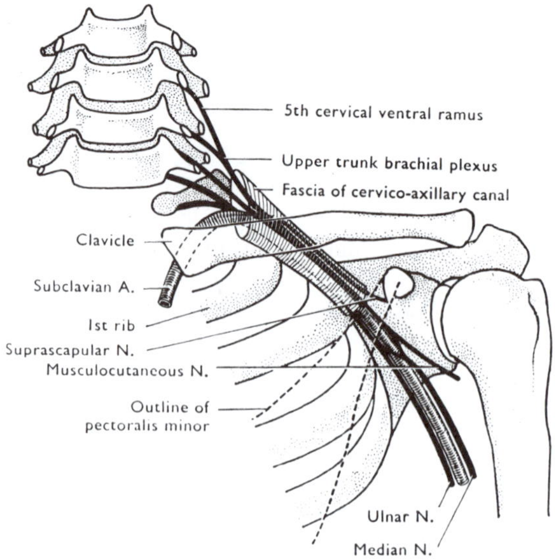

Fig. 25. A diagram to show the route of entry of the nerves and subclavian artery into the upper limb. The fascial sheath which binds these structures into a narrow bundle as they pass through the cervico-axillary canal is continuous medially with the prevertebral fascia and laterally with the axillary fascia. Compare with Fig. 128 and note how this single compact bundle is arranged close to the shoulder joint to allow free movement of the upper limb without traction on its contents.

will be found later on the deep surfaces of the rhomboid muscles.

The **suprascapular nerve** (C. 5, 6), to the supraspinatus and infraspinatus muscles, runs inferolaterally behind the clavicle and crosses the superior border of the scapula to its posterior surface [Fig. 26].

The **nerve to subclavius** (C. 5, 6) descends in front of the plexus into the back of the muscle.

The **long thoracic nerve** (C. 5, 6, 7) arises from the back of these ventral rami. It descends behind the brachial plexus and axillary artery and then on the lateral surface of the serratus anterior muscle which it supplies.

2. Branches in the axilla.

The lateral and medial **pectoral nerves** pass forwards from the corresponding cords of the brachial plexus on the lateral and medial sides of the first part of the axillary artery. They then communicate in front of the artery, and pass to supply the pectoral muscles in the anterior axillary wall. The lateral (C. 5, 6, 7) enters the deep surface of pectoralis major superior to pectoralis minor. The medial (C. 8, T. 1) supplies and pierces pectoralis minor to enter pectoralis major.

Subscapular nerves.

These two nerves (C. 5, 6) upper and lower, arise from the posterior cord to the brachial plexus with the thoracodorsal nerve. With it they supply the muscles of the posterior axillary wall. The upper passes backwards into the subscapularis muscle; the lower inclines postero-inferiorly to supply the lower fibres of subscapularis and teres major.

Thoracodorsal nerve (C. 6, 7).

This nerve passes postero-inferiorly to supply the latissimus dorsi muscle. It runs with the thoracodorsal artery on the deep surface of the muscle. For the remaining branches of the plexus see pages 49–53, 62, 69–70, 73.

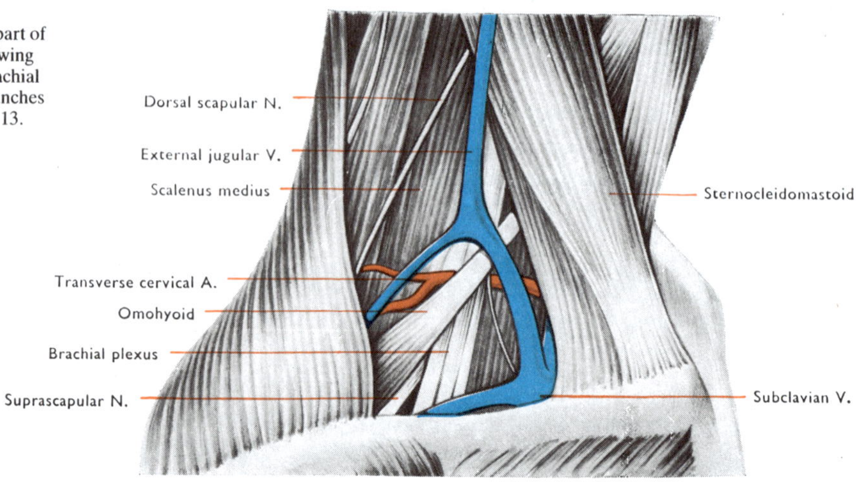

Fig. 26. Dissection of lower part of posterior triangle of neck showing the supraclavicular part of brachial plexus. For the superficial branches of the cervical plexus, see Fig 13.

The dissection of the back

Turn the body face downwards and examine the structures which connect the limb with the back of the trunk.

Surface anatomy of the back

Begin by reviewing the structure of the scapula [p. 54 and Figs. 32, 33, 49, 51].

The **scapula** is placed at a tangent to the posterolateral part of the upper thorax. It lies over the second to seventh ribs and extends into the posterior wall of the axilla. It is thickly covered with muscles, but most of its outline can be felt in the living subject. Find the acromion at the top of the shoulder. Draw your finger along the bony ridge (crest of the spine of the scapula) which runs medially and slightly downwards from the acromion to the medial border of the scapula, and trace this border to the inferior angle and, if possible, to the superior angle [Fig. 32] palpating it through the muscles that cover it. The scapula is held in position by muscles and by the clavicle. It is very movable—the scapulae being drawn apart when the arms are folded across the chest or stretched forwards, but their medial borders are brought close to the posterior median line when the shoulders are drawn back.

The rib which is palpable immediately inferior to the inferior angle of the scapula is usually the eighth; and the lower ribs may be counted from it. The **twelfth rib** is not palpable unless it projects beyond the lateral margin of the

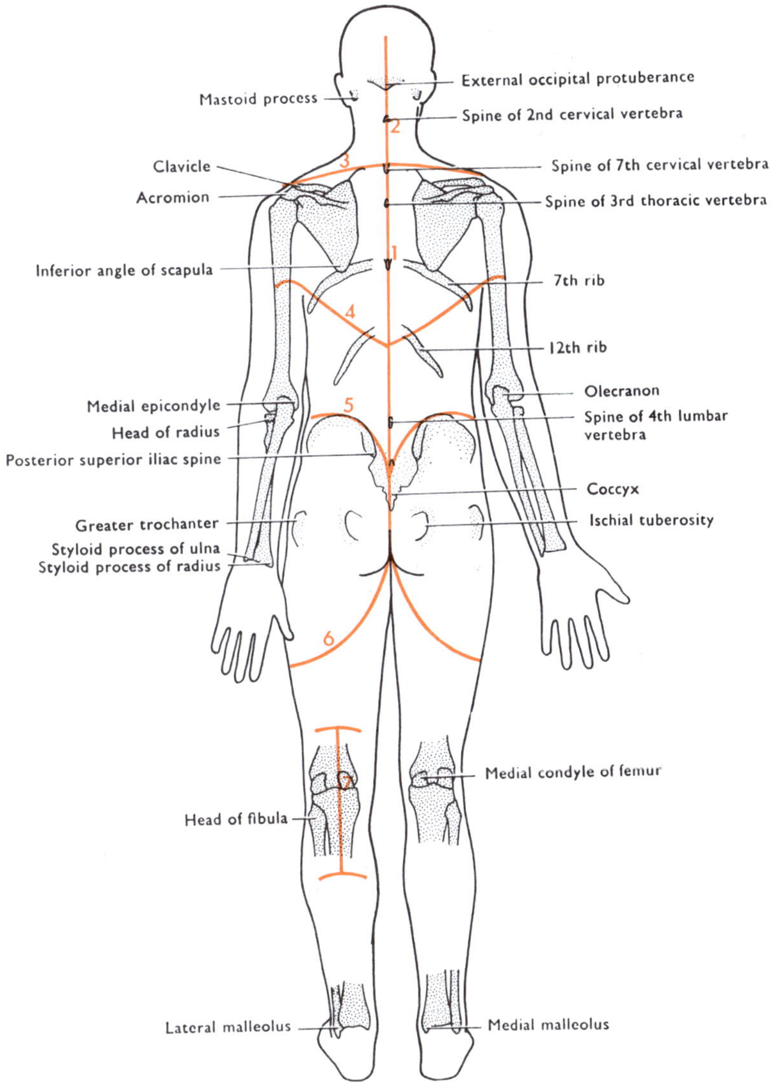

Fig. 27. Landmarks and incisions. For the bony landmarks of the upper limb, see illustrations of individual bones. Left forearm pronated, right supinated.

erector spinae, i.e. the mass of muscle in the small of the back, when its tip will be found 3 cm above the iliac crest [Figs. 27, 114].

The **iliac crest** is the curved bony ridge felt below the waist. Traced forwards and backwards it ends in the anterior and posterior **superior iliac spines** respectively. The posterior is felt in a shallow dimple in the skin above the buttock and about 5 cm from the median plane. Between the left and right dimples is the back of the **sacrum** which usually has three palpable spines in the median plane. The **coccyx** is the slightly mobile bone felt deeply between the buttocks in the median plane.

Palpate the tips of the **spines of the vertebrae** in the median furrow of the back, and note that some are deflected to one side or another. These are the only parts of the vertebral column which are readily felt. It is difficult to identify individual spines directly, but the seventh cervical (**vertebra prominens**) is the uppermost which can be readily felt at the back of the root of your neck. Below this the approximate levels of other spines are:

Spines	*Level*
Third thoracic	Where the spine of the scapula meets its medial border
Seventh thoracic	Inferior angle of the scapula
Fourth lumbar	Highest point of the iliac crest
Second sacral	Posterior superior iliac spine

Above the vertebra prominens only the **second cervical spine** can be felt easily. It is about 5 cm below the **external occipital protuberance** which is on the lower part of the back of the head where the median furrow of the neck (**nuchal groove**) meets the skull. The short cervical spines (cf. C. 7) are separated from the skin by a median fibrous partition, the **ligamentum nuchae.** Its posterior edge stretches from the external occipital protuberance to the seventh cervical spine.

The **superior nuchal line** is a curved bony ridge extending laterally from the external occipital protuberance. This line, the protuberance, the ligamentum nuchae, and the seventh cervical and thoracic spines give attachment to the upper part of the trapezius, the most superficial of the muscles of the back of the neck.

Dissection

Make the skin incisions 1, 3, 4, and 5 [Fig. 27]. Reflect the two skin flaps laterally, stripping the skin and superficial fascia from the deep fascia by blunt dissection. Find the cutaneous nerves as they pierce the deep fascia [Fig. 28]. This is more difficult than on the flexor surface because of the denser connections of the two fasciae on the back.

Cutaneous nerves

The cutaneous nerves of the back are branches of the **dorsal rami of the spinal nerves.** Each dorsal ramus divides into a medial and a lateral branch [Fig. 2]. Both of these enter and supply the erector spinae muscles, and one continues through them to supply the overlying skin. Medial branches from the cervical and upper six or seven thoracic dorsal rami form the **cutaneous branches** and pierce the deep fascia close to the median plane. Below this the lateral branches supply the skin and emerge in line with the lateral edge of the erector spinae piercing either the latissimus dorsi (upper nerves) or the dense deep fascia (thoracolumbar) of the small of the back (lower nerves). Each of these cutaneous nerves divides into a smaller medial and a larger lateral branch. In the thoracic and lumbar nerves, both these branches descend before entering the skin. Thus the area of skin supplied by the dorsal ramus of each of these nerves lies at a lower level than that at which the spinal nerve emerges. This makes the **dermatomes** [p. 6] of the trunk more nearly horizontal than would be expected from the oblique course of the ventral rami, e.g. the intercostal nerves.

The cutaneous branches of the dorsal rami of the upper three lumbar nerves pierce the deep fascia a short distance superior to the iliac crest and turn down over it to supply the skin of the gluteal region.

The **arteries** which accompany the cutaneous nerves of the back arise from the dorsal branches of the posterior intercostal and lumbar arteries.

Muscles that attach the scapula to the trunk

Two of these muscles, the **pectoralis minor** and the **serratus anterior,** have been seen already. The remaining muscles are **trapezius** [Fig. 28] with the **rhomboids** and **levator scapulae** deep to it. The latissimus dorsi will also be seen in the dissection of the back. Latissimus dorsi and pectoralis major are the two muscles which attach the humerus directly to the trunk.

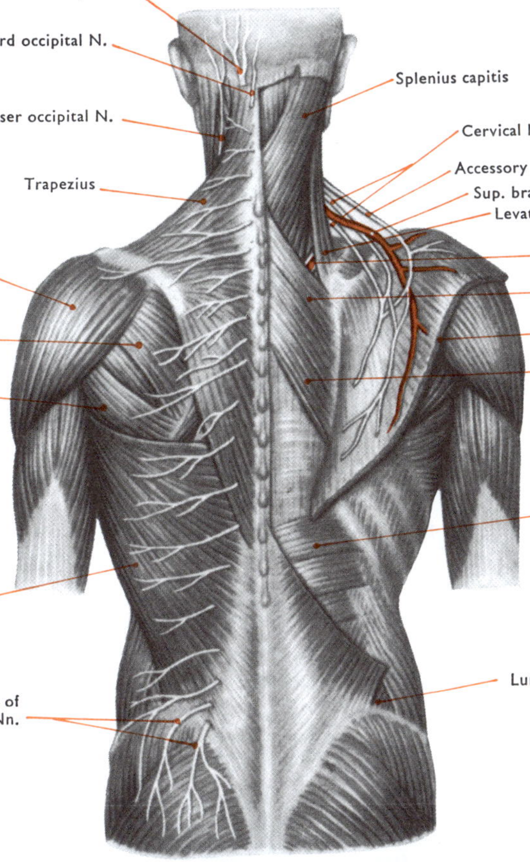

Fig. 28. Dissection of superficial muscles and nerves of the back.

Dissection

Remove the deep fascia from the surface of trapezius below the spine of the seventh cervical vertebra. The upper part of the muscle will be dissected with the head and neck.

Uncover the **latissimus dorsi** [Fig. 28]. This is difficult because of the varying direction of its fibres and the thinness of its upper part which has an ill-defined margin. Define its attachment to the thoracolumbar fascia and to the iliac crest. Expose the lateral border of the muscle and its slips from the lowest three or four ribs which interdigitate there with the external oblique muscle of the abdomen.

Reflect the lower part of **trapezius** by dividing the exposed part horizontally half way between the clavicle and the spine of the scapula, and vertically 5 cm lateral to the median plane. In the latter cut, take care not to injure the subjacent rhomboid muscles, for the trapezius is thin near its origin. Reflect trapezius and define its *attachments* to the thoracic vertebral spines, the medial border of the acromion and the superior margin of the crest of the spine of the scapula. Note the superficial branch of the transverse cervical vessels and the accessory nerve on the deep surface of the lateral part. Expose the upper part of the muscle at its attachments to the clavicle and the acromion [Fig. 30].

Define the **levator scapulae, rhomboid minor,** and **rhomboid major** muscles which are attached from above downwards, in that order, to the medial border of the scapula, deep to trapezius [Fig. 51]. The rhomboid minor is attached where the spine of the scapula meets its medial border. Only the lower part of the levator scapulae can be seen at this time. Free this part of the muscle from the underlying fat, and identify the **dorsal scapular nerve** and the **deep branch of the transverse cervical artery,** following them to the deep surface of the rhomboid muscles. Divide both rhomboid muscles midway between the vertebral spines and the medial border of the scapula. Reflect these muscles, define their attachments, and trace the dorsal scapular nerve and the deep branch of the transverse cervical artery deep to them.

Lift the medial border of the scapula from the thoracic wall. Note how easily it and the underlying **serratus anterior muscle** are lifted clear because of the loose connective tissue between them. Pass one hand between the thoracic wall and the serratus anterior, then place the other hand in the axilla from the front and slide it backwards between the subscapularis [Fig 18] and the serratus anterior which is now between your hands. Define the attachment of serratus anterior to the scapula [Fig. 33] and, turning latissimus dorsi downwards, note how the inferior digitations of serratus anterior converge on the anterior surface of the inferior angle of the scapula [Fig. 31].

Remove the fat from the suprascapular region deep to the cut edge of trapezius, and find the inferior belly of the slender **omohyoid muscle** and the **suprascapular vessels and nerve** passing to the superior border of the scapula at the scapular notch [Figs. 33, 49].

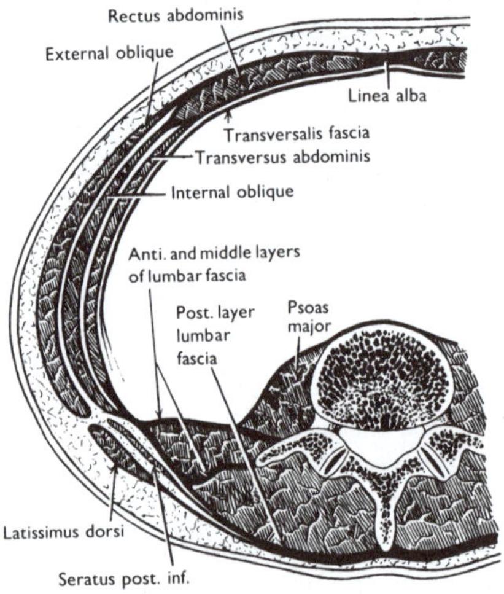

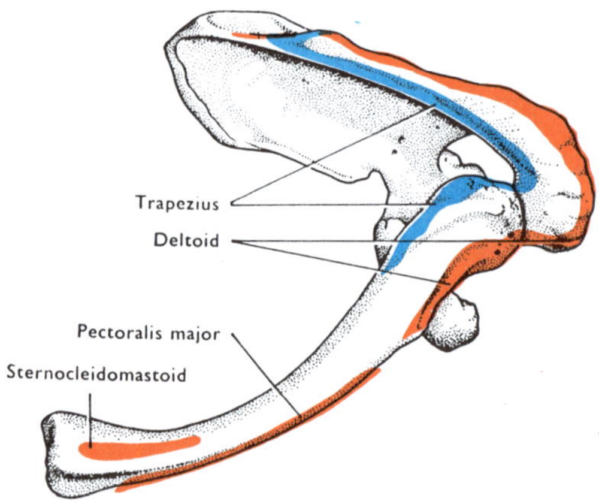

Fig. 29 (*above left*). Diagram of thoracolumbar fascia in a section through the trunk at level of second lumbar vertebra.

Fig. 30 (*above right*). Shoulder girdle from above showing muscle attachments.

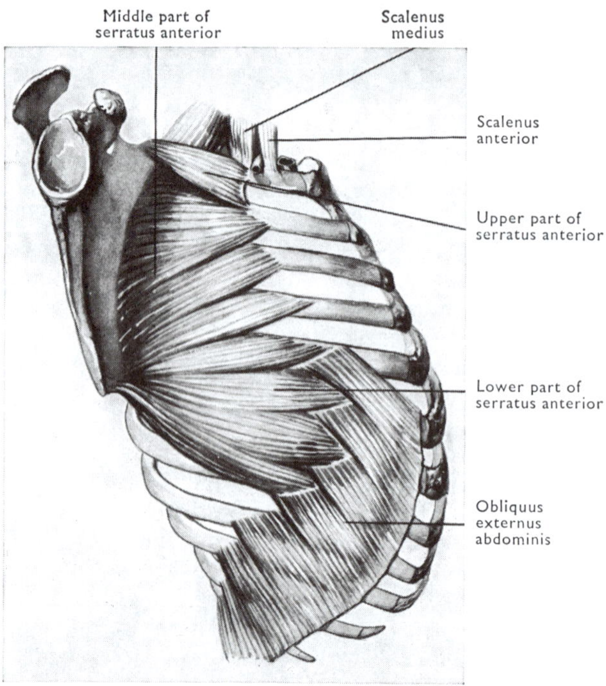

Fig. 31. Serratus anterior and origin of external oblique. The scapula is drawn away from the side of the chest.

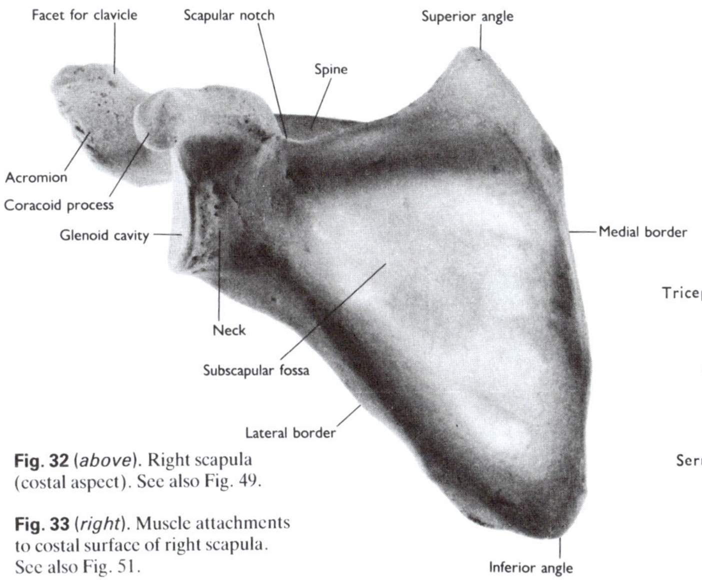

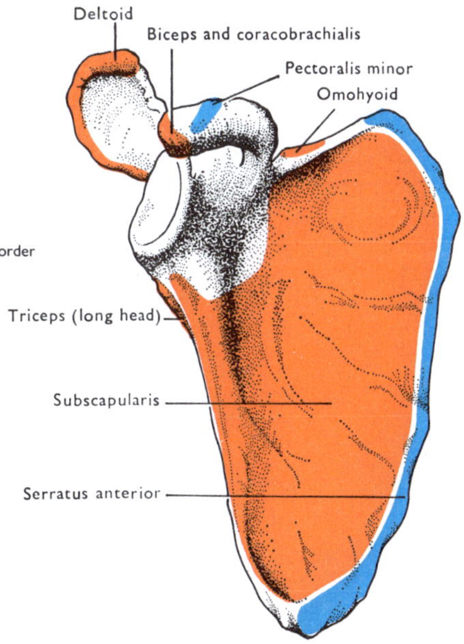

Fig. 32 (*above*). Right scapula (costal aspect). See also Fig. 49.

Fig. 33 (*right*). Muscle attachments to costal surface of right scapula. See also Fig. 51.

Movements of the scapula and the muscles which produce them

The scapula is able to slide freely over the chest wall because of the loose connective tissue between serratus anterior and that wall. Its movements are produced by the muscles which attach the scapula to the trunk and indirectly by the muscles passing from the trunk to the humerus when the shoulder joint is fixed. All these movements take place around the **sternoclavicular joint** with minor adjustments at the **acromioclavicular joint.**

Protraction

This movement of the scapula forwards on the chest wall produced by the **serratus anterior** assisted by the pectoral muscles. All eight digitations of the serratus anterior passing from the external surfaces of the ribs [Fig. 31] to the anterior surface of the medial border of the scapula contract together with **pectoralis minor** and the sternocostal fibres of **pectoralis major**. This movement is used in reaching forwards, punching, and pushing.

Retraction

This is the reverse of protraction. It draws the scapulae backwards towards the median plane and braces back the shoulders. It is produced by the contraction of the middle fibres of **trapezius** which pass horizontally from the ligamentum nuchae, and the seventh cervical and upper thoracic spines to the acromion and lateral part of the spine of the scapula. Also by the **rhomboid muscles** passing from a similar origin to the medial border of the scapula from the level of the spine to the level of the inferior angle [Fig. 28].

Elevation

Elevation, as in shrugging the shoulders, is achieved by the simultaneous contraction of the **levator scapulae** and the upper fibres of **trapezius** which descend from the skull and ligamentum nuchae to the clavicle and acromion [Fig. 30]. Levator scapulae descends from the posterior tubercles of the transverse processes of the upper four cervical vertebrae to the superior angle of the scapula.

Depression

This movement is achieved by the contraction of the pectoralis minor, the lower fibres of pectoralis major and trapezius, and by latissimus dorsi.

Rotation

This takes place around a horizontal axis passing through the middle of the scapular spine and the sternoclavicular joint [Fig. 34]. In **lateral rotation,** the upper fibres of **trapezius** raise the acromion and lateral part of the clavicle, while its lower fibres [Fig. 28] depress the medial end of the spine of the scapula. Together they act like the forces applied to a wing-nut. The lower five digitations of **serratus anterior** converge on the inferior angle of the scapula and play a powerful part in this movement by pulling that angle laterally and forwards. This lateral rotation tilts the glenoid cavity [Fig. 32] upwards and is essential in abduction of the upper limb above the horizontal—the limit of abduction at the shoulder joint [p. 59].

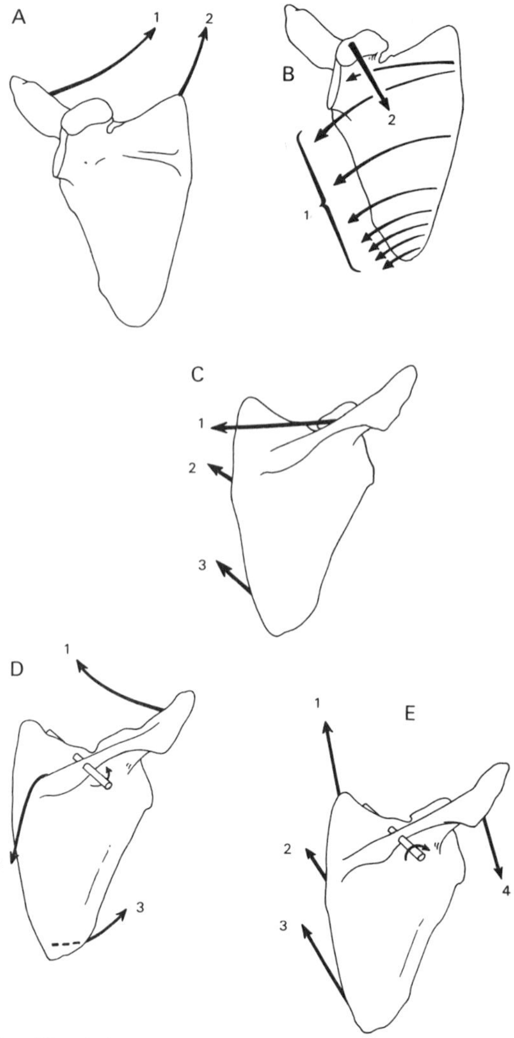

Fig. 34. Diagrams to show the direction of pull of various muscles on the scapula to produce its different movements.
A. Elevation of the scapula as in shrugging the shoulders.
1. Upper fibres of trapezius.
2. Levator scapulae.
B. Protraction of the scapula, as in punching or stretching forwards.
1. Serratus anterior pulls the entire scapula forwards on the curve of the thoracic wall.
2. Pectoralis minor assists.
C. Retraction of the scapula, as in drawing the shoulders back.
1. Middle fibres of trapezius.
2. Rhomboid minor.
3. Rhomboid major.
D. and E. Rotation of the scapula. In these figures, the axis of movement is shown as a rod piercing the scapula. The arrow shows the direction of rotation.
D. Lateral rotation.
1. Upper fibres of trapezius.
2. Lower fibres of trapezius.
3. Lower part of serratus anterior.
E. Medial rotation.
1. Levator scapulae.
2. Rhomboid minor.
3. Rhomboid major.
4. The weight of the upper limb.

Normally, scapular and shoulder joint movements occur together but, if the scapular movement is paralysed, abduction of the limb to the horizontal cannot be achieved because its weight forces the scapula into medial rotation.

Medial rotation

This is the opposite movement. Though gravity plays a large part in this movement as in depression of the scapula, combined contraction of levator scapulae, rhomboids, and latissimus dorsi produces this as an active movement which is assisted by the pectoral muscles [Fig. 55].

When all the muscles attaching the scapula to the trunk are contracted, the scapula is fixed to form a stable base on which upper limb movements can take place. It is also used in transmitting forces from the trunk to the upper limbs, as in lifting heavy weights in the hands by straightening the flexed legs.

Nerve supply of the muscles: see Table 1 [p. 114].

Latissimus dorsi

This broad sheet of muscle arises from the lower six thoracic spines and the supraspinous ligaments between them, deep to trapezius; from the thoracolumbar fascia [Figs. 28, 29]; from the posterior part of the iliac crest; and from the lower three or four ribs. It converges on the teres major and, winding round the inferior border of that muscle to its anterior surface, passes to the intertubercular groove of the humerus [Fig. 35]. **Action:** it is a powerful adductor of the humerus and depressor of the shoulder. Thus it is used to pull the arm down from its fully abducted position above the head, as in climbing or bell ringing. When the shoulder is flexed, it acts as an extensor of that joint. When the shoulder is fixed it helps with retraction and medial rotation of the scapula. **Nerve supply:** the thoracodorsal nerve.

The accessory nerve

The accessory or eleventh cranial nerve consists of cranial and spinal parts. The **spinal part** arises from the cervical spinal medulla (C. 1–5) and ascends within the vertebral column to enter the skull with the spinal medulla. Here it joins its cranial part, and emerges from the skull with the vagus (10th cranial) nerve. Leaving both, the spinal part passes postero-inferiorly through sternocleidomastoid [Fig. 13] to the deep surface of the trapezius supplying both muscles. This peculiar nerve supply to these muscles is the result of their origin from the muscles which are responsible for gill movements in the fishes.

The dorsal scapular nerve

This nerve passes postero-inferiorly in the lower part of the neck from the ventral ramus of the fifth cervical nerve. It runs deep to the lower part of the levator scapulae and the rhomboid muscles and supplies them. Here it is accompanied by the deep branch of the transverse cervical artery [pp. 38, 62].

The free upper limb

Surface anatomy

It is important for the student to know the bones of the upper limb and to be able to identify their parts and markings [Figs. 229–240], the places where they are readily palpable, the nature of the joints between them, and the movements which take place at these joints. The following points should be carefully examined on your own upper limb.

The arm

The **humerus** [Figs. 35, 36] is almost entirely covered by the muscles of the arm so that its outlines can only be felt indistinctly except in its distal quarter. Here it expands transversely and its lateral and medial **margins** (supracondylar ridges) become readily palpable. Each margin ends inferiorly in the corresponding **epicondyle** of which the medial is the more prominent. In the

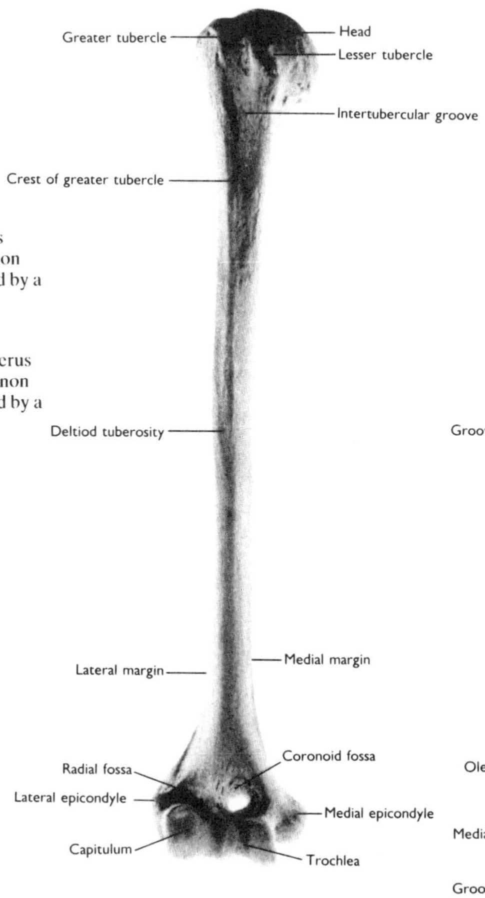

Fig. 35 (*right*). Right humerus (anterior aspect). The olecranon and coronoid fossae are united by a foramen.

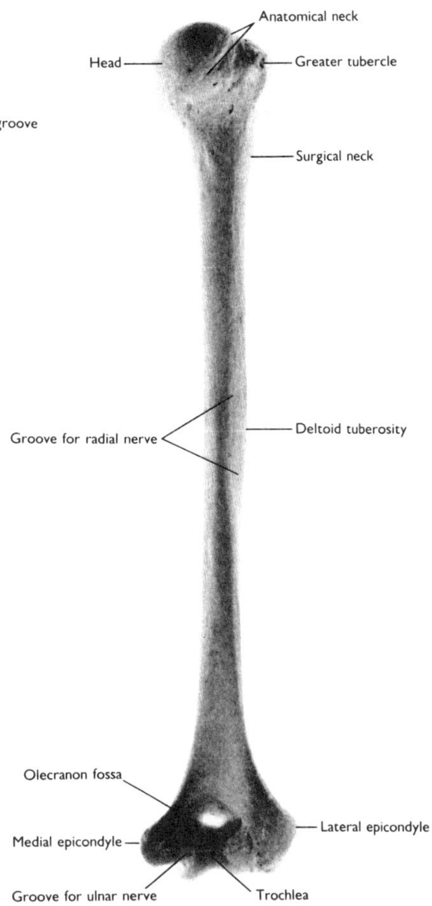

Fig. 36 (*far right*). Right humerus (posterior aspect). The olecranon and coronoid fossae are united by a foramen.

anatomical position, the epicondyles are in the positions suggested by their names and the hemispherical head of the humerus faces medially. When the palms of the hands face medially, the lateral epicondyle is more anterior in position and the head of the humerus looks posteromedially with its centre and that of the glenoid in contact.

The upper half of the humerus is covered on its anterior, lateral, and posterior surfaces by the deltoid muscle. Inferiorly, the apex of that muscle is attached to the lateral side of the middle of the humerus (**deltoid tuberosity**). The upper part of the bone consists of the **head**. This is separated by a shallow groove (**anatomical neck**) from the greater (lateral) and lesser (anterior) **tubercles**. Both head and tubercles are continuous inferiorly with the **body** of the bone through the narrowing **surgical neck.** *The greater tubercle is the most lateral bony part of the shoulder.* The lower half of the bone is covered anteriorly by the biceps and brachialis muscles and posteriorly by the triceps muscle. The anterior surfaces of the epicondyles and supracondylar ridges give rise to forearm muscles.

At the midpoint of the anterior surface of the bend of the elbow, find the **tendon of biceps muscle**. Medial to this, feel the pulsating **brachial artery** and trace it superiorly on the medial side of the arm. The **median nerve** may be palpable posteromedial to it. Lightly compress your right arm with your left hand and contract your right forearm muscles by clenching and unclenching your fist. This distends the **superficial veins** and makes them visible [Fig. 46]. Compare your superficial veins with those of the other students and note their variability and the presence of a cephalic and a basilic vein in most cases.

The forearm

The two bones of the forearm are the radius (lateral) and the ulna (medial). Proximally, the trochlear notch of the **ulna** [Fig. 37] articulates with the **trochlea of the humerus** [Fig. 35]—the larger, medial part of the continuous articular surface on the distal end of the humerus and the only part visible on the posterior surface. The superior (**olecranon**) and inferior (**coronoid process**) margins of the trochlear notch of the ulna fit into the corresponding fossae of the humerus—the olecranon in full extension, the coronoid process in full flexion of the elbow joint. The proximal part of the ulna (the olecranon) is readily palpable. On its posterior surface is a triangular, subcutaneous area which is continuous distally with the **posterior margin** (border) **of the ulna**. The entire length of this margin is palpable. It ends distally in the **styloid process** which projects from the posteromedial aspect of the cylindrical, slightly expanded **head** of the bone [Fig. 105]. This palpable line not only allows the entire length of the ulna to be examined for fractures, but also forms the line of separation between the anteromedial, flexor group of muscles of the forearm (supplied by the median and ulnar nerves) and the posterolateral, extensor group (supplied by the radial nerve).

The proximal end (**head**) of the **radius** is a short cylinder whose concave proximal surface articulates with the spherical, lateral part (**capitulum**) of the articular surface of the humerus, while its circumference articulates medially with the **radial notch of the ulna** and elsewhere with the **anular ligament**. This loop, attached to the margins of the notch on the ulna, narrows distally to fit the superior part of the **neck of the radius** [Fig. 37] and prevents the head being pulled out of the ligament. Palpate the head of the radius just distal to the lateral epicondyle of the humerus and feel it rotating within the anular ligament when you pronate and supinate your forearm [p. 20]. The **radial tuberosity** lies on the medial aspect of the radius distal to the neck. It has the tendon of biceps brachii attached to its posterior part. Beyond this the radius is markedly convex laterally and only its distal part is readily palpable through the muscles which cover it.

The wrist

Distally the radius expands into a cuboidal mass with a triangular lateral extension the apex of which is the blunt **styloid process**. When the thumb is fully extended, i.e. moved laterally, a hollow, 'the **anatomical snuff-box**', appears on the lateral side of the back of the wrist between the tendons passing to the thumb. The styloid process lies in the proximal part of the anterior margin of the hollow covered by tendons of the short extensor and

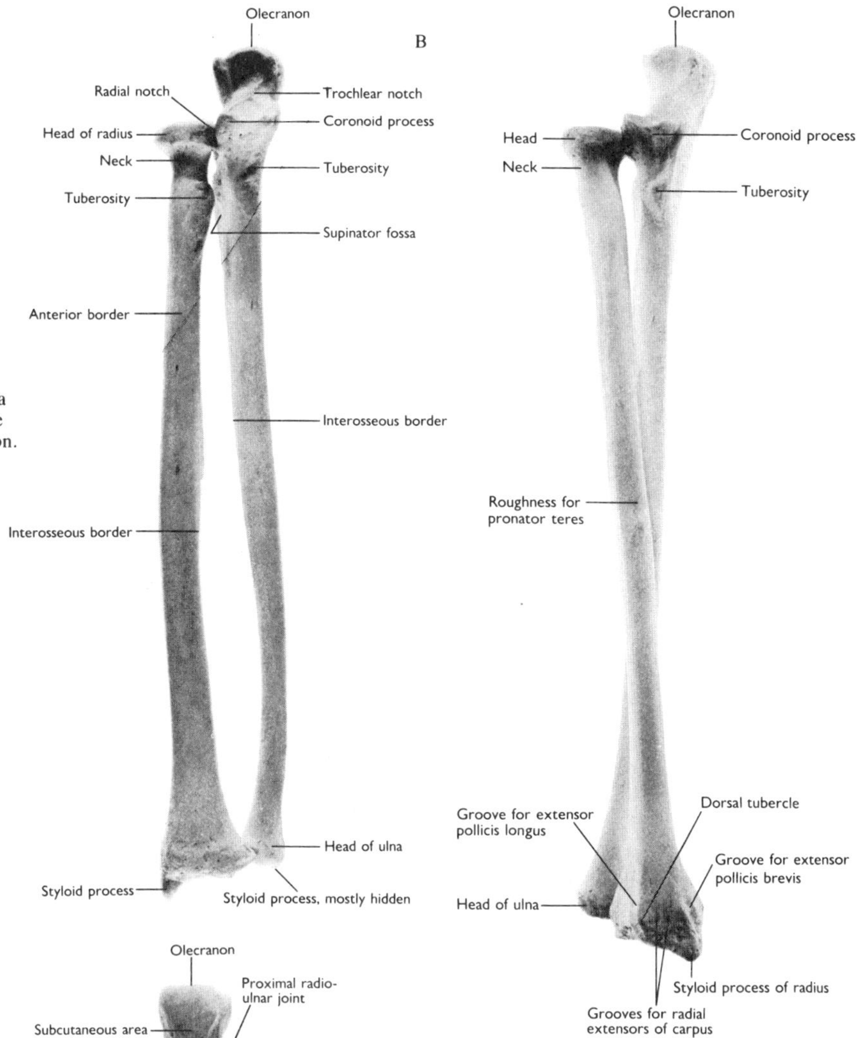

Fig. 37. Right radius and ulna (anterior surface). (A) Supine position. (B) Pronated position.

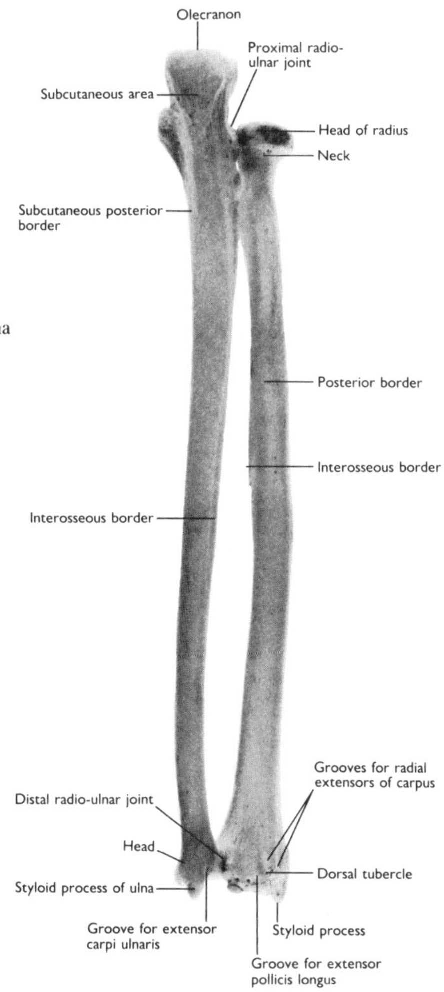

Fig. 38. Right radius and ulna (posterior surface).

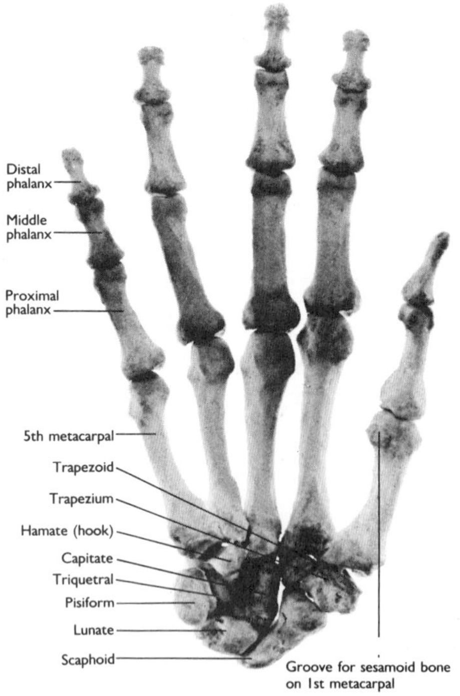

Fig. 39. Palmar aspect of bones of right hand.

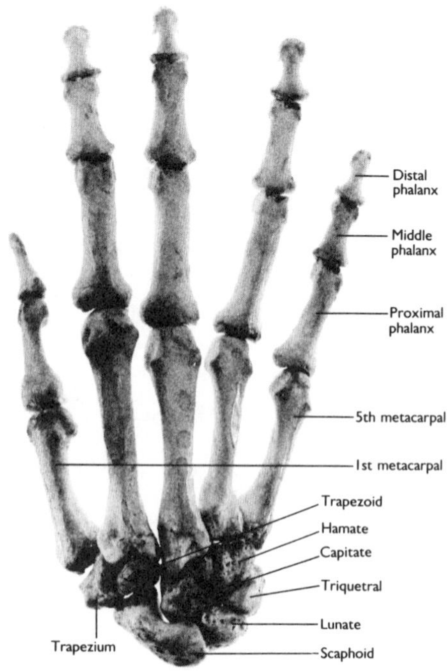

Fig. 40. Dorsal aspect of bones of right hand.

long abductor muscles of the thumb, the latter passing to the base of its metacarpal. The bones which form the lateral ends of the proximal and distal rows of the carpal bones (**scaphoid** and **trapezium** [Fig. 39]) and the base of the metacarpal of the thumb can be felt deeply in the hollow distal to the styloid process. Light pressure applied here over the trapezium reveals the pulsations of the **radial artery**. This is more easily felt as the '*radial pulse*' where the artery crosses the anterior projection of the distal end of the radius medial to the styloid process.

Feel your radial and ulnar styloid processes at the same time. Note that the radial styloid projects further distally than the ulnar—a situation which is altered when the radius is fractured. If the tendon forming the posterior boundary of the 'snuff-box' (extensor pollicis longus) is followed proximally, it curves round the medial surface of the **dorsal tubercle** of the radius which is readily palpable.

The distal end of the radius articulates medially with the ulna (**ulnar notch**) and distally with the lateral two (scaphoid and lunate) of the proximal row of **carpal** (wrist) **bones**. This forms the only direct articulation of the carpal bones with the bones of the forearm; hence any forces transmitted from the hand to the forearm pass through these bones to the radius—a feature which accounts for the fracture of the scaphoid or radius (but not the ulna) from falling on the outstretched hand.

The dorsal surfaces of both rows of carpal bones can be felt through the tendons which cover them, though the individual bones cannot be defined. The **metacarpals** (hand bones) and the **phalanges** (finger bones) are readily palpated on their dorsal surfaces. On the palmar surface of the wrist only the **pisiform bone** (medially) and the **tubercle of the scaphoid** (laterally) can be seen and felt at the level of the distal, transverse skin crease (junction of the forearm and wrist) when the wrist is fully extended. If the wrist is passively flexed, the pisiform may be gripped between finger and thumb and moved on the triquetrum bone with which it articulates, and the **tendon of flexor carpi ulnaris** can be felt passing to its proximal surface. The **hook of the hamate** and the **tubercle of the trapezium** can also be felt deeply through the proximal parts of the muscles forming the ball of the little finger (**hypothenar eminence**) and the ball of the thumb (**thenar eminence**) respectively [Fig. 77]. These four palpable bony points lying at the ends of the two rows of carpal bones are bound together by the **flexor retinaculum**—a dense layer of deep fascia—which acts like a bow-string maintaining the palmar concavity of the carpal bones (**sulcus carpi**) and converting this into a tunnel through which the flexor tendons and the median nerve pass from the forearm into the hand [Fig. 82].

The palm

The skin of the central region of the palm is firmly bound to the thickened underlying deep fascia (**palmar aponeurosis**) which is continuous distally with the deep fascia of the fingers and proximally with the flexor retinaculum and the **tendon of palmaris longus**. If present, this tendon enters the palm superficial to the retinaculum and is the most superficial tendon immediately proximal to the wrist. It and extension of the fingers tighten the palmar aponeurosis and stabilize the palmar skin to maintain a firm grip. The distal **skin crease** of the palm lies just proximal to the metacarpophalangeal joints while that at the roots of the fingers lies approximately 3 cm distal to them. The middle skin crease of each finger lies at the level of the proximal interphalangeal joint, while the distal skin crease lies proximal to the distal interphalangeal joint. When a fist is formed, the **knuckles** are the distal ends of the **heads of the metacarpal bones** uncovered by the movement of the proximal phalanges on to the palmar surfaces of these heads. The heads of the proximal and middle phalanges of the fingers are similarly exposed.

The digits

The **thumb** has only two phalanges compared with three in the fingers, and it lies at right angles to the fingers with its nail facing laterally and not posteriorly. Thus **flexion** moves the tip of the thumb medially across the palm while **extension** moves it laterally. **Abduction** swings the tip of the thumb anteriorly; **adduction** moves it to the index finger. The metacarpal of the thumb moves freely in all of these movements at the carpometacarpal joint at its base, while the metacarpal bones of the fingers are nearly rigid. To test this, grip the head of each metacarpal in turn with the thumb and index finger of your other hand on the palmar and dorsal surfaces. The metacarpal of the middle finger scarcely moves, while those of the index, ring, and little finger, in that order, have an increasing but small range of flexion and extension and slight rotation only in the little finger, but none can be abducted or adducted. Flex your thumb at the metacarpophalangeal joint and attempt to rotate its metacarpal using the phalanges as a lever. Only a tiny amount of movement is possible compared with the free flexion/extension and abduction/adduction at the carpometacarpal joint of the thumb.

Flexion of the **metacarpophalangeal joint** of the thumb is considerably less than 90 degrees while it is 90 degrees in the index and middle fingers and exceeds this in the ring and little fingers in which there is equally little rotation. Check the bones and note that there is nothing in their contours at these joints to prevent rotation—it is limited by ligaments. Also there is very little abduction or adduction at this joint in the thumb though it is relatively free in the fingers.

The **interphalangeal joint** of the thumb flexes to approximately 90 degrees while the proximal interphalangeal joints of the fingers flex to more than 90 degress and their distal interphalangeal joints to slightly less than 90 degrees.

The fingers separate on extension and come together in flexion. This is the result of the curve in which the heads of the metacarpals lie and a slight obliquity of the interphalangeal joints. Note also that the tips of all four fingers meet the palm at the same time despite the differences in their lengths. Check your interphalangeal joints for rotation. This is minimal because of the shape of the articular surfaces of the phalanges which should be checked on the bones.

Cup the palm of your hand by spreading the fingers as though to grasp a large ball. The hollow between the proximal parts of the thenar and hypothenar eminences marks the position of the **flexor retinaculum**. The furrow on the medial side of the hypothenar eminence is produced by the contraction of **palmaris brevis** which heaps up the hypothenar skin to form a pad for grasping. Note too that the thumb is slightly flexed at the carpometacarpal joint and rotated medially so that its palmar surface faces that of the little finger (opposition) which is also rotated laterally. The other three fingers are not parallel to each other, but on flexion converge to meet the tip of the thumb.

Dissection

Make incision 5 as shown in Fig. 9, but later extend the incision along the anterior surfaces of all the fingers, leaving them covered with skin at present to avoid drying of the tissues. Strip the skin and superficial fascia from the deep fascia by blunt dissection. Note and follow the large cutaneous veins and the cutaneous nerves as they pierce the deep fascia.

Superficial fascia

There are no special points about this fascia in the arm or forearm, but it contains dense bundles of fibrous tissue connecting the skin to the palmar aponeurosis in the palm and is thickened transversely in the webs of the fingers to form the **superficial transverse metacarpal ligament**. On the proximal part of the hypothenar eminence it contains **palmaris brevis** which passes from the skin on the ulnar border of the hand to the palmar aponeurosis.

Superficial veins

The main veins are extremely variable. They begin in the **dorsal venous net** of the hand—an irregular arrangement of veins, usually with a transverse element 2–3 cm proximal to the heads of the metacarpals. It receives the dorsal digital veins through the **intercapital veins** posterior to the intermetacarpal spaces, and also communicating veins from the palm which pass through the distal parts of these spaces. This net drains into a number of veins of which one or more on the medial side form the **basilic vein** and on the lateral side the **cephalic vein**. Both these veins turn round the corresponding border of the forearm as they ascend, so that they lie on the anteromedial and anterolateral surfaces of the forearm at the elbow. Here the arrangement is variable, but they are usually united anterior to the cubital fossa by a **median cubital vein** [Fig. 42] and much of the blood in the cephalic vein is transferred to the basilic vein. Another common arrangement is shown in Fig. 41. The veins then ascend on the corresponding sides of the biceps muscle. The cephalic pierces the deep fascia and runs between pectoralis major and deltoid to the infraclavicular fossa. Here it passes deeply to join the axillary vein near the apex of the axilla [Fig. 21]. The basilic vein pierces the deep fascia about the middle of the arm. It unites with the brachial veins and runs with the brachial artery to become the axillary vein at the lower border of the axilla.

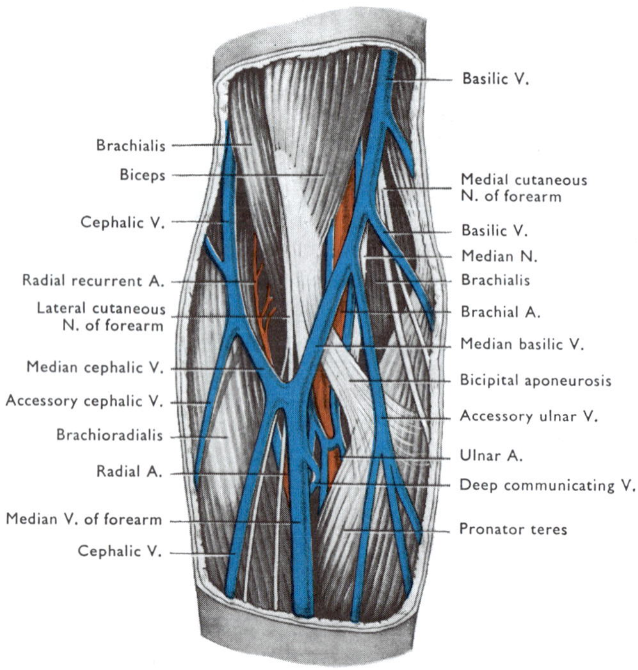

Fig. 41. Superficial veins at bend of elbow in a specimen in which the median vein was large.

Lymph vessels and lymph nodes of the upper limb

It is not possible in an ordinary dissection to display the lymph vessels in any part of the body. Lymph nodes are difficult to find especially in the elderly where they are reduced in size and scarcely distinguishable from the fat in which they lie unless involved in a disease process. It is necessary, however, to know the arrangement of the vessels and nodes because they form a common route for the spread of infection and cancer and the source of either can often be diagnosed from the nodes which are involved.

In the upper limb, as elsewhere, the lymph vessels and nodes are divided into two groups by the deep fascia.

Deep lymph vessels, which are much less numerous than the superficial vessels, drain structures which are deep to the deep fascia. They accompany the main blood vessels and drain into the axillary lymph nodes [p. 30]. Some of the lymph they contain may have passed through a small number of **deep lymph nodes** which are occasionally found on the arteries of the forearm, in the cubital fossa, and on the brachial artery.

The **superficial lymph nodes** of the upper limb are few in number. (1) One or two lie a little superior to the medial epicondyle near the basilic vein. (2) A few are scattered along the upper part of the cephalic vein.

Superficial lymph vessels of the upper limb drain the skin and subcutaneous tissues and most end in the lateral group of axillary nodes [p. 30]. The larger lymph vessels, unlike the veins, do not tend to unite into larger trunks but run individual courses directly towards the axilla. The general arrangement is shown in Figs. 42 and 43. (1) The dense palmar plexus drains mainly to the dorsum of the hand to join the posterior vessels of the forearm. (2) The vessels on the posterior surfaces of the forearm and arm spiral upwards round the medial and lateral surfaces to reach the anterior surface and approach the floor of the axilla. Some on the medial aspect enter the superficial cubital nodes, efferents from which pass through the deep fascia with the basilic

Fig. 42. Superficial lymph vessels and lymph nodes of front of upper limb.

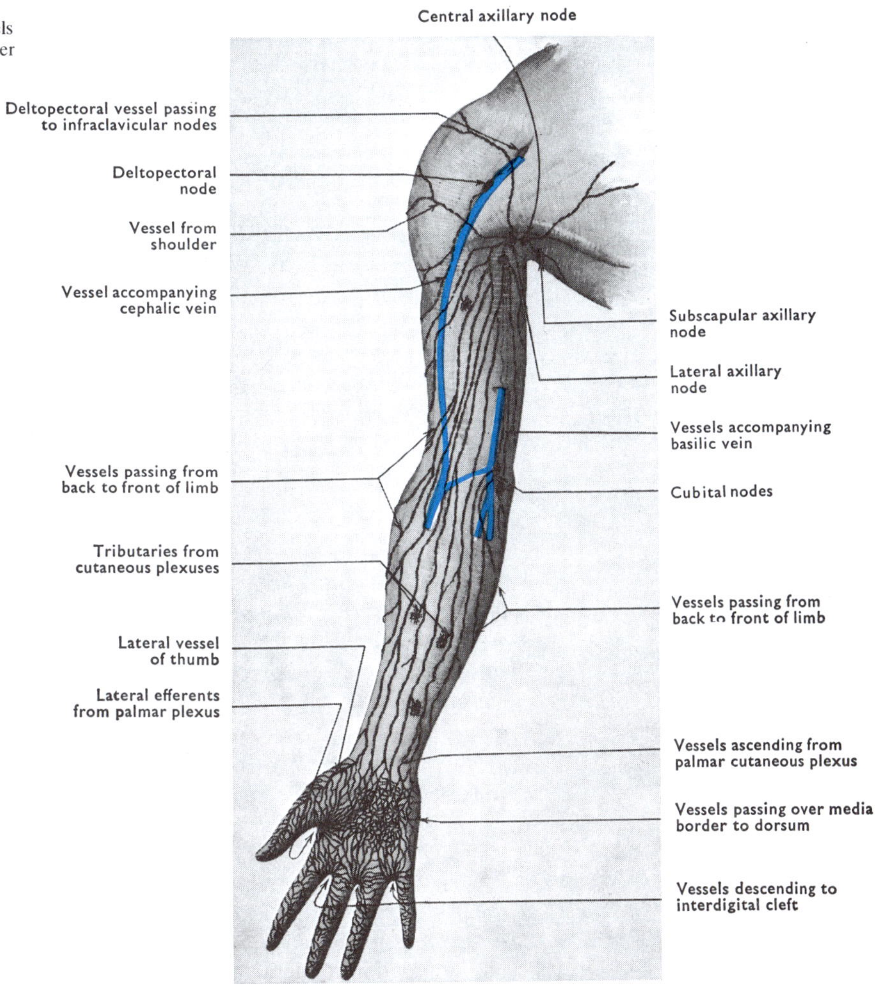

vein, but most remain superficial until they pierce the fascial floor of the axilla. (3) A few of the vessels from the lateral side of the arm and shoulder run with the cephalic vein into the apical axillary nodes. (4) Vessels from the shoulder and upper parts of the thoracic wall curve round the anterior and posterior axillary folds to enter the pectoral and subscapular groups of **axillary nodes** respectively. Those from the walls of the lower parts of the thorax and upper abdomen converge directly on the axilla.

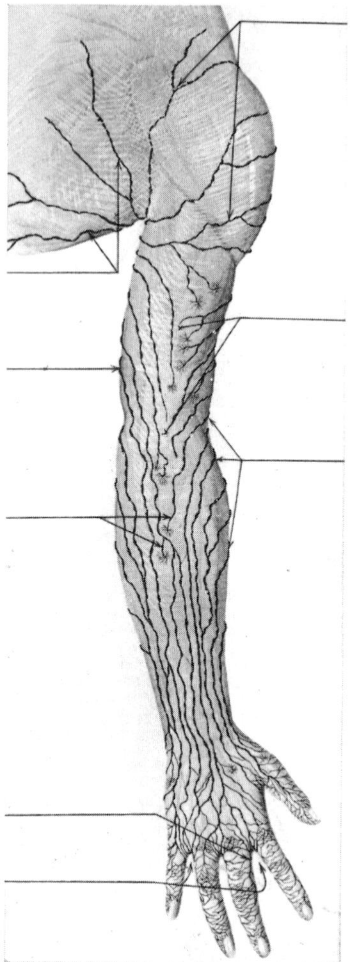

Fig. 43. Superficial lymph vessels of back of upper limb.

Cutaneous nerves of the upper limb

There are certain general points about the distribution of nerves to the skin which are of clinical importance in determining the site of a nerve injury.

1. Each nerve which passes to the skin is distributed to a circumscribed area.

2. The limb plexuses are formed by the plaiting together of the ventral rami of several spinal nerves. As a result of this: (a) *each part of the plexus and each of its branches contains nerve fibres from more than one ventral ramus;* (b) *several of these branches contain some nerve fibres from the same ventral ramus*. Thus the area of distribution of a cutaneous nerve and consequently the area of sensory loss when it is destroyed is different from that of a ventral ramus.

3. *All cutaneous nerves supplying adjacent areas of skin overlap with each other to a considerable degree*. Thus the destruction of a cutaneous nerve leads to a much smaller area of anaesthesia (total loss of sensation) than the area of distribution of the nerve surrounded by an area of altered sensation due to the presence of nerve fibres from adjacent, uninjured nerves.

Each thoracic spinal nerve (not involved in the formation of a plexus) supplies a strip of skin (**dermatome**) which overlaps those of adjacent nerves so that destruction of one thoracic spinal nerve produces only altered sensation within its dermatome. In the plexus regions, each ventral ramus

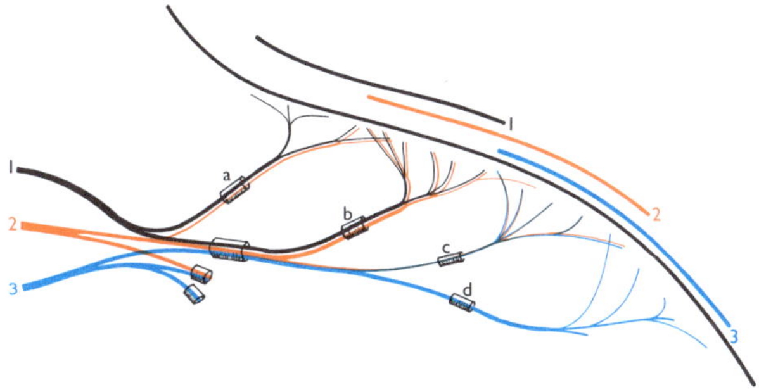

Fig. 44. Diagram to show how three spinal nerves involved in a plexus supply adjacent, overlapping dermatomes through the branches of the plexus.

supplies a circumscribed area of skin in sequence with and overlapped by the areas of adjacent ventral rami. The overlap of these dermatomes is made obvious by the presence of nerve fibres from more than one ventral ramus in every branch of the plexus.

4. Major branches of the plexus, i.e. the main nerves of a limb, give rise to several cutaneous branches which leave them at different points. Destruction of such a nerve before it has given off any branches will produce a different distribution of sensory loss to that which arises if the nerve is destroyed after giving off one or more branches. It is more important to know the total distribution of these major nerves than that of their individual cutaneous branches, but a detailed diagnosis of the site of an injury depends on knowing the distribution of the individual cutaneous nerves and the approximate site of origin of these nerves from the major nerves.

The diagrams of nerve distribution in this book take no account either of the overlap or of the fact that nerve fibres may sometimes pass to their destinations by unusual routes and hence modify the expected clinical effects of destruction of a particular nerve.

5. *In both upper and lower limbs, the nerves which pass to the anterior surface supply a greater area of the skin than those which pass to the posterior surface.* In the upper limb, this means that the greater part of the skin is supplied by nerves arising from the medial and lateral cords of the brachial plexus which are formed from the anterior divisions of the trunks of the plexus.

Dissection

Many of the cutaneous nerves will have been found when the skin and superficial fascia were removed from the upper limb, but their distribution is best determined by reference to Figs. 46–48, since they are very difficult to follow through the superficial fascia. Retain those that have been found piercing the deep fascia so that they can later be traced to their parent nerves.

(1) *Cutaneous nerves which arise from the ventral rami of the spinal nerves immediately adjacent to those forming the brachial plexus.*

(a) The **supraclavicular nerves** (C. 3,4) descend from the neck, cross the superficial surface of the clavicle and acromion, and supply the skin over the upper part of the front of the chest and deltoid muscle to the level of the sternal angle [Fig. 13].

(b) The **intercostobrachial nerve** (T. 2). This lateral cutaneous branch of the second intercostal nerve, enters the axilla from the second intercostal space. It descends obliquely across the axilla, communicates with the medial cutaneous nerve of the arm, and sends branches to the floor of the axilla. It pierces the deep fascia below the axilla to supply skin on the upper, posteromedial part of the arm.

(2) *Cutaneous nerves containing fibres from the posterior cord of the brachial plexus.* These supply the posterior surface of the limb.

(a) Via the axillary nerve.

The **upper lateral cutaneous nerve of the arm** (C. 5, 6) pierces the deep fascia at a variable point posterior to the lower half of the deltoid muscle. It

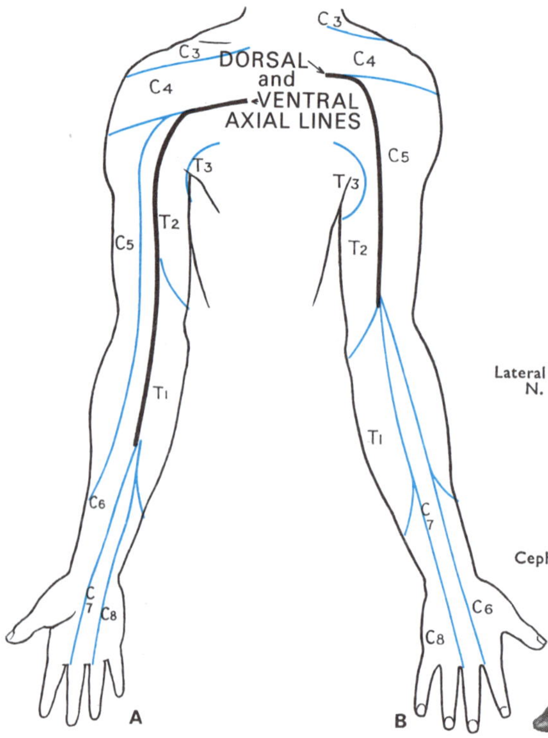

Fig. 45. Dermatomes of upper limb, showing segmental cutaneous distribution of spinal nerves (C–T) on A, the front, and B, the back of the limb. (After Head, 1893, and Foerster, 1933.)

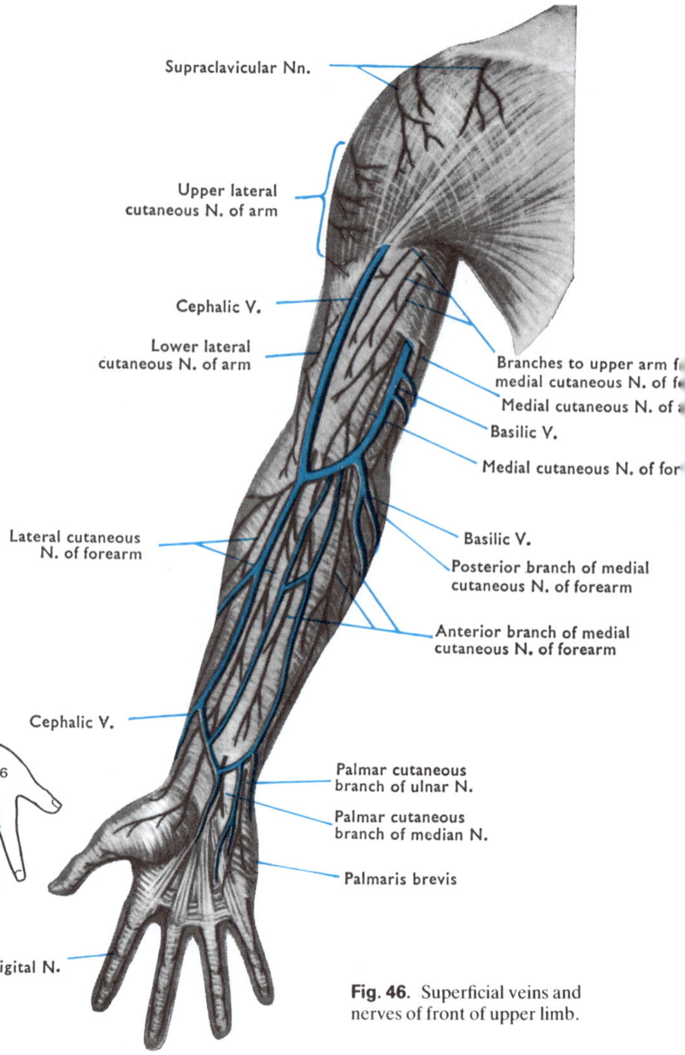

Fig. 46. Superficial veins and nerves of front of upper limb.

curves round the posterior border of that muscle, and supplies skin over its lower half [Fig. 58].

(b) Via the radial nerve [Fig 58].

(i) The **posterior cutaneous nerve of the arm** (C. 5) arises in the axilla, pierces the deep fascia below the posterior axillary fold, and supplies the skin of the back of the arm from the insertion of the deltoid to the olecranon.

(ii) The **lower lateral cutaneous nerve of the arm** (C. 5, 6) arises posterior to the humerus, and pierces the deep fascia below the insertion of deltoid. It supplies the skin of the lateral side of the arm below that insertion.

(iii) The **posterior cutaneous nerve of the forearm** (C. 6, 7, 8) arises with the previous nerve and pierces the deep fascia below it. It gives some branches to the lateral side of the arm, descends posterior to the lateral epicondyle, and lies on the middle of the back of the forearm. It supplies the skin there to the level of the wrist or occasionally on to the dorsum of the hand.

(iv) The **superficial branch of the radial nerve** (C. 6, 7, 8) arises anterior to the elbow [Fig. 84] and, descending in the forearm between the extensor and flexor muscle groups, passes posteriorly, deep to brachioradialis, in the distal half of the forearm to pierce the deep fascia 5 cm superior to the styloid process of the radius. It supplies the lateral two-thirds of the dorsum of the hand and the dorsal surfaces of the thumb and lateral two and a half fingers through five **dorsal digital nerves**. These do not supply the terminal parts of the fingers. The area supplied by the nerve varies reciprocally with the other nerves with which it communicates on the dorsum of the hand (ulnar, posterior cutaneous nerve of the forearm, and median), presumably as a result of variation in the course of fibres through the brachial plexus.

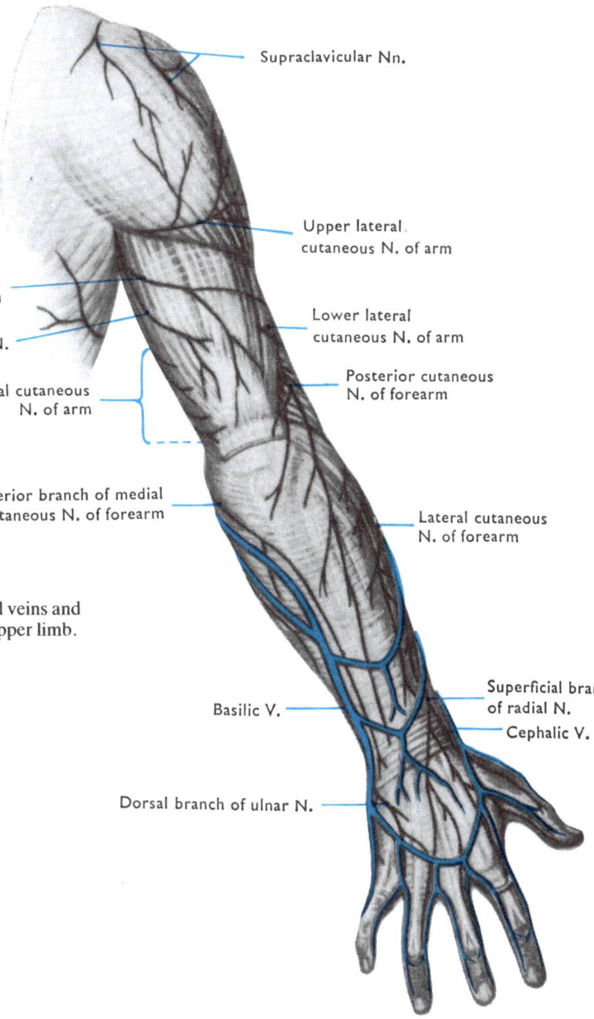

Fig. 47. Superficial veins and nerves of back of upper limb.

(3) *Cutaneous nerves containing fibres from the lateral cord of the brachial plexus* (C. 5, 6, 7).

(a) Via the musculocutaneous nerve (C. 5, 6).

The **lateral cutaneous nerve of the forearm** (C. 5, 6) pierces the deep fascia just lateral to the biceps 2–3 cm proximal to the bend of the elbow. It divides into anterior and posterior branches which supply the anterolateral and posterolateral surfaces of the forearm, the anterior extending on to the ball of the thumb [Fig. 46].

(b) See median nerve (C. 5, 6, 7).

(4) *Cutaneous nerves containing fibres from the medial cord of the brachial plexus* (C. 8, T. 1, (2)).

(a) The **medial cutaneous nerve of the arm** (T. 1, 2) pierces the deep fascia on the medial side of the middle of the arm. It supplies skin on the medial side of the inferior half of the arm, posterior to the basilic vein [Fig. 46].

(b) The **medial cutaneous nerve of the forearm** (C. 8, T. 1) pierces the deep fascia with the basilic vein. Descending, it divides into anterior and posterior branches which traverse the anteromedial and posteromedial surfaces of the forearm to the wrist. The anterior branch supplies skin of the distal part of the front of the arm, and together they supply the skin of the medial half of the forearm [Fig. 48].

(c) Via the **ulnar nerve** (C. 8, T. 1, with fibres of C. 7 received from the median nerve in the axilla). *This nerve supplies skin only in the hand and fingers* (Fig. 85).

(i) The **dorsal branch of the ulnar nerve** (C. 7, 8) arises at the middle of the forearm and descends with the ulnar nerve almost to the pisiform bone. It

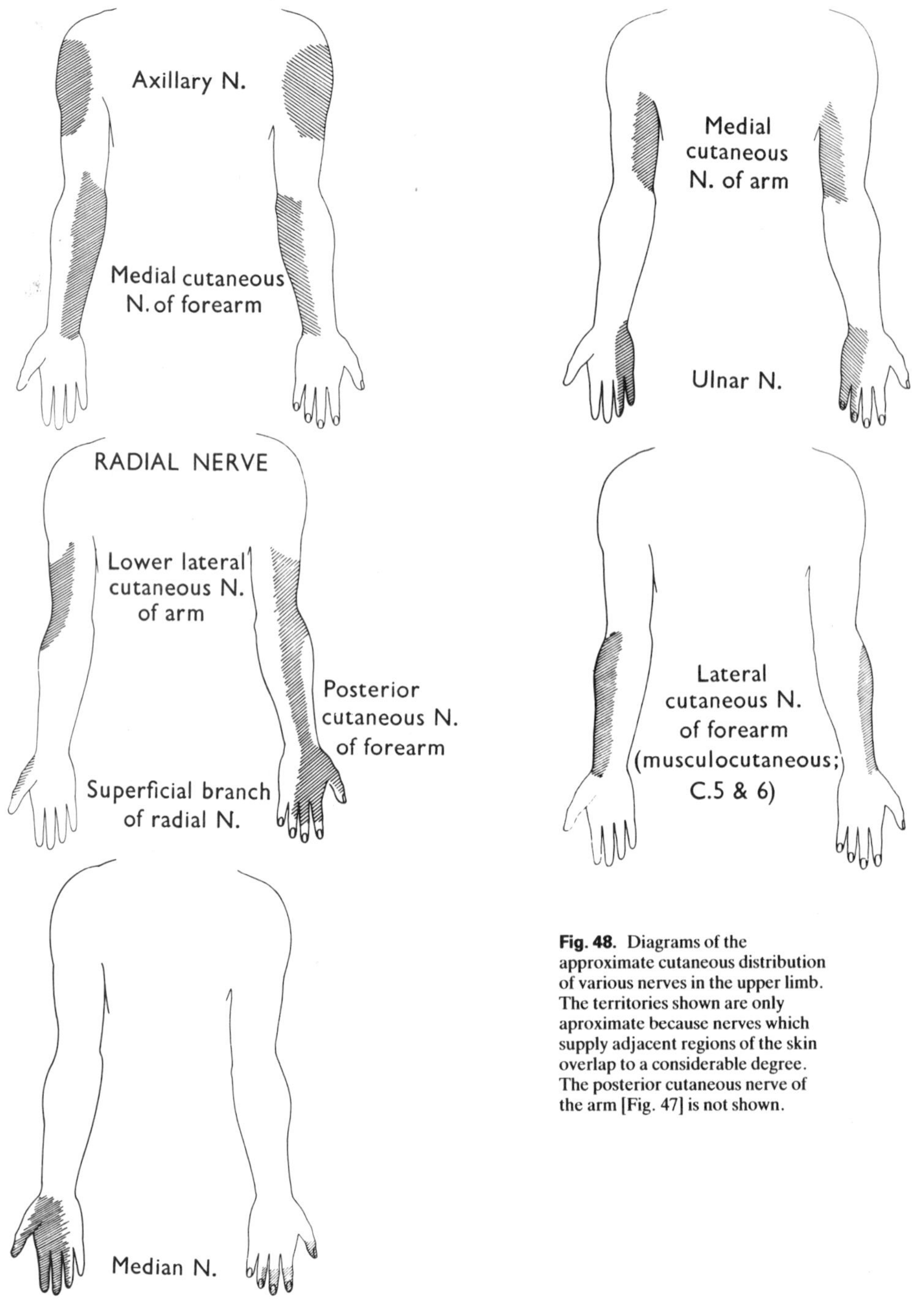

Fig. 48. Diagrams of the approximate cutaneous distribution of various nerves in the upper limb. The territories shown are only aproximate because nerves which supply adjacent regions of the skin overlap to a considerable degree. The posterior cutaneous nerve of the arm [Fig. 47] is not shown.

then passes obliquely backwards across the medial surface of the carpus to divide into two **dorsal digital nerves**. These supply the skin of the medial third of the back of the hand and the dorsal surfaces of the little and medial half of the ring fingers, except their terminal parts which are supplied by palmar digital branches of the ulnar nerve.

(ii) The **palmar (cutaneous) branch** (C. 7, 8) arises in the distal half of the forearm, pierces the deep fascia anterior to the wrist, and supplies the medial third of the palmar skin.

(iii) **Palmar digital nerves** (C. 7, 8) arise distal to the pisiform bone from the superficial branch of the ulnar nerve. The medial nerve is the proper palmar digital nerve to the medial side of the little finger. The lateral nerve is a common palmar digital nerve which divides near the cleft between the little and ring fingers to give a proper palmar digital nerve to the contiguous sides of each. Palmar and plantar digital nerves and arteries are called '**proper**' when each is distributed only to one finger or toe. The term '**common**' indicates that the nerve or artery is distributed to two adjacent fingers or toes as two proper digital branches.

(d) Via the **median nerve** (C. 5, 6, 7 from lateral cord, C. 8, T. 1 from medial cord) the branches of which supply skin only in the hand and fingers [Fig. 83].

(i) The **palmar (cutaneous) branch** (C. 6, 7, 8) arises a little superior to the wrist, pierces the deep fascia just above it, and descends to supply the lateral two-thirds of the palmar skin.

(ii) The **palmar digital branches** (C. 6, 7, 8) arise in the palm. The medial two are common palmar digital nerves, the more medial of which communicates with that of the ulnar nerve and each divides near the cleft on the corresponding aspect of the middle finger [Fig. 90] to form a proper palmar digital nerve to each side of that cleft. The next is the proper palmar digital nerve to the lateral side of the index finger. The lateral two curve round the distal border of the thenar eminence as proper palmar digital nerves to the sides of the thumb. The proper palmar digital nerves not only supply the corresponding parts of the fingers but send branches to the dorsal skin on the middle and terminal phalanges.

Lamellated corpuscles are minute, ovoid bodies found throughout the deeper parts of the skin. They are sensitive to deformation and hence act as pressure recorders. Commonly enlarged in the fingers, they are often visible along the course of the proper palmar digital nerves.

Dissection

Expose the palmar aponeurosis by removing the superficial fascia from the palm. Follow it proximally into continuity with the deep fascia of the forearm and the palmaris longus tendon and distally to the slip which it sends to the palmar surface of each finger. Look between these slips for the three common palmar digital nerves and follow them and their branches (proper palmar digital nerves) into the fingers. Identify and follow the proper palmar digital arteries which accompany the nerves. Find the proper palmar digital nerve to the medial side of the little finger on the hypothenar eminence [Fig. 75] and follow it distally. Find the corresponding nerve to the lateral side of the index finger immediately lateral to the slip of the palmar aponeurosis to that finger. Find the digital nerves of the thumb at the distal margin of the thenar eminence [Fig. 75] and trace them into the thumb.

Remove the fat from the medial side of the wrist distal to the ulnar styloid process and expose the dorsal branch of the ulnar nerve. Follow it and its dorsal digital branches, thus confirming the presence of four digital nerves (two palmar and two dorsal) in the little finger as in each of the digits. Expose the deep fascia on the lateral surface of the lower end of the radius and find the superficial branch of the radial nerve. Trace its branches to the thumb and fingers and note its communication with the dorsal branch of the ulnar nerve.

Deep fascia of the upper limb

On the dorsal surface of the scapula a very dense layer of fascia extends downwards from the spine of the scapula to the margins of the infraspinous fossa [Fig. 49] covering the infraspinatus muscle. Superolaterally it splits to enclose the deltoid muscle and below this it surrounds the teres major and minor muscles [Fig. 54] passing between them to the underlying lateral border of the scapula to which the teres muscles are attached [Fig. 51]. All these muscles arise partly from this fascia when they are well developed.

In the arm, the deep fascia is strongest posteriorly where it covers the triceps muscle. Below the insertion of deltoid it is thickened on each side where it sends a strong **intermuscular septum** to the corresponding supracondylar line and epicondyle of the humerus. These lie between the triceps muscle, posteriorly, and the muscles attached to the anterior surface of the distal half of the humerus [Fig. 53] and give attachment to both.

At the elbow, the deep fascia is thickened by extensions into it from the triceps and biceps muscles and by the origin of the forearm muscles from its deep surface and from the extensions which it sends between them. The **bicipital aponeurosis** is a strong slip which extends medially from the tendon of biceps into the deep fascia. Thus it is indirectly attached to the subcutaneous, posterior border of the ulna which is fused with the deep fascia. The aponeurosis is readily felt by sliding a finger down the medial side of the taut biceps tendon.

The wrist is surrounded by a thickened band (retinaculum) of deep fascia attached to all the subcutaneous bony points [p. 44]. The extensor retinaculum binds down the extensor tendons posteriorly and laterally, and the flexor retinaculum, the flexor tendons and median nerve anteriorly. Both parts of the band act as pulleys for the corresponding tendons which slide freely in synovial sheaths on the retinacula when the wrist is moved.

The **flexor retinaculum** [Figs. 76, 77] is a very strong band (approx. 2 x 2 cm) which is continuous with the deep fascia of the forearm at the distal flexor skin crease of the wrist. Here it is attached to the tuberosity of the scaphoid and the pisiform bone. Distally it is attached to the tubercle of the trapezium and the hook of the hamate bone and is continuous with the palmar aponeurosis. It completes the carpal tunnel [p. 78] but is partly hidden by the origin of the thenar and hypothenar muscles from its superficial surface.

The **extensor retinaculum** extends from the lateral aspect and styloid process of the radius to the ulna. Its deep surface is attached to all the subcutaneous parts of these bones, thus dividing the space deep to it into a number of tunnels through which the extensor tendons pass [Fig. 79]. Distally it is continuous with the thin deep fascia of the dorsum of the hand which fuses, in its turn, with the extensor tendons of the fingers.

In the palm, the deep fascia is thin over the thenar and hypothenar eminences but is thickened between them to form the **palmar aponeurosis**. The edges of the slip of the palmar aponeurosis passing to each finger turn backwards to form a tunnel [Fig. 98] containing the long flexor tendons of the finger. This is continuous with a dense fibrous tunnel in the finger—the **fibrous flexor sheath**. The posterior margins of this sheath are attached to the lateral and medial edges of the palmar surfaces of the phalanges producing a fibro-osseous tube through which the long flexor tendons of the fingers pass to the phalanges. Here too the tendons are enclosed in synovial sheaths to facilitate their movement in the tube.

The shoulder

Begin by reviewing the scapula and proximal part of the humerus [Figs. 225–232].

The **scapula** is a thin, triangular plate of bone which lies at a tangent to the posterolateral surface of the thorax. It has a long, slightly thickened, medial border which meets the thin, concave, superior border at the **superior angle** and the markedly thickened lateral border (margin) at the **inferior angle**. The lateral angle is the thickest part of the bone. It is truncated, the end forming the shallow, pear-shaped **glenoid cavity** which is continuous with the rest of the scapula through its **neck,** and faces anterolaterally to articulate with the hemispherical head of the humerus.

The **scapular notch** [Fig. 49] separates the coracoid laterally from the remainder of the superior border. The **coracoid,** which develops separately from the remainder of the scapula, is a thick buttress extending antero-superiorly from the neck of the scapula and the upper part of the glenoid cavity to end in a thick process which projects anterolaterally, the **coracoid process**.

The dorsal surface of the scapula is divided into **supraspinous** and **infraspinous fossae** (which lodge the corresponding muscles) by the **spine of the scapula**. This runs from the medial border of the scapula to its neck increasing rapidly in height. The posterior surface of the spine widens laterally to become continuous with the flattened **acromion** which projects

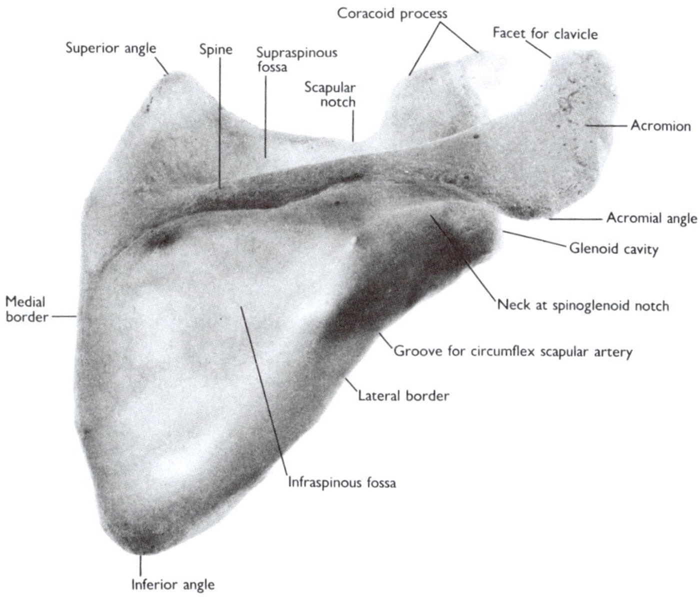

Fig. 49. Dorsal surface of right scapula.

forwards from it at the palpable **acromial angle** [Fig. 49]. Viewed from the anterolateral aspect [Fig. 66], the acromion and coracoid are seen to form two parts of an incomplete bony arch above the glenoid cavity and the head of the humerus which articulates with it. This **coraco-acromial arch** is completed by the **coraco-acromial ligament** and above that by the lateral end of the clavicle articulating directly with the acromion and indirectly with the coracoid process through the powerful **coracoclavicular ligaments**. In the same view, it can be seen that the acromion and the coracoid process arch forwards, each leaving a space beneath it which transmits a muscle to the humerus. The subscapularis passes from the subscapular fossa of the scapula beneath the coracoid process. The supraspinatus passes from the supraspinous fossa beneath the acromion. The thick **lateral border of the scapula** gives attachment to the two teres muscles which also pass to the humerus.

The expanded proximal end of the **humerus** consists of the hemispherical, articular **head,** the centre of which faces medially, upwards, and backwards. Its superior surface forms the greater part of the proximal surface of the humerus. The remainder of the expanded end is formed by the **tubercles**—the greater lying laterally, the lesser anteriorly. The tubercles are separated by the **intertubercular sulcus** which transmits the tendon of the long head of the biceps muscle passing from the upper margin of the glenoid cavity, the **supraglenoid tubercle**. The sulcus continues inferiorly on the surgical neck and upper part of the body of the humerus as a shallow groove bounded by the **crests of the tubercles** [Fig. 35]. The crest of the greater tubercle is continuous inferiorly with the anterior limb of the V-shaped **deltoid tuberosity**. The lesser tubercle is the site of insertion of the subscapularis. The greater tubercle has three facets (superior, posterosuperior, and posterior) for the insertion of supraspinatus, infraspinatus, and teres minor respectively. The tubercles are separated from the head by a shallow sulcus, the **anatomical neck** while all three are united to the body by the **surgical neck**.

Muscles attaching the humerus to the scapula

[Table 2, p. 115]

(a) Those which have considerable mechanical advantage over the shoulder joint by being attached at some distance from it—deltoid, teres major, coracobrachialis, and biceps brachii (short head).

(b) Those which lie close to the shoulder joint and have a smaller mechanical advantage over it. They help to stablize the joint in any position and act as the main ligaments of the joint—subscapularis, supraspinatus, infraspinatus, teres minor, and the long heads of biceps and triceps brachii.

Dissection

Remove the fascia from the surface of the **deltoid muscle.** It has a V-shaped origin from the outer border of the subcutaneous bony arch formed by the lateral third of the clavicle, the acromion, and the crest of the spine of the scapula. It is inserted into the deltoid tuberosity of the humerus [Fig. 52]. Note that the long anterior and posterior fibres run parallel to each other on the corresponding surfaces of the shoulder joint. The lateral fibres are short and multipennate to increase the power of this part. Separate the muscle from the spine of the scapula and turn this part downwards. Remove the dense deep fascia from the surface of the **infraspinatus muscle** thus exposed. Define its attachments to the infraspinous fossa and the greater tubercle of the humerus. Find the inferior border of infraspinatus and separate it from the two **teres muscles** which arise from the lateral margin of the scapula [Fig. 54]. Turn the detached part of deltoid forwards; identify the **axillary nerve** (from which the upper lateral cutaneous nerve of the arm arises) and the posterior humeral circumflex vessels supplying its deep surface. Trace these on the surgical neck of the humerus through the **quadrangular space** [Fig. 54], inferior to teres minor and the articular capsule of the shoulder joint.

Expose the **long head of triceps** medial to the quadrangular space. It descends from the **infraglenoid tubercle** beside the inferior part of the capsule of the shoulder joint and passes between the teres minor and major muscles as they approach the humerus. Find the branch of the axillary nerve to the **teres minor** and follow this muscle to its attachments, separating it from teres major.

Divide the remainder of **deltoid** close to its origin and turn it downwards. It lies on the proximal end and surgical neck of the humerus with the anastomosis of the circumflex humeral vessels deep to it [Fig. 59]. On the anterior surface, follow the **subscapularis**

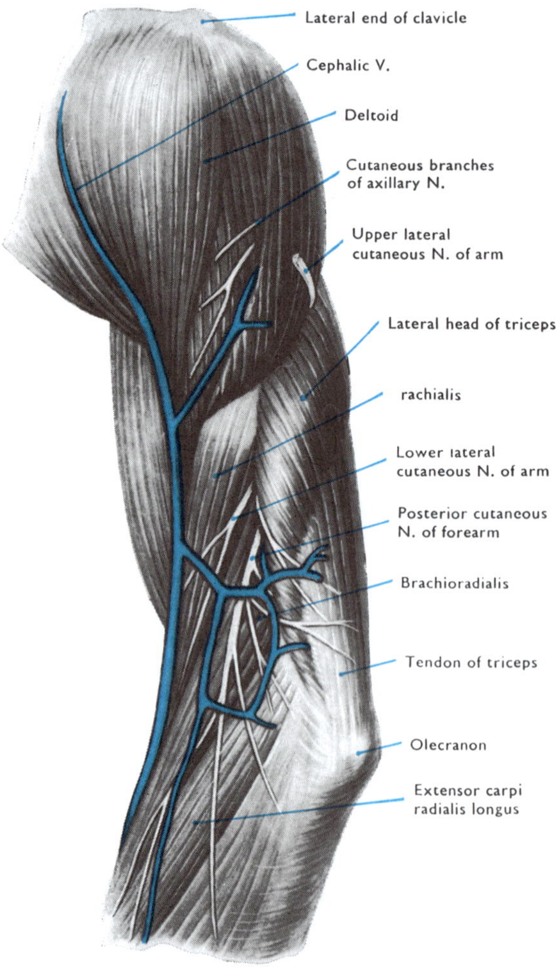

Fig. 50. Deltoid muscle and lateral aspect of arm.

Fig. 51. Muscle attachments to dorsal surface of right scapula.

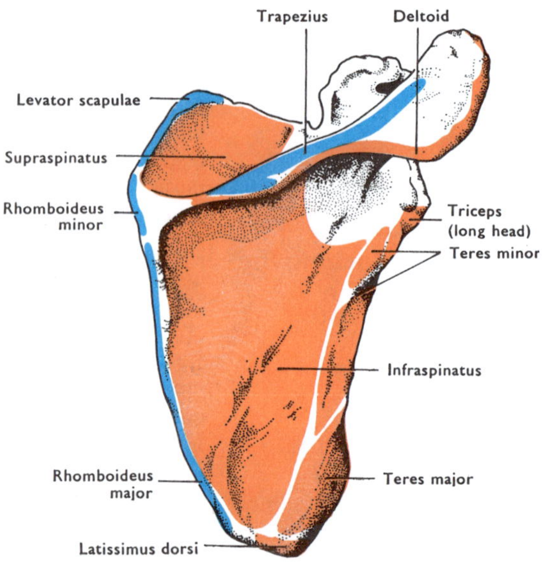

Fig. 52 (*left*) Posterior aspect of humerus to show muscle attachments.

Fig. 53 (*right*) Muscle attachments to anterior surface of right humerus.

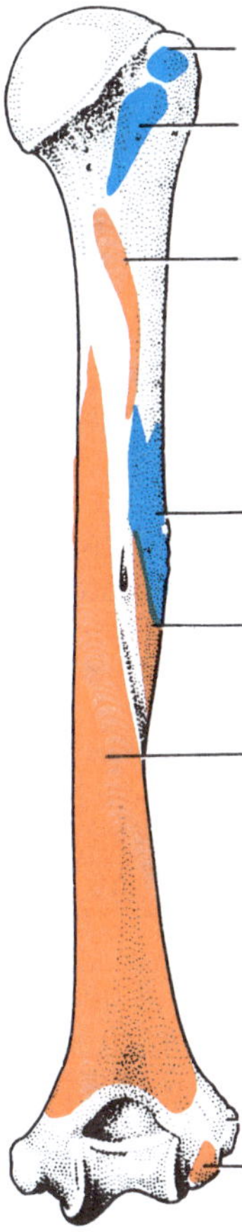

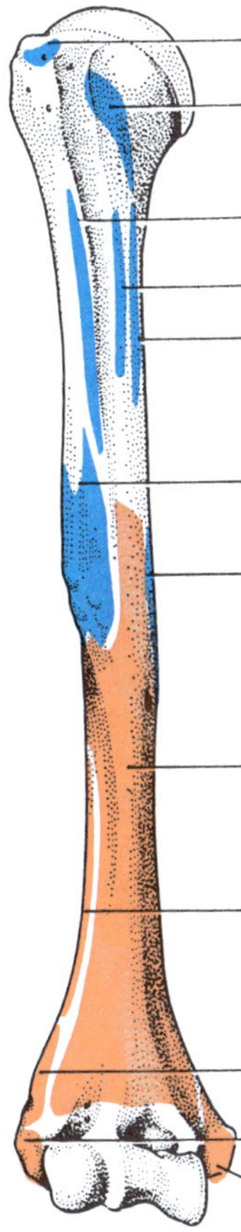

muscle from the subscapular fossa to the lesser tubercle. Separate it inferiorly from the **teres major** and trace that muscle to its insertion on the crest of the lesser tubercle of the humerus immediately behind the insertion of the tendon of **latissimus dorsi.** Both these insertions are lateral to the coracobrachialis and short head of biceps which descend in front of them from the coracoid process [Fig. 22]. Find the **axillary nerve** arising from the posterior cord of the brachial plexus and follow it to the quadrangular space which, when seen from in front, is between subscapularis and teres major. The **radial nerve** continues from the posterior cord. It passes anterior to latissimus dorsi and teres major and then posterolaterally between the parts of triceps muscle after giving branches to the long and medial heads of that muscle.

Remove the fascia covering the **coracobrachialis** and the **short head of biceps** from the coracoid process to the insertion of coracobrachialis on the medial aspect of the body of the humerus [Fig. 53]. Follow the **musculocutaneous nerve** from the lateral cord of the brachial plexus into the medial aspect of coracobrachialis and find the branch which it gives to that muscle. Pull these muscles medially and identify the tendon of the **long head of biceps.** It lies in the intertubercular sulcus posterolateral to the short head. Follow the long head upwards to the level of the lower border of the lesser tubercle where it disappears deep to the articular capsule of the shoulder joint.

Move the fascia covering the superior surface of the greater tubercle of the humerus. It slides easily on the tubercle because of the **subacromial bursa** deep to the fascia. Open the bursa and explore its limits with a blunt seeker. Then open it widely. The bursa separates the superior surface of the humerus and the capsule of the shoulder joint from the acromion and coraco-acromial ligament and makes a secondary synovial socket for the humerus with the coraco-acromial arch.

The **coraco-acromial ligament** is a strong, triangular band. Its base is attached to the lateral border of the coracoid process and its apex to the tip of the acromion. It lies between the subacromial bursa and the deltoid muscle [Figs. 63, 64, 66].

Remove the subacromial bursa and expose the **supraspinatus** passing from the supraspinous fossa, beneath the coraco-acromial arch and bursa, to the superior surface of the greater tubercle. The tendon of supraspinatus is firmly fused to this part of the capsule of the shoulder joint.

Cut across the infraspinatus and teres minor muscles at the level of the neck of the scapula. Turn their parts medially and laterally. Find the **suprascapular** and **circumflex scapular arteries** passing deep to the muscles and anastomosing on the posterior surface of the scapula [Fig. 61]. The **suprascapular nerve** also enters the deep surface of infraspinatus from supraspinatus. The tendons of teres minor and infraspinatus fuse with the capsule of the shoulder joint as they pass to the greater tubercle of the humerus, but there may be a bursa deep to the tendon of infraspinatus, and this may open into the cavity of the shoulder joint [Fig. 64].

Follow the tendon of the **long head of triceps** to its attachment on the infraglenoid tubercle [Fig. 51] and find the dependent part of the capsule of the shoulder joint lateral to it. The **axillary nerve** passes posteriorly on the surgical neck of the humerus immediately inferior to this part of the capsule and sends a branch to it.

Cut across the **subscapularis** at the neck of the scapula and reflect its parts. Though fused with the capsule of the shoulder joint laterally, it is separated from it medially and from the neck of the scapula and the root of the coracoid process by the **subscapular bursa** which facilitates its movement over these structures. This bursa is commonly continuous with the cavity of the shoulder joint through an aperture in its capsule [Figs. 63, 64].

Expose the powerful **coracoclavicular ligament** in the space between the coracoid process and the clavicle [Fig. 66]. It is attached to the upper surface of the posterior part of the coracoid process. The posteromedial part (**conoid ligament**) is an inverted cone attached above to the **conoid tubercle** of the clavicle [Fig. 11]. The anterolateral,

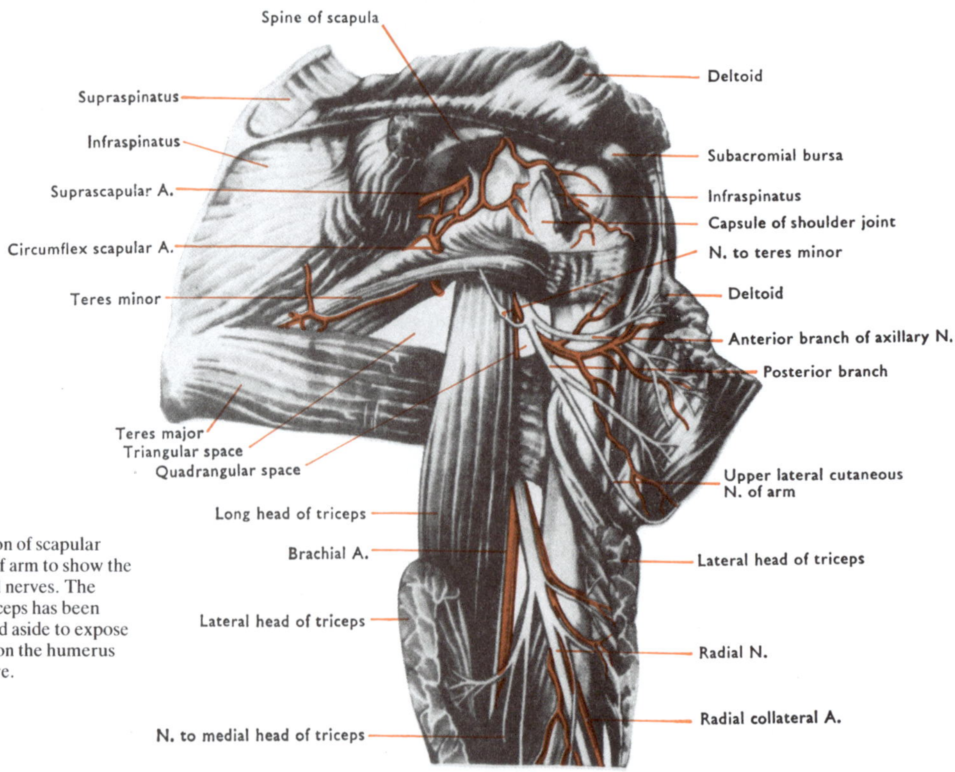

Fig. 54. Dissection of scapular region and back of arm to show the axillary and radial nerves. The lateral head of triceps has been divided and turned aside to expose the spiral groove on the humerus for the radial nerve.

triangular part (**trapezoid ligament**) passes superolaterally to the trapezoid line on the clavicle and meets the conoid ligament at an angle which is open anteriorly. This is the main structure suspending the scapula and hence the upper limb from the clavicle. It supports the acromioclavicular joint and helps to transmit to the trunk forces which are applied to the upper limb. If the clavicle is broken medial to this ligament, the upper limb at once drops—a sign which is characteristic of this common fracture.

Acromioclavicular joint

Remove the trapezius and the remainder of the deltoid from the capsule of the acromioclavicular joint. Cut away the superior part of the capsule (acromioclavicular ligament) of this joint and note the articular disc partly or completely separating the two bones. The bony articulating surfaces slope upwards and laterally; thus any compression force tends to make the clavicle override the acromion—a movement which is prevented by the coracoclavicular and acromioclavicular ligaments. The slight gliding and rotatory movements at this joint permit sufficient adjustment of the relative positions of the scapula and clavicle to keep the scapula in apposition to the chest wall during shoulder girdle movements.

Medial to the coracoclavicular ligament and coracoid, identify the **suprascapular artery and nerve** crossing the superior margin of the scapula at the scapular notch [Fig. 61].

Movements of the limb at the shoulder

[Table 2, p. 116]

The very wide range of movements which is possible at the shoulder joint is the result of (1) the nature of the articular surfaces (the large, hemispherical head of the humerus fitted to the small, shallow glenoid cavity); (2) a loose-fitting articular capsule [p. 64]; and (3) the replacement of ligaments by a group of muscles (subscapularis, supraspinatus, infraspinatus, teres minor, and the long heads of triceps and biceps). They closely surround the joint and can maintain its stability by tension at all phases of movement and in any position of the joint. The **glenoid cavity** faces anterolaterally at rest and its plane is parallel to the axis around which the scapula is rotated in movements of the shoulder girdle. Movement of the shoulder joint can take place independently, but is accompanied by movements of the shoulder girdle in almost every case, thus increasing the complexity of the group of muscles involved. Even if the scapula is not moved, the muscles which would move it have to be in tension to maintain a stable scapula on which the limb may be moved.

Flexion

This is carried out by muscles which pass anterior to the shoulder joint (short head of biceps, coracobrachialis, and the clavicular parts of deltoid and pectoralis major) but the arm can be flexed to the horizontal only if the inferior angle of the scapula is also pulled forwards on the chest wall (lateral rotation) by **serratus anterior,** thus tipping the glenoid cavity upwards.

Extension

Extension from the anatomical position is more restricted. It is produced by the posterior fibres of **deltoid** assisted initially by latissimus dorsi and finally by the elevation of the scapula on the convex thoracic wall by trapezius and levator scapulae. Extension of the flexed shoulder joint to the anatomical position against resistance is produced by latissimus dorsi, teres major, and the sternocostal part of pectoralis major, assisted by the rhomboid major and pectoralis minor both of which rotate the scapula medially [p. 40].

Abduction

This is produced by the middle fibres of **deltoid** and by the **supraspinatus** both of which pass superior to the joint. The supraspinatus is said to be responsible for initiating the movement, but it is not essential. The contracting deltoid is prevented from pulling the humerus upwards against the coraco-acromial arch (and thus blocking abduction) by the simultaneous contraction of teres minor and the lower fibres of subscapularis. These do not prevent abduction because of their attachment to the humerus on the axis around which this movement takes place [Fig. 55]. The failure of this mechanism is shown by attempting to abduct the arm from the side when it is fully medially rotated (the palm of the hand facing posterolaterally). Then abduction beyond the horizontal is impossible even with full scapular rotation. Theoretically the deltoid can abduct the humerus on the scapula to the horizontal, but this movement is associated from the beginning with **lateral rotation of the scapula**. It is this rotation (produced by serratus anterior and trapezius) which permits the humerus to be carried upwards to the vertical position by turning the glenoid cavity to face superiorly. This is readily confirmed by noting the elevation of the shoulder and the lateral projection of the inferior angle of the scapula.

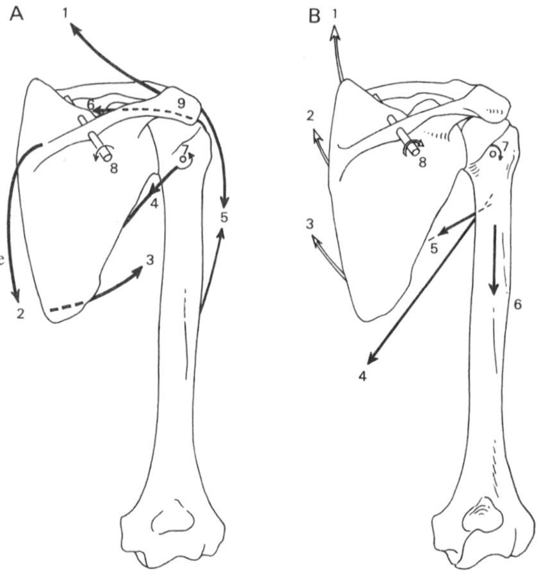

Fig. 55. Diagrams to show the direction of pull of various muscles concerned in producing abduction (A) and adduction (B) of the arm. This movement is produced at the shoulder joint combined with rotation of the scapula on the thoracic wall.
A. Abduction of the arm. Lateral rotation of the scapula is produced by the upper (1) and lower (2) fibres of trapezius, combined with the lower fibres of serratus anterior (3). Abduction at the shoulder joint is produced by supraspinatus (6) and deltoid (5). When deltoid contracts, it tends to pull the humerus upwards against the acromion (9). This is prevented by teres minor (4) which does not interfere with the abduction of the humerus because it is attached to the humerus on the axis of abduction (7). 8 is the axis of scapular rotation.
B. Adduction of the arm to the side. This movement is normally produced by gravity. In this case, the arm is lowered to the side by the muscles which produce abduction. When adduction is produced against resistance, the scapula is rotated medially by rhomboid major (3) and minor (2) and levator scapulae (1) around the axis (8). The humerus is drawn towards the scapula by teres major (5) and towards the trunk by latissimus dorsi (4) and pectoralis major (not shown). These act around the axis of abduction of the humerus (7). The weight of the limb (6) assists.

Adduction

Adduction against resistance of the arm abducted above the head is first produced by **latissimus dorsi** and the lowest sternocostal fibres of **pectoralis major** assisted by teres major and the medial rotators of the scapula [p. 55]. Once the horizontal position has been passed, progressively higher fibres of pectoralis major are involved. When this movement is not resisted, the

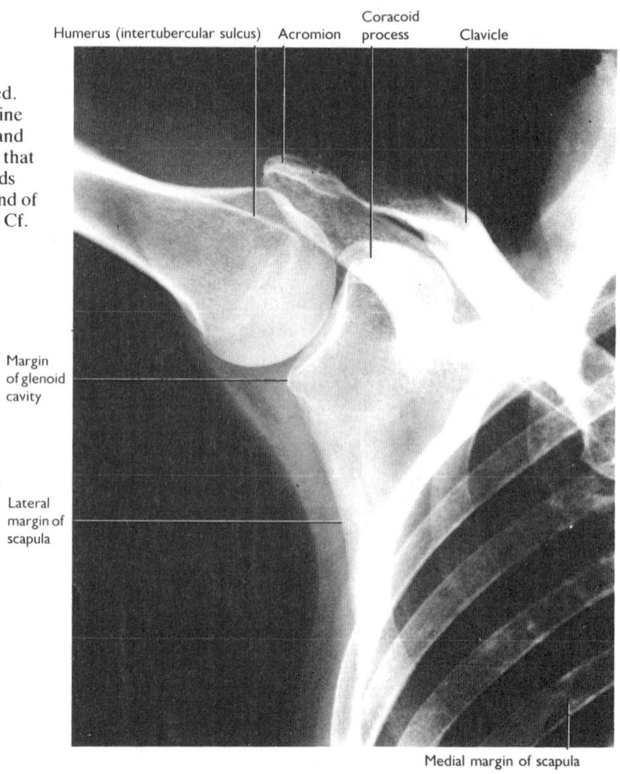

Fig. 56. Radiograph of the shoulder with the arm abducted. Note that the humerus lies in line with the spine of the scapula, and that the scapula has rotated so that the glenoid cavity faces upwards and laterally, and the lateral end of the clavicle has been elevated. Cf. Fig. 57.

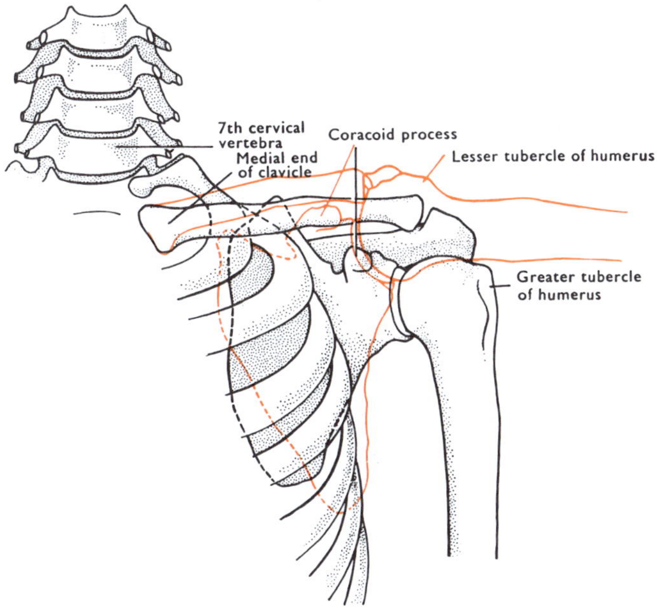

Fig. 57. A diagram prepared from tracings of two radiographs of the same individual to show the change in position of the various bones during abduction of the arm to the horizontal. Note the rotation of the scapula, the elevation of the clavicle, and the elevation and rotation of the humerus laterally.

muscles which are active are the same as for abduction for they act excentrically [p. 9] to control the gravitational descent of the limb—a situation which is common to every movement where gravity is the driving force. It can be demonstrated in this case by the continuing firmness (contraction) of deltoid as the arm is lowered to the side and its immediate flaccidity when the movement encounters resistance.

Rotation of the humerus

This may occur in any position but is best shown with the arm by the side and the elbow flexed to a right angle. The hand is then swung laterally (lateral rotation) or medially (medial rotation). In this position *medial rotation* is produced by muscles passing from the trunk (pectoralis major, latissimus dorsi) or scapula (subscapularis, teres major, anterior fibres of deltoid) to the anterior surface of the humerus. *Lateral rotation* results from the contraction

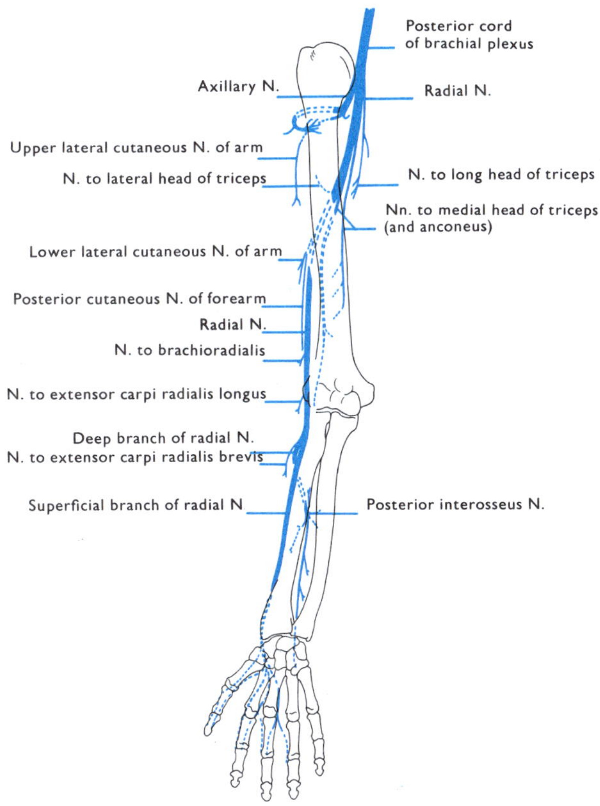

Fig. 58. A diagram of the course and distribution of the axillary and radial nerves.

of muscles passing from the scapula to the posterior surface of the humerus (infraspinatus, teres minor, the posterior fibres of deltoid).

The axillary nerve [Figs. 54, 58]

The axillary and radial nerves are the terminal branches of the posterior cord of the brachial plexus formed near the lower border of subscapularis. The axillary nerve curves backwards on the lower border of subscapularis and passes through the quadrangular space with the posterior circumflex humeral artery. Here they lie on the medial side of the surgical neck of the humerus, immediately inferior to the capsule of the shoulder joint. The nerve gives a branch to the **shoulder joint** and then divides into anterior and posterior branches.

The **posterior branch** supplies teres minor and the posterior part of deltoid. It then descends over the posterior border of deltoid and supplies skin over the lower half of that muscle as the **upper lateral cutaneous nerve of the arm** [Fig. 48].

The **anterior branch** continues horizontally between the deltoid muscle and the surgical neck of the humerus with the artery. They supply deltoid and send a few branches through it to the overlying skin.

The axillary nerve is at risk in downward dislocation of the head of the humerus from the shoulder joint and in fractures of the surgical neck of the humerus because of its close relation to the joint and the bone [Fig. 62]. When it is damaged, the deltoid and teres minor muscles are paralysed. Thus abduction of the shoulder is seriously impaired. There is also an area of altered sensation over the lower part of the deltoid muscle (upper lateral cutaneous nerve of the arm).

Circumflex humeral arteries

These branches of the third part of the axillary artery together form a circular anastomosis on the surgical neck of the humerus [Fig. 59]. They supply the surrounding muscles, the shoulder joint, and the upper end of the humerus. They also anastomose with the profunda brachii artery by a descending branch.

Anastomosis around the scapula

This anastomosis [Fig. 61] ensures an adequate arterial supply to the mobile scapula and forms a subsidiary route through which blood can pass from the proximal (first) part of the subclavian artery to the third part of the axillary artery when either the subclavian or axillary artery is blocked between these two points. The **suprascapular** and **transverse cervical arteries** arise from the first part of the subclavian artery and they anastomose freely with the branches (circumflex scapular and thoracodorsal) of the **subscapular artery** [p. 31].

Suprascapular nerve

This nerve arises from the upper trunk of the brachial plexus (C. 5, 6: Fig. 24]. It passes downwards and backwards, superior to the plexus, to meet the suprascapular vessels and pass into the supraspinous fossa through the scapular notch. Here it supplies the supraspinatus and gives branches to the

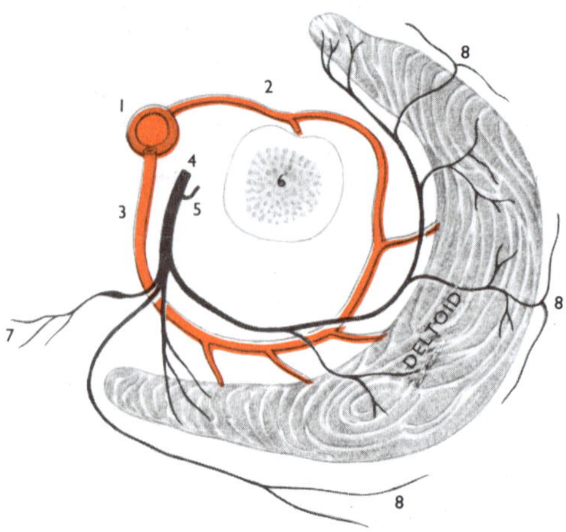

Fig. 59. Diagram of circumflex arteries and axillary nerve.
1. Axillary A.
2. Anterior circumflex humeral A.
3. Posterior circumflex humeral A.
4. Axillary N.
5. Articular branch.
6. Transverse section of humerus immediately below the tubercles.
7. Branch to teres minor.
8. Cutaneous branches.

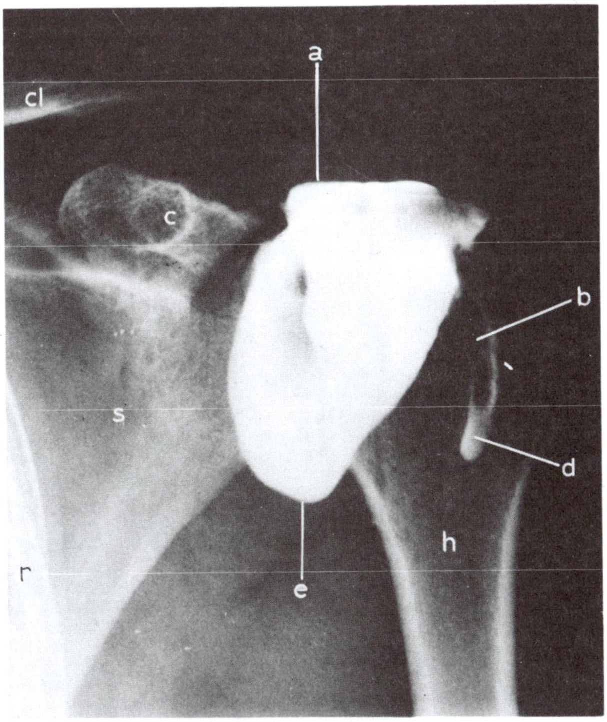

Fig. 60. Arthrogram of the shoulder joint. The synovial cavity has been filled with an X-ray-opaque medium and an oblique radiograph taken with the humerus laterally rotated. The dark central area is due to the protruding head of the laterally rotated humerus.
a. Flat upper margin of capsule inferior to the tendon of supraspinatus.
b. Tendon of the long head of biceps (dark) within the extension of the synovial membrane (d) which surrounds it in the intertubercular groove.
c. Coracoid process.
cl. Clavicle.
e. Dependent part of joint cavity.
h. Humerus.
r. Ribs.
s. Scapula.

acromioclavicular and shoulder joints. The nerve then descends immediately lateral to the root of the spine of the scapula. It enters the infraspinous fossa and supplies infraspinatus and the shoulder joint.

The shoulder joint

The disproportionate sizes of the head of the humerus and the small, shallow glenoid cavity combined with a lax articular capsule give this joint a wide range of movements but make the joint inherently unstable. This instability is overcome by the powerful muscles which immediately surround the joint [p. 59 and Fig. 64]. These muscles are capable of supporting the joint in any position without the restriction of movement which ligaments would inevitably produce. However, this arrangement brings with it an increased risk of displacement of the head of the humerus from the glenoid cavity (dislocation) when the joint is suddenly wrenched—a displacement which not infrequently occurs through the lower part of the capsule which is

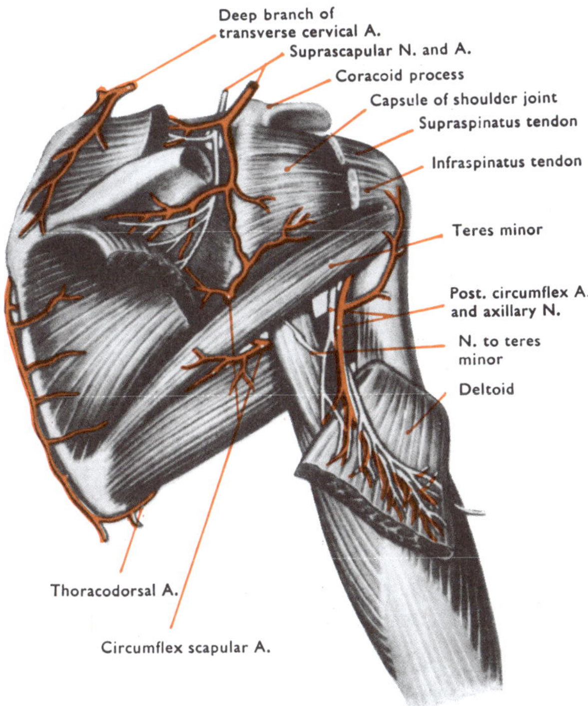

Fig. 61. Anastomosing arteries around the scapula. The acromion has been removed to expose the suprascapular A and N.

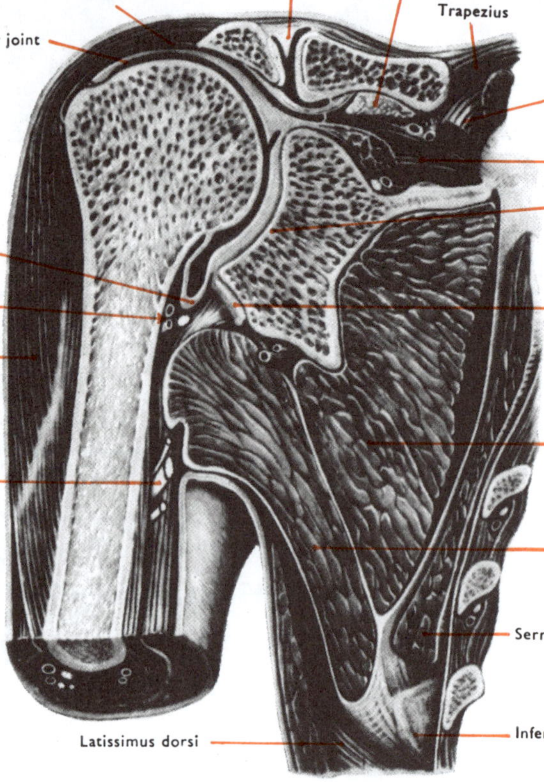

Fig. 62. Coronal section through right shoulder joint. The inferior part of serratus anterior has been cut away (Viewed from the front. Cf. Fig. 65.)

inadequately supported by the long head of triceps. This can result in damage to the adjacent axillary nerve [Fig. 62].

Articular capsule

Most of the surface of the thin capsule has already been exposed by the removal of the muscles which closely surround it. These muscles are partly fused to the fibrous membrane so that they prevent it from passing between the joint surfaces when they contract.

The outer, **fibrous membrane** of the articular capsule is a thin but relatively strong, tubular structure. It is attached to the margin of the glenoid cavity

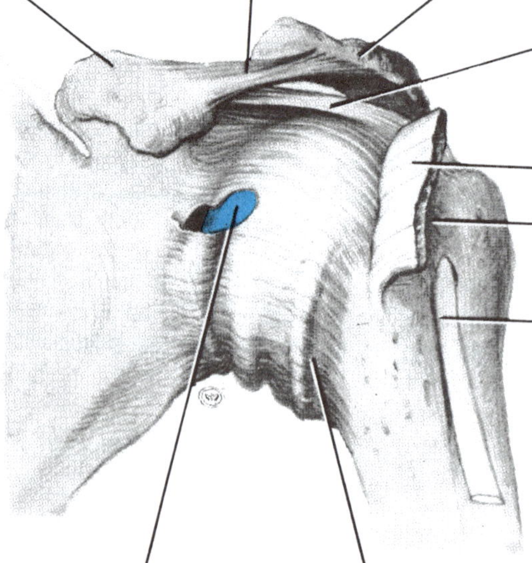

Fig. 63. Anterior aspect of left shoulder joint. The clavicle has been removed.

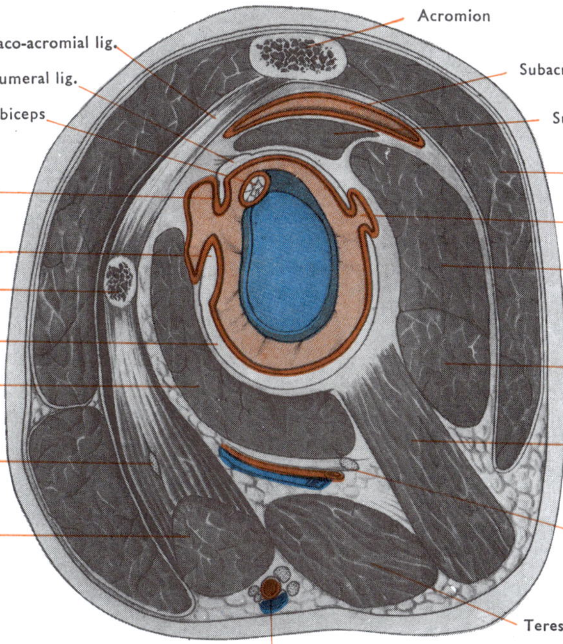

Fig. 64. Dissection of sagittal section through left shoulder (semi-diagrammatic). The subscapular bursa protrudes between the superior and middle glenohumeral ligaments. Red = arteries and synovial membrane.

and to the anatomical neck of the humerus except inferiorly where it extends downwards 1.5 cm or more on the surgical neck of the bone [Fig. 65]. With the arm by the side, this inferior part of the membrane hangs downwards in a redundant fold between the teres major and minor muscles, but it is tensed when the arm is abducted to a right angle. In the latter position the lower part of the articular surface of the head of the humerus lies on this part of the articular capsule with the long head of triceps and the teres major muscles stretched beneath it. Anteriorly, the attachment of the fibrous membrane extends inferiorly between the tubercles of the humerus bridging over the upper part of the intertubercular sulcus and forming a synovial-lined tunnel through which the tendon of the long head of biceps muscle escapes from the interior of the joint [Fig. 65]. This is one of three apertures in the fibrous membrane; the other two are also extensions of the synovial membrane through the fibrous membrane to form the subscapular and infraspinatus

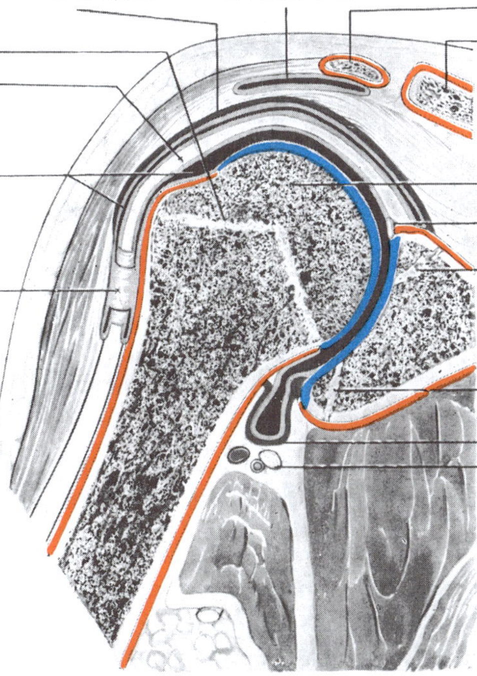

Fig. 65. Coronal section through the right shoulder joint. The parietal and visceral layers of the synovial sheath of the biceps tendon have been partially left in place. Red = periosteum. Blue = articular cartilage.

Fig. 66. Left shoulder joint. The articular capsule has been cut across and the humerus removed together with the surrounding muscles. Articular cartilage and labrum glenoidale, blue.

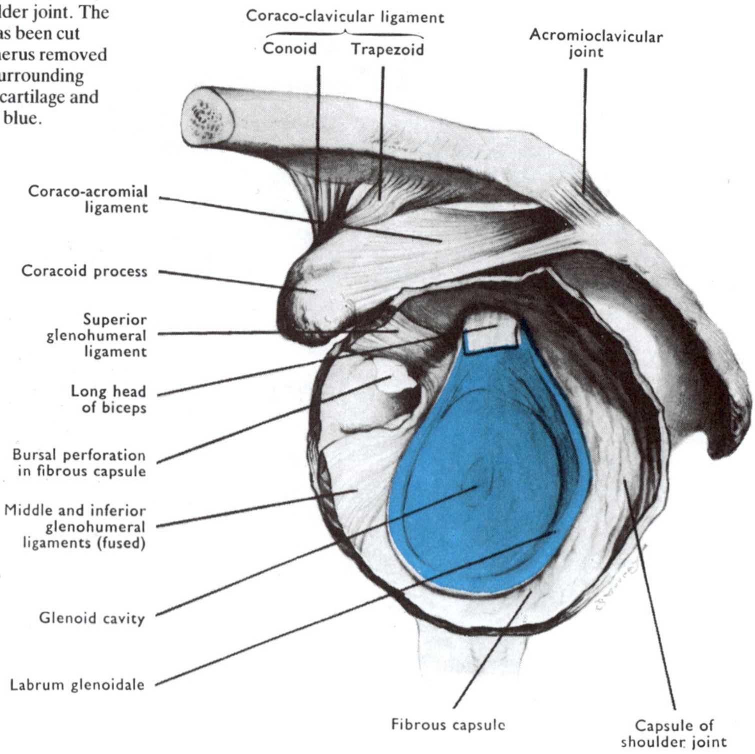

bursae [Figs. 63, 64]. Of these, the **subscapular bursa** is larger and more commonly present. It lies close to the root of the coracoid process and occasionally allows dislocation of the head of the humerus at this point.

There are four slight thickenings of the fibrous membrane. (1) The **coracohumeral ligament** [Fig. 63] lies obliquely across the upper surface from the base of the coracoid process to the superior surface of the greater tubercle of the humerus. Part of the tendon of pectoralis minor may pass over the coracoid process and, piercing the coraco-acromial ligament, become continuous with the coracohumeral ligament. (2) Two or three **glenohumeral ligaments** [Fig. 66] may be visible as thickenings of the anterior part of the membrane when viewed from the interior of the joint.

The **synovial membrane** lines the fibrous membrane and covers the part of the surgical neck of the humerus which lies within the fibrous membrane. Synovial membrane also forms a sheath round the tendon of the long head of biceps and is continuous with the lining of the bursae which are extensions of the joint.

The **nerve supply** of the shoulder joint is by the axillary, suprascapular, and lateral pectoral nerves.

Movements See p. 59.

Dissection

Make a vertical incision through the posterior part of the articular capsule of the shoulder joint. Rotate the arm medially and dislocate the head of the humerus through the cut in the capsule. Identify the **tendon of the long head of biceps** passing over the superior surface of the head of the humerus within the capsule to reach the supraglenoid tubercle [Fig. 66]. Note that it becomes continuous here with a fibrocartilaginous ring, the **labrum glenoidale,** which is attached to the margin of the glenoid cavity and the internal surface of the articular capsule. By surrounding the glenoid cavity, the labrum slightly deepens it, and is continuous inferiorly with fibres of the tendon of the long head of triceps through the capsule. Try to expose the glenohumeral ligaments on the deep surface of the anterior part of the capsule and note the aperture of the subscapular bursa between them. If necessary, cut through the tendon of the long head of biceps to increase the mobility of the humerus.

The arm

The deep fascia which encloses the arm sends septa between the various groups of muscles to allow them to slide on each other and to give an increased area of origin for their fibres. Two of these, the lateral and medial intermuscular septa, pass to the corresponding epicondyles and supracondylar lines of the humerus, thus dividing the distal part of the arm into anterior and posterior compartments.

The anterior compartment

Dissection

Cut vertically through the deep fascia on the anterior surface of the arm as far as the elbow, and cut transversely through it at this level. Reflect the flaps to uncover biceps brachii. Lift this muscle forwards and find the musculocutaneous nerve in the delicate septum which separates biceps from the brachialis muscle posteriorly. Follow the musculocutaneous nerve and the biceps and coracobrachialis muscles proximally and distally. Neither the tendon of origin of the long head of biceps nor its tendon of insertion can be followed to their insertions.

Remove the fascia from brachialis and define the forearm muscles, brachioradialis and extensor carpi radialis longus. They arise from the lateral supracondylar line and the lateral intermuscular septum and appear to be part of brachialis but are separated from it by a thin septum which contains the radial nerve and a terminal branch of the profunda brachii artery [Fig. 69]. Find the nerve in this situation and its branches to brachioradialis, extensor carpi radialis longus, and brachialis [Fig.84]. Trace the radial nerve proximally to the point where it passes posterior to the humerus and the lower lateral

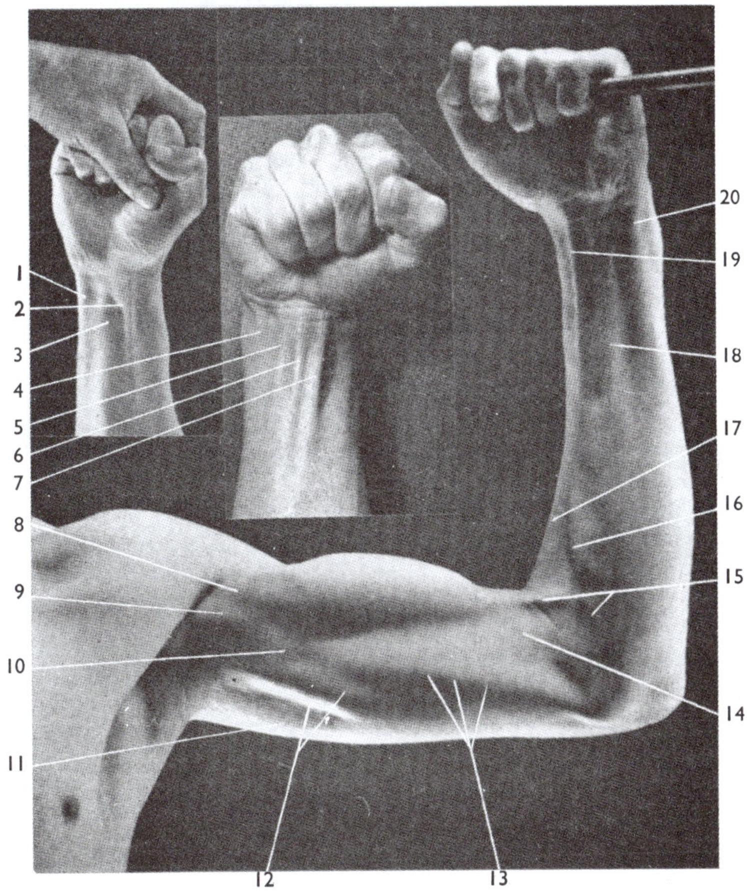

Fig. 67. Flexors of wrist and elbow in action. In the top left figure the median nerve, escaping from under flexor carpi radialis to lie upon flexor digitorum superficialis tendons, is seen well because palmaris longus is absent. (From *Living anatomy* by R. D. Lockhart, 6th edn. Faber and Faber, London (1963).)

1. Flexor carpi ulnaris.
2. Median nerve.
3. Flexor digitorum superficialis.
4. Flexor carpi ulnaris.
5. Flexor digitorum superficialis, ring finger tendon.
6. Palmaris longus.
7. Flexor carpi radialis.
8. Biceps, short head.
9. Coracobrachialis.
10. Neurovascular bundle.
11. Triceps, long head.
12. Triceps, medial head.
13. Intermuscular septum.
14. Brachialis.
15. Bicipital aponeurosis.
16. Pronator teres.
17. Brachioradialis.
18. Flexor digitorum superficialis.
19. Flexor carpi radialis.
20. Flexor carpi ulnaris.

cutaneous nerve of the arm and the posterior cutaneous nerve of the forearm arise from it [Fig. 50].

Find the principal neurovascular bundle of the arm immediately deep to the deep fascia, medial to biceps. Trace its contents proximally into continuity with the structures in the axilla, and distally to the level of the elbow.

Biceps brachii and coracobrachialis

The biceps muscle arises from the scapula by two heads. The **short head** arises with coracobrachialis from the coracoid process. The muscles descend together. Coracobrachialis then leaves the short head to be inserted into the middle of the medial surface of the humerus. The **long head** of biceps arises from the supraglenoid tubercle within the shoulder joint. Its tendon runs superior to the head of the humerus and emerges from the joint through the intertubercular groove. The two heads of biceps fuse in the distal third of the arm, and form a short tendon which gives off the **bicipital aponeurosis** [Fig. 74]. This thickened part of the deep fascia forms a secondary insertion through which biceps is indirectly attached to the posterior border of the ulna. The **tendon** then passes deeply into the proximal part of the forearm to the posterior surface of the tuberosity of the radius. **Nerve supply:** musculocutaneous. **Action:** see below.

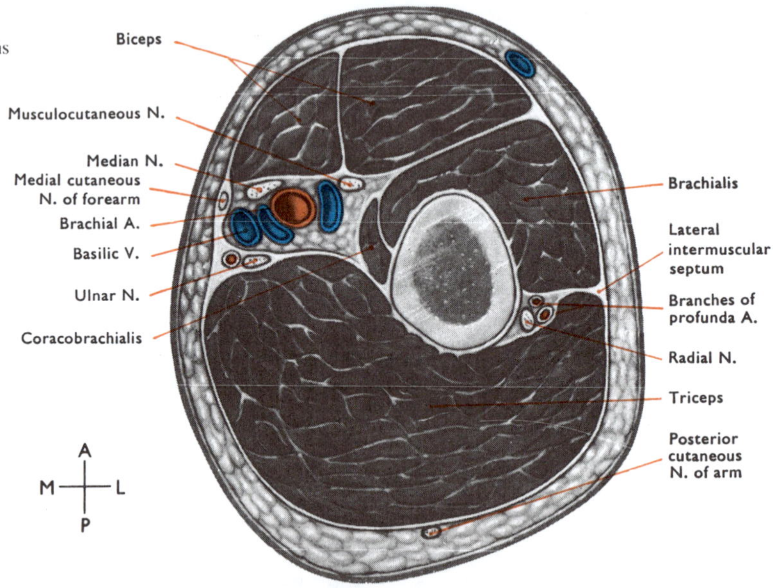

Fig. 68. Section through the middle of right arm. Note positions of neurovascular bundles and intermuscular septa.
A. Anterior.
P. Posterior.
M. Medial.
L. Lateral.

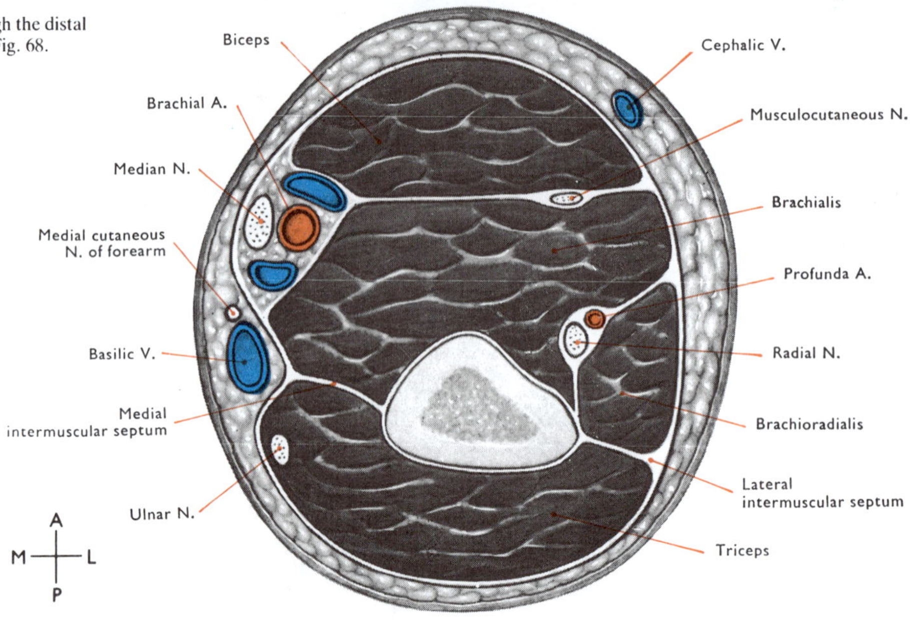

Fig. 69. Section through the distal third of right arm. Cf. Fig. 68.
A. Anterior.
P. Posterior.
M. Medial.
L. Lateral.

Brachialis

This muscle arises from the anterior surface of the distal half of the humerus [Fig. 53]. It descends across the anterior surface of the elbow joint to the coronoid process of the ulna [Fig. 86]. **Nerve supply:** musculocutaneous; some sensory fibres from the radial nerve. **Action:** see below.

Cubital fossa

This triangular fossa forms the hollow at the front of the elbow. The base of the fossa is a line drawn between the two epicondyles of the humerus. The medial border, pronator teres muscle, meets the lateral border, the brachioradialis muscle, where that muscle overlaps the pronator teres. The floor is formed by the brachialis and supinator muscles. The median nerve, brachial artery, and tendon of biceps enter the fossa. Here the artery divides into radial and ulnar arteries. The radial artery leaves the fossa at the apex, the ulnar passes deep to pronator teres. The median nerve supplies the muscles medial to it and leaves the fossa through pronator teres. The tendon of biceps passes backwards between the forearm bones to reach the tuberosity of the radius. If the elbow is flexed and the margins pulled apart, the contents of the fossa can be displayed after the deep fascia covering it has been removed.

Musculocutaneous nerve (C. 5 and 6)

This nerve arises from the lateral cord of the brachial plexus. It passes inferolaterally to supply and then pierce coracobrachialis [Fig. 20]. It then descends between biceps and brachialis, sending branches to both, and emerges from beneath the lateral border of the tendon of biceps [Fig. 41] as the lateral cutaneous nerve of the forearm [p. 51].

Principal neurovascular bundle of the arm

Superior to the insertion of coracobrachialis, this bundle consists of the brachial artery, the basilic and brachial veins, and the following nerves: the median, the ulnar, the radial, and the medial cutaneous of the forearm. The **radial nerve** is the first to leave the bundle. It passes inferolaterally from the posterior surface of the brachial artery to the sulcus for the radial nerve on the posterior surface of the humerus [Fig. 36] accompanied by the **profunda brachii artery**. Its continuity with the nerve already exposed on the lateral side of the arm can be confirmed by slight traction on that nerve. The **ulnar nerve** is the next to leave the bundle. It sinks backwards through the medial intermuscular septum into the posterior compartment. Below this, the **basilic**

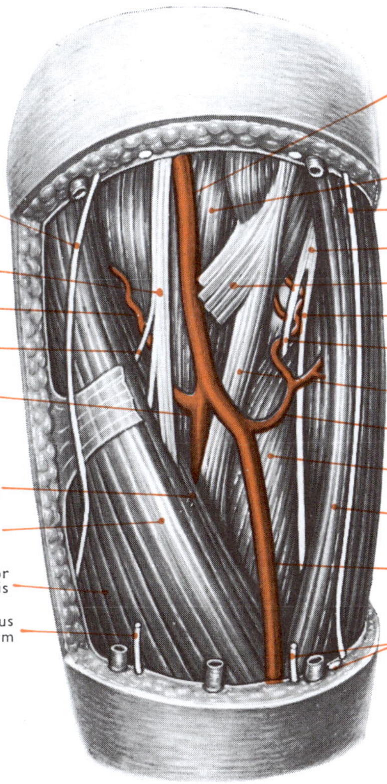

Fig. 70. Dissection of left cubital fossa. The fat has been removed and the bicipital aponeurosis cut away with the rest of the deep fascia.

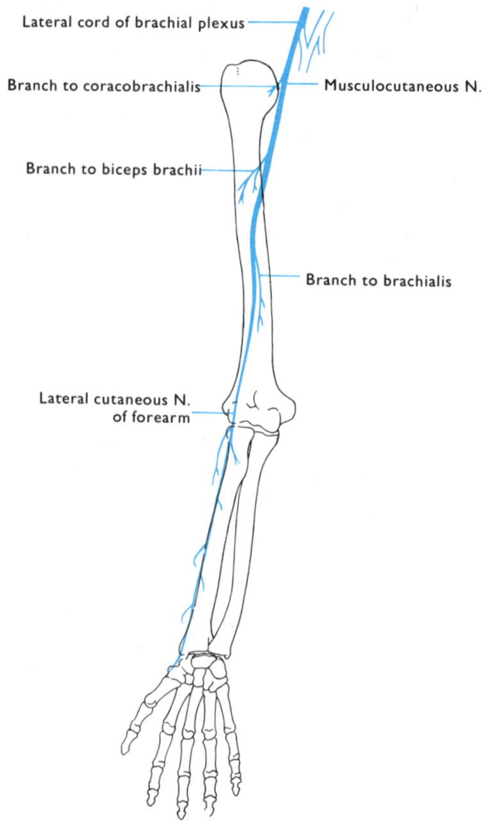

Fig. 71. The course and distribution of the musculocutaneous nerve.

vein and the **medial cutaneous nerve of the forearm** pass into the superficial fascia. Thus the bundle contains only the **median nerve** and **brachial artery** and veins in the lower third of the arm. These structures incline forwards, in front of brachialis, to lie just medial to the tendon of biceps at the elbow.

Median nerve (C. 5, 6, 7, 8; T. 1)

This nerve is formed in the axilla by one root each from the medial and lateral cords of the brachial plexus. It descends anterior to the axillary and upper part of the brachial arteries to reach the medial aspect of the brachial artery in the distal half of the arm. It supplies most of the flexor muscles in the anterior aspects of the forearm and the thenar and two lumbrical muscles in the hand [Fig. 83]. It also supplies skin in the hand and fingers [Fig. 48] but only sympathetic postganglionic fibres to the axillary and brachial arteries in the axilla and arm.

Ulnar nerve (C. 8 and T. 1)

This nerve is concerned principally with the supply of the small muscles of the hand, flexor carpi ulnaris, and the medial half of flexor digitorum profundus in the forearm [Fig. 85] and some skin in the hand and fingers [Fig. 48]. It supplies no structures in the axilla or arm. It arises from the medial cord of the brachial plexus and descends posteromedial to the distal part of the axillary artery and the proximal part of the brachial artery. At the middle of the arm it pierces the medial intermuscular septum and passes distally in the posterior compartment of the arm to enter the forearm by passing over the posterior surface of the medial epicondyle.

Brachial artery

This continuation of the axillary artery supplies the structures of the arm distal to the axilla mainly by branches which accompany the major nerves. Smaller branches pass from its lateral aspect directly into the muscles of the arm.

The **profunda brachii artery** accompanies the radial nerve and gives a descending branch on each side of the lateral intermuscular septum [Fig. 73].

The superior **ulnar collateral artery** accompanies the ulnar nerve, while the inferior ulnar collateral artery arises 5 cm above the elbow and sends descending branches on each side of the medial intermuscular septum. These vessels supply adjacent muscles and take part in the anastomosis around the elbow joint [Fig. 80].

The **nutrient artery to the humerus** arises near the middle of the humerus.

Action of muscles of front of arm

The short head of **biceps** and **coracobrachialis** are flexors of the shoulder joint, while the long head of biceps helps to hold the head of the humerus against the glenoid cavity, especially when the arm is abducted. **Brachialis** is a pure flexor of the elbow joint, while biceps is also a supinator of the forearm [p. 73] by virtue of its attachment to the posterior surface of the tuberosity of the radius.

The musculocutaneous nerve is the motor supply to all these muscles. Thus damage to this nerve interferes with flexion at the shoulder and elbow joints, especially the elbow, and causes weakening of supination [p. 121].

Posterior compartment of the arm

Dissection

Remove the deep fascia from the back of the arm to expose the triceps muscle which fills the posterior compartment. Superiorly, separate the medially placed long head of triceps, which arises from the infraglenoid tubercle of the scapula [Fig. 51], from the lateral head, which has a linear origin from the posterior surface of the humerus between the insertions of teres minor and deltoid [Fig. 52].

Find the radial nerve in the axilla posterior to the axillary artery. Trace the nerve as far as triceps, and separate the parts of triceps by passing a blunt seeker along the line of the nerve in that muscle. Divide and reflect the parts of the lateral head of triceps where it overlies the radial nerve to expose that nerve and the profunda brachii

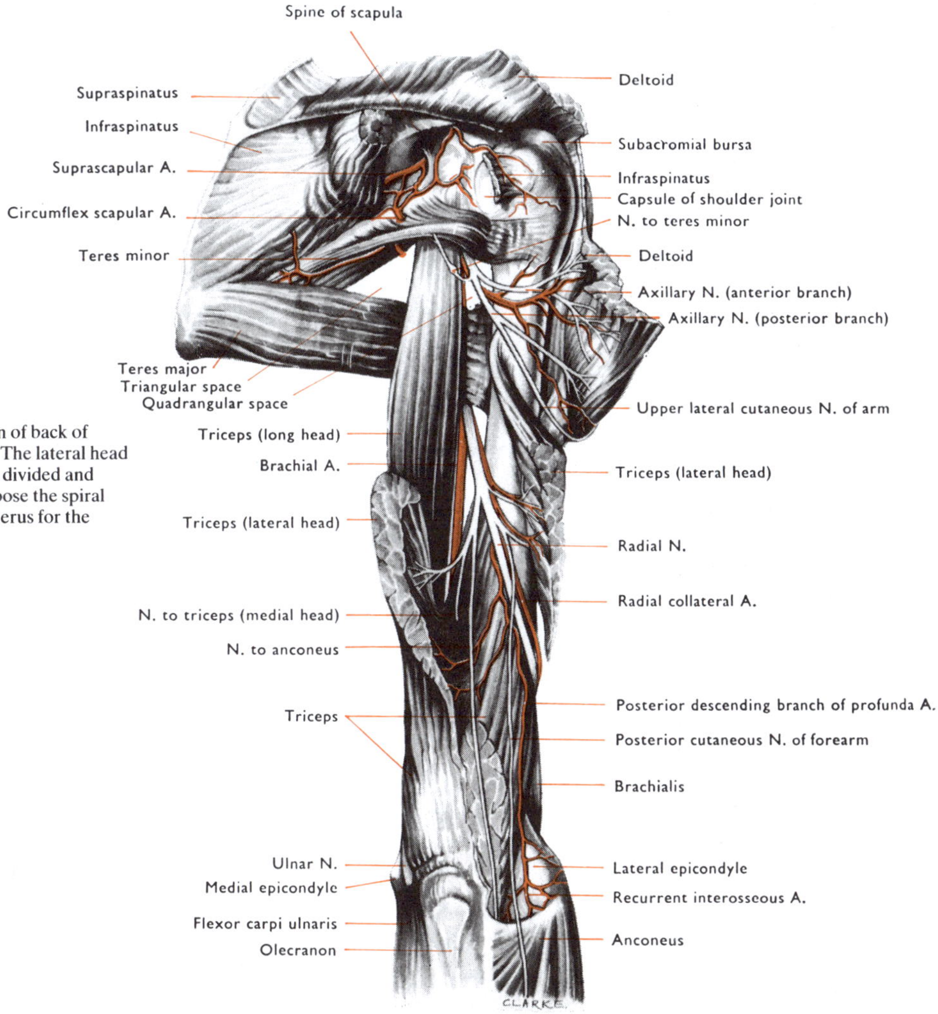

Fig. 72. Dissection of back of shoulder and arm. The lateral head of triceps has been divided and turned aside to expose the spiral groove on the humerus for the radial nerve.

artery in the groove for the radial nerve on the back of the humerus, with the medial head of triceps inferior to the groove. Follow the branches of the radial nerve and check its continuity with the part of the radial nerve already seen between brachialis and brachioradialis. Follow this part of the nerve distally. Check its branches to brachioradialis, extensor carpi radialis longus, and brachialis (sensory), and find its division into superficial (anterior) and deep (posterolateral) branches at the level of the elbow joint.

Follow the ulnar nerve into the posterior compartment of the arm with the superior ulnar collateral artery and the branch of the radial nerve to the medial head of triceps. Trace the ulnar nerve to the back of the medial epicondyle. Remove the connective tissue from the posterior surface of the medial intermuscular septum and find the posterior branch of the inferior ulnar collateral artery [Figs. 73, 80].

Triceps brachii

The **long head** of this muscle, which arises from the infraglenoid tubercle of the scapula, together with the **lateral head** from the upper third of the posterior surface of the humerus [Fig. 52] form the superficial part of the muscle. They descend, posterior to the groove for the radial nerve [Fig 36], and, fusing with one another, are joined on their deep surfaces by the **medial head** which arises from the posterior surface of the humerus distal to that groove. The three heads form a common tendon which is inserted into the superior surface of the olecranon [Fig. 93] and the surrounding deep fascia. Some of the deep fibres pass to the articular capsule of the elbow joint. They pull up the redundant part of the capsule to avoid it being caught between the olecranon and the humerus in extension of the joint. **Nerve supply:** the radial nerve. **Actions:** all three heads of triceps are extensors of the elbow joint. The long head also acts on the shoulder joint. It is mainly responsible for steadying the humerus in the glenoid cavity, especially when it is stretched across the inferior surface of the joint in abduction of the arm. Then the long heads of triceps and biceps lie like guy ropes inferior and superior to the joint, and the long head of triceps is the main structure supporting the joint inferiorly.

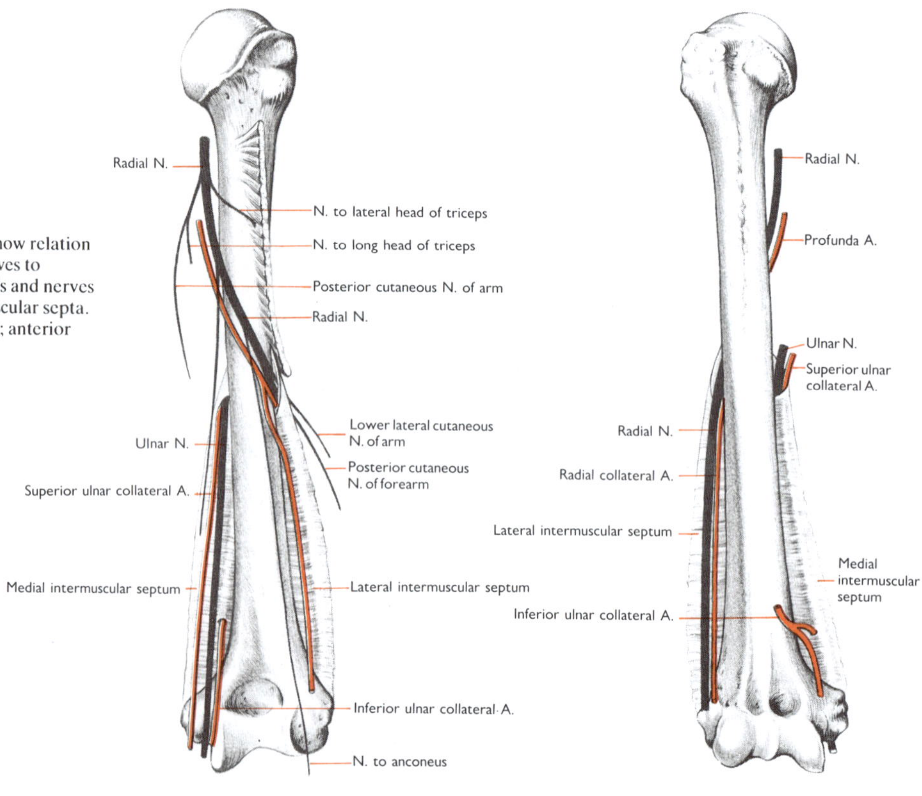

Fig. 73. Diagram to show relation of radial and ulnar nerves to humerus, and of vessels and nerves (black) to the intermuscular septa. Posterior surface—left; anterior surface—right.

Radial nerve

This nerve is the continuation of the posterior cord of the brachial plexus in the axilla. Here it gives off the **nerve to the long head of triceps** and then passes into the arm posterior to the brachial artery. Almost immediately it gives off the **posterior cutaneous nerve of the arm** and a branch to the **medial head of triceps** (which accompanies the ulnar nerve into the posterior compartment), then passes inferolaterally into the groove for the radial nerve on the posterior surface of the humerus [Fig. 36], winding spirally round the posterior surface of the humerus with the profunda brachii artery, in contact with the periosteum. Thus it is liable to be damaged in fractures of the middle third of the humerus in the same manner as the axillary nerve may be in fractures of the surgical neck. In the groove, the nerve gives off branches to the lateral head and a long slender branch which descends through the medial head of triceps of the muscle anconeus [Fig. 72] distal to the lateral epicondyle. Two cutaneous branches, lower lateral of the arm and posterior of the forearm, are also given off here.

The nerve then pierces the lateral intermuscular septum and descends in the anterior compartment between brachialis (medially) and brachioradialis and extensor carpi radialis longus (laterally). It divides into superficial and deep branches. The **superficial branch** is a sensory nerve to the back of the fingers and hand [Fig. 48]. The **deep branch** supplies the muscles of the back of the forearm and the joints at the wrist. The radial nerve also is sensory to the elbow joint, principally through its branches to anconeus and the medial head of triceps, and to the radio-ulnar joints.

The forearm and hand

Begin by revising the palpable parts of the **radius** and **ulna** [p. 42] in your own forearm and compare these with the bones themselves. Articulate a radius and ulna parallel to one another with the head of the radius lying in the radial notch of the ulna and the head of the ulna in the ulnar notch of the radius [Fig. 233]. Note the following points:

1. The ulna extends further proximally than the radius. This extension of the ulna is formed by the **trochlear notch** and the **olecranon**.

2. The radius projects slightly beyond the distal end of the ulna. The distal end of the radius is marked by the lateral two (**scaphoid** and **lunate**) of the proximal row of carpal bones—the only direct articulation between forearm and carpal bones. Because of this, (a) the carpal bones (and hence the hand) move with the radius; (b) forces applied to the hand are transmitted to the radius through these carpal bones which are therefore subject to injury.

3. The radius is markedly convex laterally. Only its ends articulate with the ulna. The two bones are held together by an interosseous membrane attached to the sharp, **interosseous borders** on their adjacent surfaces.

4. The anterior surface of the radius is crossed obliquely in its proximal half by its **anterior border,** and the distal end of this surface curves forwards to form a sharp margin against which the pulsations of the radial artery may be felt (**radial pulse**).

5. Rotate the head of the radius medially in the radial notch of the stationary ulna. When this is done, the distal end of the radius describes an arc of a circle around the head of the ulna so that it comes to lie medial to the ulna with its posterior surface facing anteriorly and the body of the radius crossing that of the ulna. This movement is **pronation**. The reverse movement is **supination**. These are the only movements at the radio-ulnar joints. The axis of movement passes through the centre of the head of the radius proximally and the centre of the head of the ulna distally. Any muscle which is so placed that it can rotate the radius medially produces pronation, while those that rotate it laterally, e.g. biceps brachii, produce supination. In pronation and supination only the radius moves. Hence this is not rotation of

the forearm on the arm—a movement which is impossible because the humerus is fitted into the ulna. Since the hand is carried with the radius, its palm faces posteriorly in pronation (elbow extended). If medial rotation of the humerus is combined with pronation, the palm faces posterolaterally. Hence testing of the range of pronation is carried out with the elbow flexed.

6. Identify the **subcutaneous posterior border of the ulna**. The flexor muscles are attached to the bones anterior and medial to this and are supplied by the median and ulnar nerves. The extensor muscles are attached lateral to this border and are supplied by the radial nerve. These two groups of muscles abut on each other anteriorly along a line from the lateral side of the tendon of biceps to the styloid process of the radius.

Muscles of the forearm

These are complex, but as a general rule both the flexor and extensor groups are arranged in two layers. (1) Each superficial layer consists of long muscles which arise principally from the humerus and pass either to the hand (acting on elbow and wrist joints) or to the digits (acting on elbow, wrist, and digital joints). (2) Each deep layer consists of muscles which arise from the forearm bones and pass to the digits, thus crossing and acting on wrist and digital joints. (3) In addition, there is (a) an intermediate layer in the flexor group which passes to the digits (flexor digitorum superficialis) from the humerus and the forearm bones, and (b) muscles which pass from the humerus to the forearm bones (pronator teres, brachioradialis, anconeus, and supinator) and between the forearm bones (pronator quadratus and supinator).

The front of the forearm and hand

Dissection

Divide the deep fascia of the forearm from the cubital fossa to the proximal margin of the flexor retinaculum. Make a transverse incision just proximal to the retinaculum, avoiding the structures deep to the fascia, and reflect the flaps of fascia. The muscles uncovered consist of the flexor group medially and the extensor group laterally. Separate the most superficial muscle [**brachioradialis**; Fig. 74] on the lateral side of the front of the forearm. Follow it to its insertion on the lateral surface of the distal end of the radius. Push aside the tendons of abductor pollicis longus and extensor pollicis brevis which overlie the tendon of insertion of brachioradialis as they pass to the base of the thumb, but avoid injury to the superficial branch of the radial nerve which crosses their superficial surfaces. Pull brachioradialis laterally. This exposes extensor carpi radialis longus and separates the extensor and flexor groups of muscles. In the groove between these groups, identify the **radial artery** and the **superficial branch of the radial nerve.** Follow them distally and proximally [Fig. 84]. In this way find the origin of the artery from the brachial artery in the cubital fossa (occasionally high in the arm) and the branch from the **deep branch of the radial nerve** which supplies extensor carpi radialis brevis—a muscle deep to extensor carpi radialis longus. Deep to the brevis is the supinator muscle which the deep branch of the radial nerve supplies before entering it.

Separate the **superficial group of flexor muscles.** These arise from the distal part of the medial supracondylar line and the medial epicondyle of the humerus. Most also have a minor attachment to the coronoid process of the ulna [Figs. 53, 234]. These superficial muscles diverge from the medial epicondyle as a narrow fan with a vertical, medial edge—**flexor carpi ulnaris**. The most lateral muscle, **pronator teres,** arises furthest superiorly and passes obliquely across the proximal half of the forearm to the point of maximum convexity of the radius [Fig. 86] by passing deep to the radial artery, the superficial branch of the radial nerve, and the extensor muscles overlying the anterolateral surface of the radius [Fig. 84]. Medial to pronator teres is **flexor carpi radialis** (the radial flexor of the wrist) which also takes an oblique course across the forearm. Its tendon disappears deep to the lateral part of the flexor retinaculum, medial to the **radial artery.**

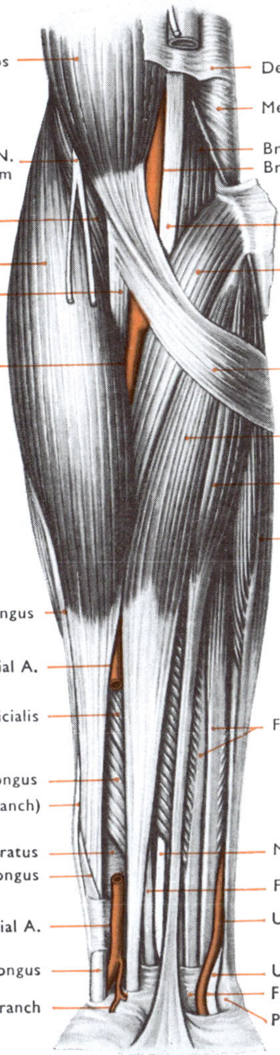

Fig. 74. Dissection of superficial muscles, arteries, and nerves of front of forearm. Part of the radial artery was removed to show the muscles deep to it.

Identify this tendon in your own wrist [Fig. 67] and feel the pulsation of the radial artery (**radial pulse**) lateral to it on the distal margin of the radius. Medial to flexor carpi radialis is **palmaris longus** (if present). Follow its tendon superficial to the flexor retinaculum to join the palmar aponeurosis. Beneath the tendon and between it and that of flexor carpi radialis the median nerve becomes superficial just proximal to the flexor retinaculum.

The **flexor carpi ulnaris** is immediately medial to palmaris longus in the proximal third of the forearm. Further distally they separate and flexor digitorum superficialis appears between them [Fig. 74]. Find the **ulnar artery and nerve** which become superficial between the tendon of flexor carpi ulnaris and those of flexor digitorum superficialis, just proximal to the flexor retinaculum. Here the artery and nerve pierce the deep fascia and enter the hand superficial to the retinaculum, immediately lateral to the insertion of flexor carpi ulnaris to the **pisiform** bone. They then pass deep to the palmaris brevis and divide into their terminal branches.

Palmaris brevis is a thin cutaneous muscle which arises from the palmar aponeurosis and flexor retinaculum. It passes transversely across the proximal 2–3 cm of the hypothenar eminence and is inserted into the skin on its medial side. When it contracts, it bunches up the skin over the eminence, thus deepening the concavity of the palm and producing a cushion of skin against which the handle of a tool can be held steady. It is supplied by the ulnar nerve.

Expose the superficial surface of **flexor carpi ulnaris.** Note its origin from the medial epicondyle, the olecranon, and the proximal two-thirds of the posterior (subcutaneous) border of the ulna. Follow the

ulnar nerve from the arm posterior to the medial epicondyle and between the attachments of flexor carpi ulnaris to the humerus and ulna to reach the deep surface of that muscle. Pull flexor carpi ulnaris medially and expose the ulnar nerve on its deep surface lying on flexor digitorum profundus which covers the ulna. Trace the nerve and the ulnar artery into continuity with the parts exposed at the wrist. Note the branches of the nerve to flexor carpi ulnaris and flexor digitorum profundus, the **dorsal branch** arising near the middle of the forearm, and the small **palmar branch** [p. 52] which arises in the distal half of the forearm. Trace the dorsal branch to the medial side of the forearm.

Cut through the middle of flexor carpi radialis, palmaris longus, and pronator teres muscles and reflect their parts. Identify the branches of the median nerve entering them proximally. **Flexor digitorum superficialis** is now exposed. Identify the radial head of this muscle attached to the anterior border of the radius deep to the distal part of pronator teres [Figs. 84, 86]. Follow the **median nerve** from the cubital fossa between the radial and humero-ulnar heads of flexor digitorum superficialis. Lift the medial edge of the muscle and find the nerve attached by fascia to its deep surface. Note its branches to the muscle. A short distance proximal to the wrist, the nerve curves round the lateral surface of the tendons of the muscle and becomes superficial to them between the tendons of flexor carpi radialis and palmaris longus, before entering the hand deep to the flexor retinaculum [Fig. 76]. Identify this position in your own wrist and note how easily the nerve could be injured by a relatively superficial cut at this point. It is here that the **palmar branch** of the median nerve arises. It enters the palm superficial to the flexor retinaculum.

Turn the tendon of palmaris longus distally. Note its attachment to the flexor retinaculum and its continuity with the apex of the palmar aponeurosis. Complete the exposure of the superficial surface of the **palmar aponeurosis** and the slips which pass from its distal margin to each of the fingers. Note that the edges of each slip turn posteriorly

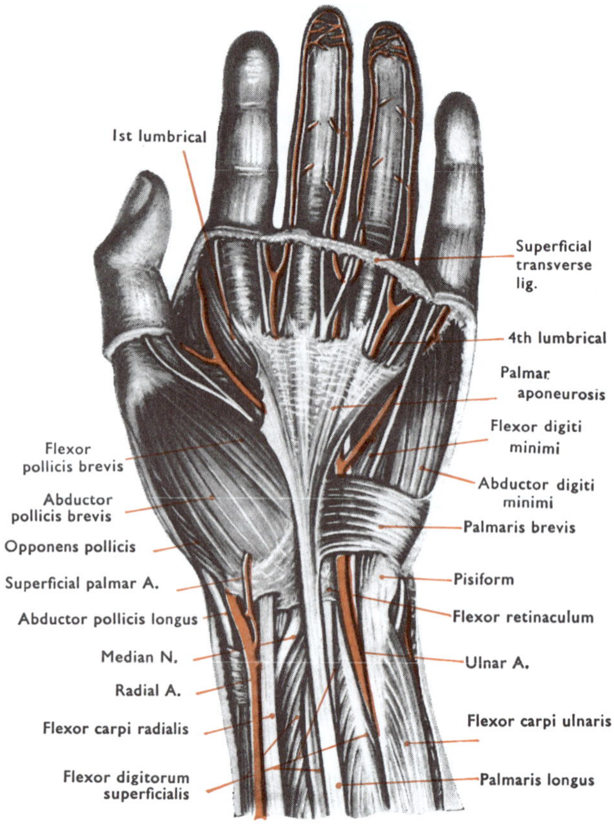

Fig. 75. Superficial dissection of palm to show the palmar aponeurosis. The deep fascia has been removed from the thenar and hypothenar eminences. Cf. Fig. 76.

into the palm leaving spaces between the slips through which the digital vessels and nerves (and lumbrical muscles) escape from beneath the palmar aponeurosis into the fingers [Fig. 75]. Each slip of the aponeurosis is attached to the phalanges by fusing (a) with the fibrous flexor sheath (the fibrous tunnel attached to the palmar surfaces of the phalanges in which the tendons of the long flexor muscles of each finger slide); (b) with the deep transverse metacarpal ligament (q.v.) and the fascia with which it is continuous covering the palmar surfaces of the metacarpal bones and the interosseous muscles between them.

Separate the palmaris longus tendon and the aponeurosis from the surface of the flexor retinaculum. Turn the aponeurosis distally by separating its edges from the thinner deep fascia covering the thenar and hypothenar muscles and divide the septum which passes backwards from each edge to fuse with the fascia anterior to the interosseous and adductor pollicis muscles [Fig. 88]. Avoid injury to the vessels and nerves immediately deep to the aponeurosis.

Palmar aponeurosis

This thick, triangular portion of the deep fascia lies in the central region of the palm with its apex at the flexor retinaculum and its base near the level of the heads of the metacarpals. It stabilizes the palmar skin which is firmly adherent to it. At each side the aponeurosis is continuous posteriorly with the layer of fascia with covers the anterior surfaces of the metacarpals, the interosseous muscles between them, and the adductor pollicis [Fig. 88]. Together these fascial layers form a sort of mitten which surrounds the central palmar space and encloses the vessels and nerves, the long flexor tendons to the fingers, and the lumbrical muscles which arise from them. Distally this mitten is turned into a glove by sheets of fascia which pass from the aponeurosis and both edges of each of its digital slips to the metacarpal fascia. Thus each slip forms a tunnel around the flexor tendons to its digit [Fig. 98] but adjacent tunnels are not united, the spaces between them allowing the nerves, vessels, and lumbrical muscles to emerge into the superficial tissues. Confirm this by pushing a blunt instrument proximally between any two fingers—it passes readily into the palm deep to the aponeurosis without having to pierce it. Remove the fat from this interdigital region and expose the **digital nerves and vessels** with a **lumbrical muscle** posterior to them [Fig. 75]. The loose tissue in which these lie gives ready access for infection to spread from the superficial tissues of the fingers to the central palmar region whence it can extend behind the flexor retinaculum into the forearm.

Progressive shortening of the palmar aponeurosis—a condition known as Dupuytren's contraction—produces flexion of the fingers because the aponeurosis is attached to the proximal phalanges through the deep transverse metacarpal ligament [p. 101]. The shortening usually affects the medial part of the aponeurosis and hence the little and ring fingers. It requires surgical division of the aponeurosis to straighten them.

Dissection

Remove any remnants of palmaris brevis and follow the **ulnar nerve** and **artery** distally, superficial to the flexor retinaculum. Note, but do not follow, the deep branch of the nerve (motor) and the deep palmar branch of the artery entering the hypothenar muscles. Follow the superficial palmar arch which the artery forms and trace its branches and those of the ulnar nerve (sensory and sympathetic) to the fingers [Fig. 76]. The superficial palmar arch is immediately deep to the palmar aponeurosis and has the branches of the median and ulnar nerves between it and the long flexor tendons [Fig. 88].

Pull gently on the **median nerve** proximal to the flexor retinaculum. This demonstrates its position at the distal edge of the retinaculum. Carefully follow the branches of the median nerve distal to the retinaculum, but do not disturb the flexor tendons. The nerve gives a short, thick, recurrent (motor) branch into the thenar muscles close to

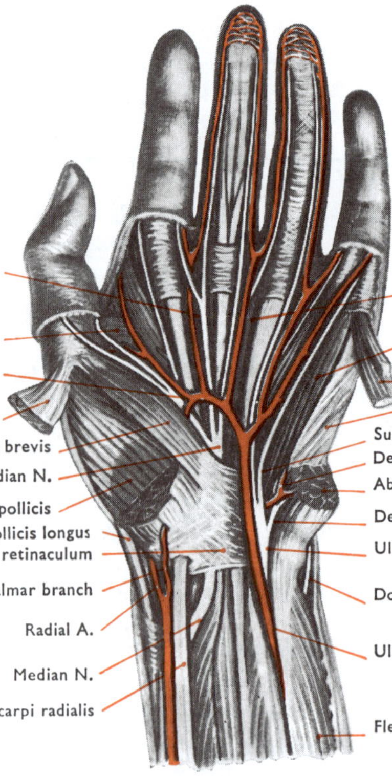

Fig. 76. Structures in palm displayed by removal of palmar aponeurosis. In this specimen the radialis indicis and the princeps pollicis arteries took origin from the superficial palmar arch.

the distal edge of the retinaculum. It then divides into **common** and **proper palmar digital nerves** (mainly sensory and sympathetic) which pass to the thumb and lateral two and one half fingers [Fig. 90]. The most medial digital branch communicates with the most lateral digital branch of the ulnar nerve. The branch to the lateral side of the index finger sends a twig posteriorly into the first lumbrical muscle, while the branch medial to this supplies the second lumbrical. Follow the digital branches at least to the roots of the fingers and trace them to the tip of one finger. Note the branches which pass dorsally in the distal part of the finger. Through these the skin on the dorsal surfaces of the distal two phalanges is supplied by these palmar digital nerves.

Expose the surface of the **fibrous flexor sheath** in one finger at least, but avoid damage to the tissue surrounding the flexor tendons at its proximal end. Note that the sheath is thick where it lies opposite the bodies of the phalanges but is thinner and has a cruciate arrangement of its fibres at the levels of the interphalangeal joints.

Superficial palmar arch

This arterial arch is variable. Normally, it begins as a terminal branch of the ulnar artery on the flexor retinaculum distal to the pisiform bone. It then crosses the hook of the hamate bone and turns laterally deep to the palmar aponeurosis to join one or other of the branches of the radial artery [Figs. 76, 90] which may form a significant portion of an incomplete arch. The distal point of the arch lies at the same level as the distal border of the thenar eminence when the thumb is fully extended.

Branches

The principal branches are four palmar digital arteries. The most medial is the proper palmar digital artery to the medial side of the little finger. The other three—**common palmar digital arteries**—pass to the interdigital clefts where each receives the corresponding palmar metacarpal artery from the deep palmar arch and divides into two **proper palmar digital arteries** to the adjacent sides of two fingers [Figs. 75, 76, 90]. The proper palmar digital arteries to each finger form a rich anastomosis in the pulp of the finger and in the nail bed.

Flexor retinaculum

This dense fibrous band unites the ends of the arch of carpal bones and thus converts that arch into an osteofibrous **carpal tunnel.** The median nerve and long flexor tendons of the fingers and thumb pass through this tunnel—the flexor retinaculum acting as a pulley for these tendons in flexion of the wrist. The retinaculum is part of the deep fascia and is therefore continuous with the deep fascia of the forearm and the palmar aponeurosis in the hand.

Attachments are to the pisiform bone and the hook of the hamate medially and to the tubercle of the scaphoid and the front of the trapezium laterally. The attachment to the trapezium is to either side of the groove which lodges the tendon of flexor carpi radialis, thus forming a separate tunnel for this tendon [Fig. 78].

The superficial surface of the retinaculum gives partial origin to the thenar and hypothenar muscles and has the ulnar nerve and vessels, the palmar cutaneous branches of the median and ulnar nerves, and the tendon of palmaris longus on it.

Fibrous flexor sheaths

These are thickened tunnels of deep fascia within which the long flexor tendons slide in the digits. These tunnels are attached to the sides of the palmar surfaces of the phalanges and of the palmar ligaments of the metacarpophalangeal and interphalangeal joints. The sheath is composed of a thick layer of transverse fibres where it is attached to the phalanges. At the level of the joints it is thinner and consists mainly of oblique, cruciform fibres to allow free flexion at the joints. Together with the phalanges each sheath forms an osteofascial tube which prevents the tendons from springing away from the digits during flexion.

Synovial sheaths of flexor tendons

Synovial sheaths surround tendons wherever they pass through fascial or osteofascial tunnels. They consist of two concentric tubes of smooth synovial membrane joined together at their ends. They are separated by a capillary interval (the cavity of the sheath) which contains only sufficient synovial fluid to lubricate the opposed surfaces and to allow them to slide on each other. The inner tube surrounds and is adherent to the tendon (or tendons), the outer tube lines the fibrous or bony canal and is fused with it. Tendons may be completely surrounded by the synovial space or suspended in the sheath by a fold of synovial membrane (**mesotendon**). The mesotendon allows blood vessels to reach the tendon at any point along the sheath; otherwise they must enter at the ends or run across the cavity of the sheath in a tube of synovial membrane (see vincula). The cavity of a synovial sheath forms a route for rapid spread of infection along its length. When thus inflamed, the cavity becomes distended with fluid, tense, and painful and the pressure may rise within the sheath sufficiently to interfere with the blood supply of the tendon.

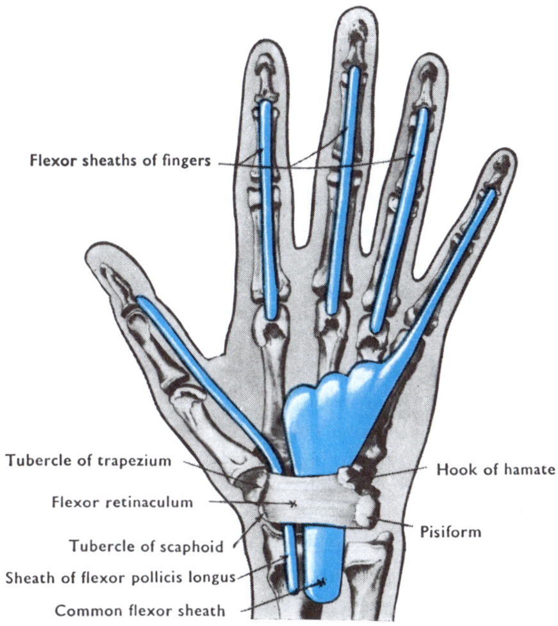

Fig. 77. Synovial sheaths of flexor tendons of digits.

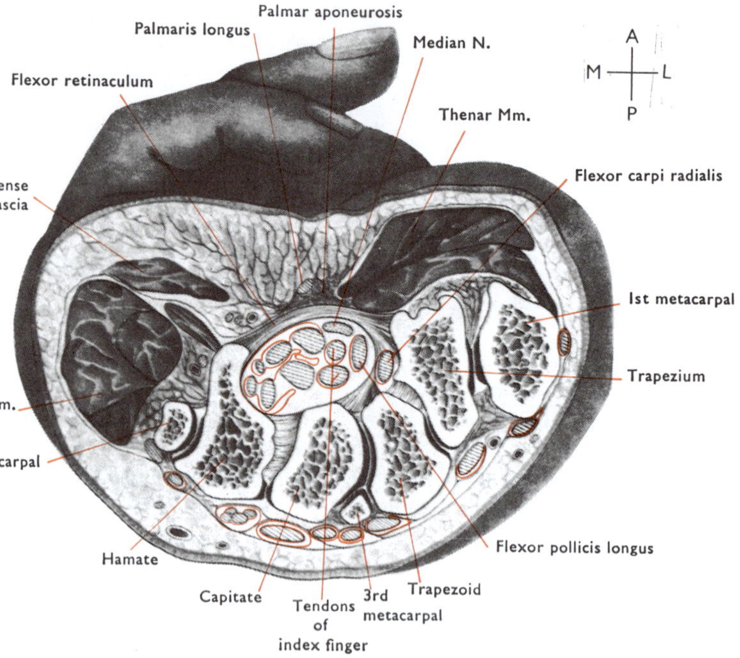

Fig. 78. Drawing of transverse section through distal row of carpal bones to show position of long flexor tendons and their synovial sheaths (red). At this level the tendons to the index and middle fingers are leaving the common synovial sheath, which still surrounds those to the ring and little finger.
A. Anterior.
P. Posterior.
M. Medial.
L. Lateral.

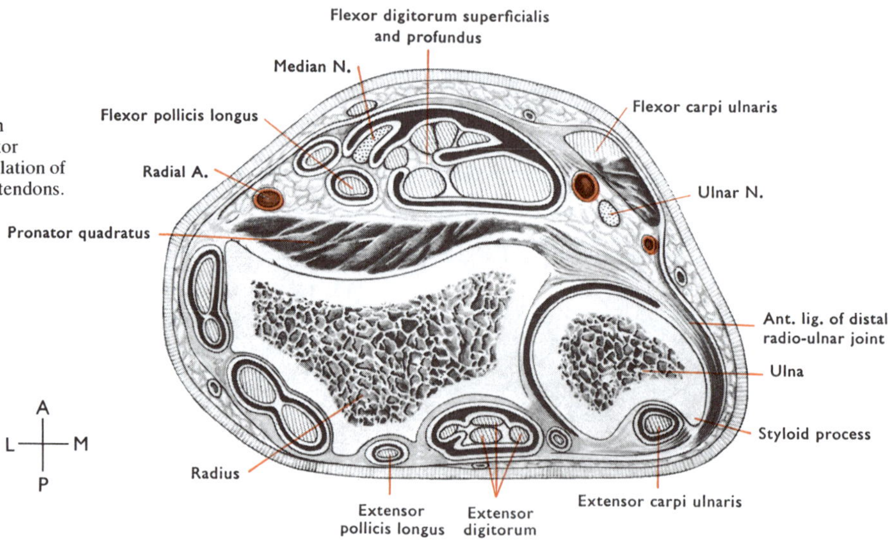

Fig. 79. Transverse section through forearm above flexor retinaculum showing the relation of the synovial sheaths to the tendons.
A. Anterior.
P. Posterior.
M. Medial.
L. Lateral.

In the carpal tunnel [Fig. 77], the tendons of flexor digitorum superficialis and profundus are enclosed in a common sheath beside the sheath containing the tendon of flexor pollicis longus. These two sheaths may communicate and both extend 2–3 cm proximally into the forearm posterior to the tendons and distally to the terminal phalanx only in the thumb and little finger. The synovial sheaths in the fibrous flexor sheaths of the middle three digits are separated from the common sheath and that in the little finger is incomplete to allow the lumbrical muscles which are attached to the tendons of flexor digitorum profundus to emerge from the sheath. The continuity of the common synovial sheath with that in the little finger and sometimes with that in the thumb allows infection to spread rapidly from these digits to the carpal tunnel. The tight packing of tendons, sheath, and median nerve in the carpal tunnel results in compression of the median nerve when any swelling arises there. Hence there is loss of function of that nerve in the hand (*carpal tunnel syndrome*) and even death of the tendons due to interference with their blood supply in extreme cases. The tendon of flexor carpi radialis has only its own synovial sheath.

Dissection

Synovial sheaths are difficult to demonstrate though they may be injected with air or water through a hypodermic needle introduced into the sheath. Attempt to do this by lifting the loose connective tissue (external layer of sheath) which surrounds the tendons of flexor digitorum superficialis close to the flexor retinaculum and introducing the needle along the surface of one tendon. If this proves unsatisfactory, divide the loose connective tissue down to the tendon and note the smooth, slippery, internal surface of the sheath and external surface of the tendon. Introduce a blunt probe into the sheath and try to define its extent. Note that it allows the probe to pass easily into the hand deep to the flexor retinaculum, but also that the structures here are tightly packed in the carpal tunnel. Divide the fibrous flexor sheath longitudinally in one finger. Note its thickness at the level of the bodies of the phalanges and its relative thinness opposite the joints. Examine the extent of the digital synovial sheath.

Lift the tendons of flexor digitorum superficialis and profundus within the digital sheath and note the vinculae [Fig. 87] passing between them and the outer layer of the synovial sheath on the phalanges.

Divide the flexor retinaculum by a sagittal cut between the thenar and hypothenar muscles. Take care not to damage the median nerve. Establish the continuity of the trunk of the median nerve with the branches found in the hand.

Follow the tendons of flexor digitorum superficialis distally to the fingers. Note how each tendon divides to enclose the corresponding tendon of flexor digitorum profundus and is then inserted on the palmar aspect of the middle phalanx after reuniting dorsal to the profundus tendon [Fig. 87].

Cut transversely through the humero-ulnar head of flexor digitorum superficialis. Reflect the distal part of the muscle laterally to uncover the deep muscles of the forearm, the median nerve, and the ulnar artery.

Separate the **median nerve** from the deep surface of flexor digitorum superficialis and trace it proximally. Find its branches to the muscle and the **anterior interosseous nerve** arising from it in the distal part of the antecubital fossa. Follow the **ulnar artery** to its origin from the brachial artery and trace its principal branches [Fig. 80]. Do not follow the posterior interosseous artery at this stage. Trace the anterior interosseous artery and nerve on the interosseous membrane between the deep flexor muscles of the forearm. These are (medially) **flexor digitorum profundus**, (laterally) **flexor pollicis longus** (which arise from the proximal two-thirds of the ulna and radius respectively [Figs. 84, 86]), and (distally) **pronator quadratus,** a rectangular muscle which passes transversely between the anterior surfaces of the distal quarters of the radius and ulna. Expose these muscles and find the branches of the artery and nerve to them and the artery passing posteriorly through the interosseous membrane at the proximal border of pronator quadratus. Cut across flexor digitorum superficialis distal to the origin of its radial head and turn its tendons distally. Follow the tendons of flexor digitorum profundus and flexor pollicis longus through the carpal tunnel into the palm. Note the separation of the tendons of flexor digitorum profundus in the palm, and the four small muscles (**lumbricals**) arising from them there. Follow the lumbrical muscles to their tendons which pass with the proper digital vessels and nerves to the lateral side of the base of each finger. Their tendons will be traced later.

Reconfirm the supply to the medial part of flexor digitorum profundus from the ulnar nerve and the origin of that muscle from the medial and anterior surface of the ulna. If possible, follow the anterior interosseous nerve through the pronator quadratus to the anterior surface of the **wrist joint.** It supplies this joint and the **distal radio-ulnar joint.**

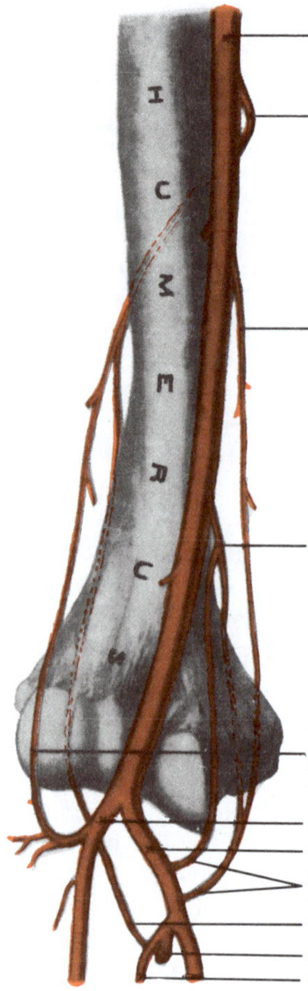

Fig. 80. Diagram of anastomosis around elbow joint.

Arteries of the flexor compartment of the forearm

The brachial artery normally divides into the radial and ulnar arteries at the level of the neck of the radius in the cubital fossa. The smaller **radial artery** passes inferolaterally between brachioradialis and flexor carpi radialis to reach the anterior surface of the distal end of the radius between the tendons of these muscles. Here the artery can be felt readily (radial pulse) against the bone. Except in the initial part of its course the artery is immediately deep to the deep fascia. It crosses the superficial surface of pronator teres with the superficial branch of the radial nerve [Fig. 84].

The **ulnar artery** passes inferomedially deep to the median nerve and the muscles arising from the medial epicondyle of the humerus and the coronoid process of the ulna. It lies on brachialis and flexor digitorum profundus, meets the ulnar nerve above the middle of the forearm, and descends vertically with it to pierce the deep fascia just proximal to the flexor retinaculum, between the tendons of flexor carpi ulnaris and flexor digitorum superficialis.

The ulnar artery is the principal source of supply to the forearm; the radial is usually the main artery of the hand. Both arteries send **recurrent branches** to anastomose with those of the brachial (**ulnar collateral arteries**) and profunda brachii (**radial collateral artery**) arteries in the rich anastomosis around the elbow joint [Fig. 80]. Both arteries supply the muscles adjacent to them and give **palmar** and **dorsal carpal arteries** at the wrist. These anastomose on and supply the carpal bones, the surrounding joint tissues, and the adjacent parts of the hand [p. 98]. At the wrist, the radial artery sends a **superficial palmar branch** of very variable size into the thenar muscles. It lies superficial to the flexor retinaculum and may anastomose with the superficial palmar arch of the ulnar artery [Fig. 90] occasionally forming a large or separate part of it.

The **common interosseous artery** is the principal branch of the ulnar artery in the forearm [Fig. 80]. It passes to the upper border of the interosseous

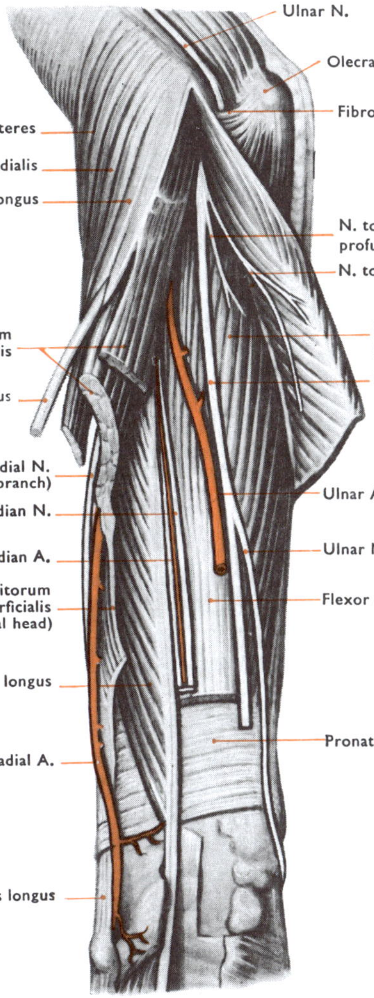

Fig. 81. Deep dissection of the front of forearm. The elbow is partially flexed, the forearm semi-pronated. The superficial muscles are cut short and turned aside. The deeper parts are still further displayed by the separation of the flexor digitorum superficialis from the flexor carpi ulnaris.

membrane. Here it divides into anterior and posterior **interosseous arteries**. The posterior passes above the membrane to the back of the forearm [p. 98]. The anterior interosseous artery gives off the long, slender median artery to the median nerve and then descends on the front of the interosseous membrane between flexor pollicis longus and flexor digitorum profundus to pronator quadratus. It supplies these muscles, sends nutrient arteries to the radius and ulna, and pierces the interosseous membrane at the upper border of pronator quadratus to enter the back of the forearm [p. 98].

Nerves of the flexor compartment of the forearm and hand

These are the median and ulnar nerves. Neither of these nerves supplies any structures proximal to the elbow except a vascular branch (sympathetic and sensory) from the median nerve to the brachial artery in the arm, and articular branches from both to the elbow joint.

Median nerve [Fig. 83]

The median nerve gives branches to the pronator teres, flexor carpi radialis, palmaris longus, flexor digitorum superficialis, and the elbow joint as it lies on brachialis in the cubital fossa. As it leaves the fossa on the anterior surface of the ulnar artery it gives off the **anterior interosseous nerve**. This nerve runs with the corresponding artery, supplies flexor digitorum profundus (lateral half), flexor pollicis longus, and pronator quadratus. It passes posterior to pronator quadratus to end on the front of the wrist and distal radio-ulnar joints.

The median nerve descends on the deep surface of flexor digitorum superficialis and, near the wrist, curves round the lateral side of its tendons to lie between them and the tendon of flexor carpi radialis deep to the tendon of palmaris longus [Fig. 74]. Here it gives off the palmar cutaneous branch

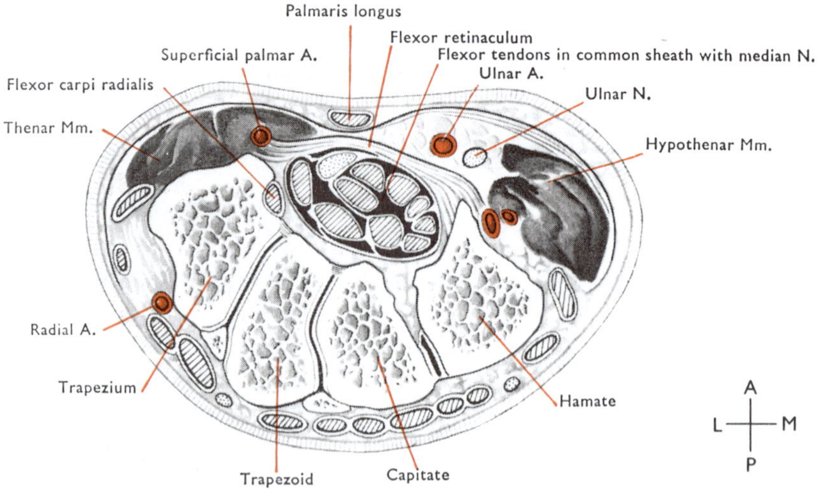

Fig. 82. Transverse section at the level of distal row of carpal bones. The flexor pollicis longus, the median nerve, and the tendons of the two flexors (superficial and deep) of the digits are seen in the carpal tunnel. The sheath of flexor pollicis longus is continuous with the common sheath at this level.
A. Anterior.
P. Posterior.
M. Medial.
L. Lateral.

[p. 53]. It then traverses the carpal tunnel between the flexor retinaculum and the lateral margin of the tendons of flexor digitorum superficialis and divides into six branches near the distal border of the retinaculum. The most lateral branch turns proximally on to the retinaculum and enters the thenar muscles to supply abductor pollicis brevis, flexor pollicis brevis, and opponens pollicis. Medial to this the mode of division is variable but commonly three **proper palmar digital nerves** pass one to each side of the thumb and the radial side of the index finger [Fig. 90], the last supplying the first lumbrical muscle. A **common palmar digital nerve** passes towards each side of the middle finger, the lateral one supplying the second lumbrical muscle, the medial communicating with the common palmar digital nerve from the ulnar nerve. Proximal to the division of the corresponding common palmar digital arteries, each of these nerves divides into two **proper palmar digital nerves** which pass between the slips of the palmar aponeurosis [Fig. 75] to enter the subcutaneous tissue of the index, middle, and ring fingers [Fig. 76]. Here they are anterior to the corresponding arteries.

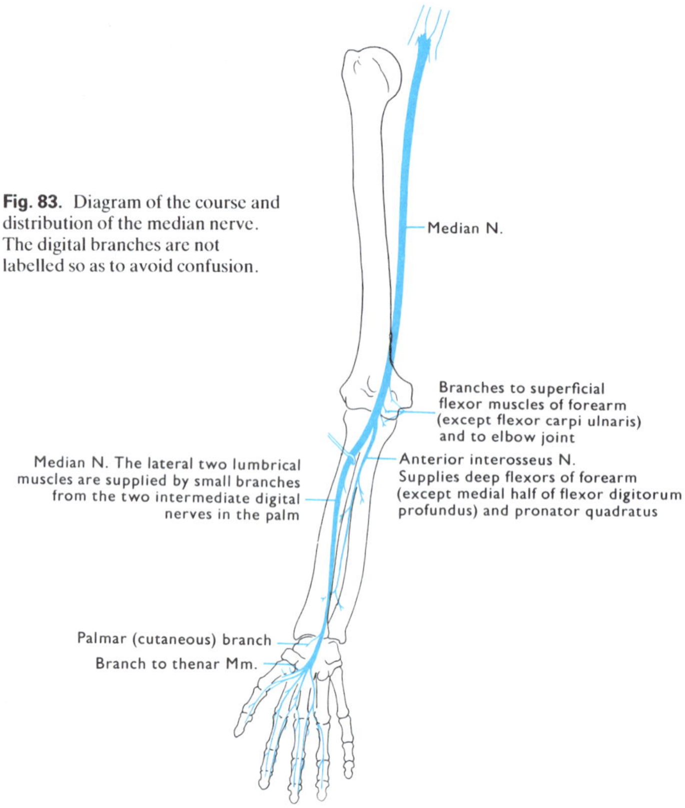

Fig. 83. Diagram of the course and distribution of the median nerve. The digital branches are not labelled so as to avoid confusion.

The distribution of these proper palmar digital nerves is to all structures on the palmar aspects of the finger but is also to the dorsal structures at the level of the distal 1½–2 phalanges through dorsal branches. In the thumb, they frequently supply dorsal structures in the region of the terminal phalanx. All the digital nerves communicate and their territories overlap to such an extent that the total destruction of one of the nerves (median, ulnar, or radial) which give rise to them produces an area of total sensory loss much smaller than that to which the individual branches of the destroyed nerve are distributed.

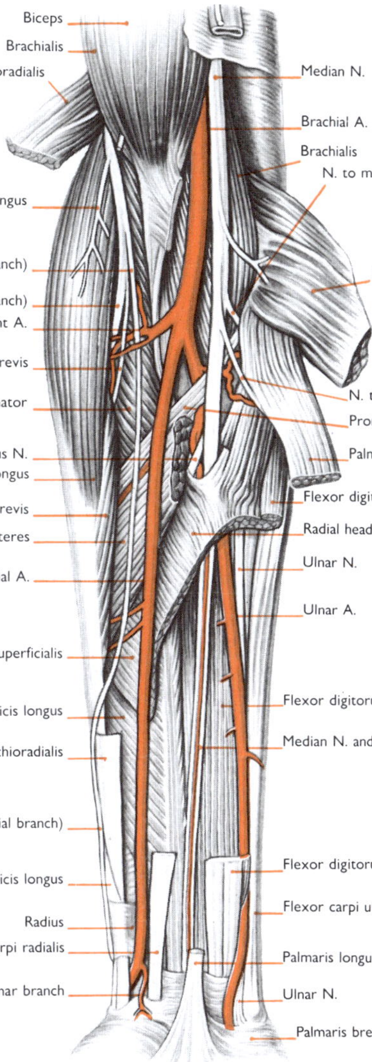

Fig. 84. Deep dissection of muscles and nerves of front of forearm. The division of the brachial artery is slightly lower than usual.

Ulnar nerve [Fig. 85]

The ulnar nerve enters the forearm on the posterior surface of the medial epicondyle of the humerus. It supplies a branch to the elbow joint, and passing deep to the flexor carpi ulnaris [Fig. 81] gives a branch to it and one to the medial half of flexor digitorum profundus. It then descends between these two muscles in the medial part of the front of the forearm and is joined by the ulnar artery and gives off its **dorsal branch** [Fig. 81 and p. 51] above the middle of the forearm. It emerges on the lateral side of the tendon of flexor carpi ulnaris close to the pisiform bone. Here it pierces the deep fascia with its palmar cutaneous branch and the ulnar artery, and passing on to the flexor retinaculum divides into deep [p. 92] and superficial branches.

The **superficial branch** supplies palmaris brevis and, passing deep to it, divides into a **proper palmar digital nerve** to the medial side of the little finger and a **common palmar digital nerve** to the medial interdigital cleft. This communicates with the adjacent common palmar digital nerve from the median nerve, and divides into proper palmar digital nerves to the adjacent sides of the ring and little fingers [Fig. 90].

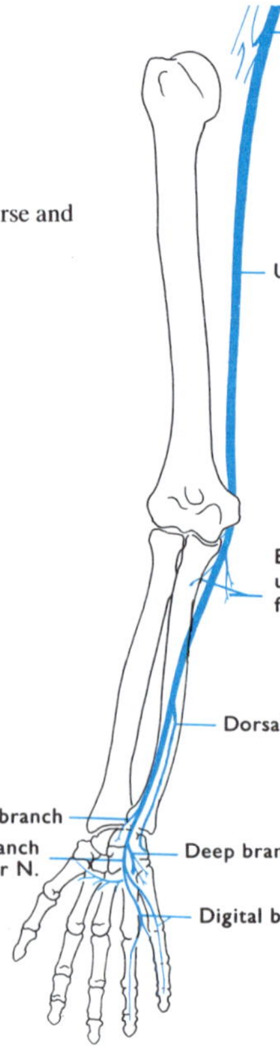

Fig 85. Diagram of the course and distribution of the ulnar N.

The ulnar nerve may transmit nerve fibres from the seventh cervical ventral ramus to the skin of the hand. It receives these either through a communication with the median nerve in the forearm or through a branch from the lateral cord of the brachial plexus in the axilla. *Occasionally the ulnar nerve supplies the thenar muscles*, presumably because it transmits fibres which normally enter the median nerve through its medial root [p. 70].

Muscles of the front of the forearm and hand

Extensor muscles

Brachioradialis arises high on the lateral supracondylar line of the humerus. It descends in front of the elbow joint with extensor carpi radialis longus [p. 95] which arises inferior to it [Fig. 53]. Thus both are flexors of the elbow joint though they belong to the extensor group of muscles supplied by the radial nerve. Brachioradialis is inserted into the lateral surface of the distal end of the radius [Fig. 86]. In addition to flexing the elbow joint, it also partially supinates the fully pronated forearm because of its spiral course through the forearm in this position.

Flexor muscles

There are superficial and deep groups. The flexor digitorum superficialis is considered with the superficial group although it lies in a somewhat intermediate position.

The *superficial group* consists of pronator teres, flexor carpi radialis, palmaris longus, flexor carpi ulnaris, and flexor digitorum superficialis. All arise from the medial epicondyle of the humerus and the fascia between them, and some have a subsidiary attachment to the coronoid process of the ulna [Fig. 86]. All pass anterior to the elbow joint and are weak flexors of that joint though each has other specific actions. All are supplied by the median nerve in the cubital fossa *except* flexor carpi ulnaris which is supplied by the ulnar nerve.

Flexor carpi ulnaris arises from the olecranon and posterior border of the ulna in addition to the humeral origin. It passes vertically to the pisiform at the anteromedial side of the carpus. It is a flexor of the wrist and an adductor (ulnar deviator) of the hand. The force which it applies to the pisiform is transmitted to the hook of the hamate bone [Fig. 89] by the **pisohamate ligament**, and to the base of the fifth metacarpal by the **pisometacarpal ligament**. Both ligaments are essentially continuations of the tendon of flexor carpi ulnaris.

Palmaris longus expands into and therefore tenses the palmar aponeurosis. Thus it stabilizes the palmar skin in grasping an object. It passes anterior to the wrist joint and so may assist in its flexion. The muscle is frequently absent.

Flexor carpi radialis runs obliquely across the anterior surface of the forearm to the anterolateral surface of the wrist. Here it passes through a separate compartment in the lateral end of the flexor retinaculum, grooving the trapezium [Fig. 78] to the bases of the second and third metacarpals (that of the thumb is the first). It is a flexor of the wrist and abductor (radial deviator) of the hand [p. 108]. Acting with flexor carpi ulnaris it produces pure flexion of the wrist joint. Because of its oblique course in the forearm, it tends to rotate the hand and radius medially and so assists pronation.

Pronator teres is the most lateral and most oblique of these muscles. It is mainly a medial rotator of the radius on the ulna (pronation) and has increased mechanical advantage by being attached to the most lateral part of the convex radius [Fig. 86].

Flexor digitorum superficialis lies deep to the other muscles of this group. The thin **radial head** [Figs. 84, 86] straightens the pull of the muscle so that it passes vertically down the middle of the front of the forearm. Its four tendons enter the palm through the carpal tunnel (the tendons to the middle and ring fingers are anterior) in the same synovial sheath as those of flexor digitorum profundus. One tendon passes into the fibrous flexor sheath of each finger. At the proximal phalanx, each tendon flattens and splits into two bands which curve posteriorly one on each side of the tendon of flexor digitorum profundus and are inserted into the sides of the palmar surface of the middle phalanx. The most posterior fibres of each band pass behind the profundus tendon to intermingle with the corresponding fibres of the other band (**chiasma tendinum**) and end in its insertion. Thus they form an oblique sling around the profundus tendon. The tendons of flexor digitorum superficialis cross the anterior surfaces of all the joints from the wrist to the proximal interphalangeal and so may flex all of these (the range of movement at the carpometacarpal joints is so small that it may be ignored). Usually they act

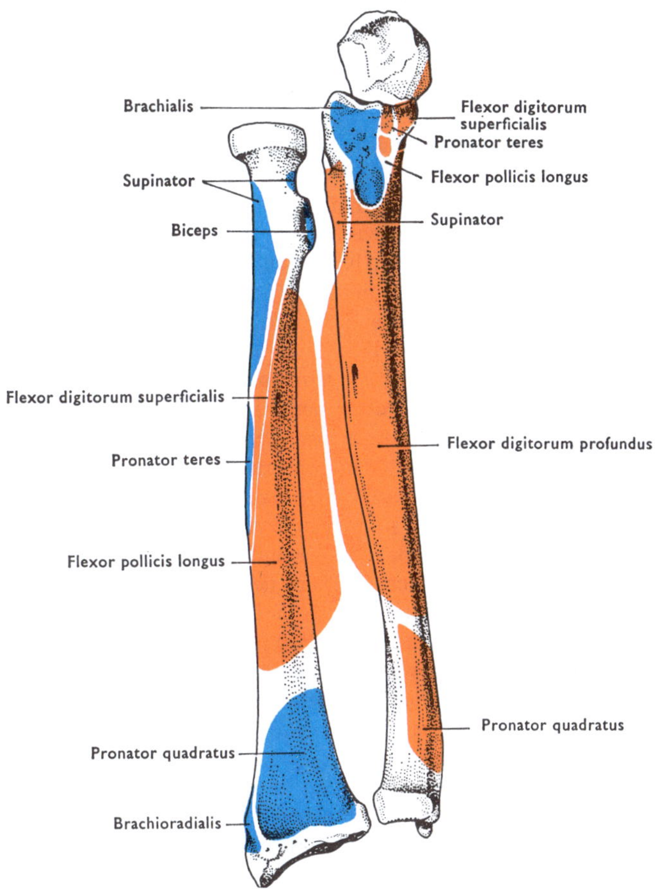

Fig. 86. Muscle attachments to anterior surface of right radius and ulna.

on the metacarpophalangeal and proximal interphalangeal joints, the wrist being fixed by its extensors. The tendon to the little finger is occasionally missing.

The deep group arises from the ulna and radius [Fig. 86] and consists of flexor digitorum profundus, flexor pollicis longus, and pronator quadratus.

Flexor digtorum profundus arises distal to the coronoid process from the medial and anterior surfaces of the proximal three-quarters of the ulna and the adjacent interosseous membrane. When the fist is clenched it may be felt contracting through the aponeurotic origin of flexor carpi ulnaris from the posterior border of the ulna by placing your fingers medial to that border. The four tendons pass through the carpal tunnel, but the medial three only separate when they enter the palm and give origin to the **lumbrical muscles** from their radial or adjacent sides. Each tendon then enters the fibrous flexor

Fig. 87. Flexor tendons of finger with vincula tendinum.

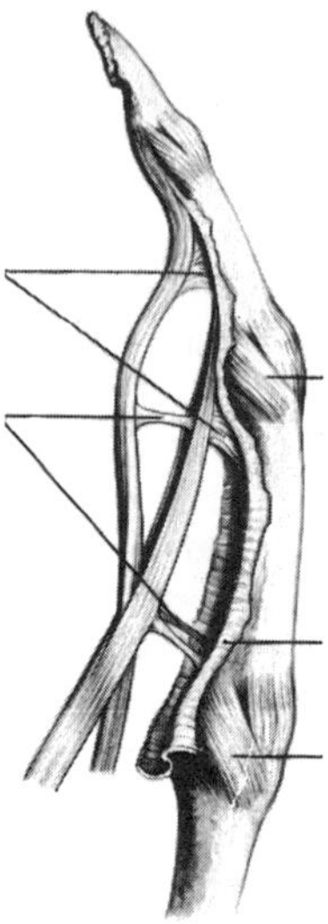

sheath of the corresponding finger, traverses the aperture in the tendon of flexor digitorum superficialis, and is inserted into the palmar surface of the base of the distal phalanx. **Nerve supply:** the lateral half, which passes to the index and middle fingers, is supplied by the median nerve through its anterior interosseous branch; the medial half, which acts on the ring and little fingers, is supplied by the ulnar nerve. **Action:** this muscle has the same actions on the wrist and fingers as flexor digitorum superficialis, but also flexes the terminal interphalangeal joints and forms the structure from which the lumbricals act [p. 101]. *When the muscle is paralysed, the obvious effect is the absence of the flexion of the terminal phalanges.*

Vincula tendinum [Fig. 87]. These thin fibrous slips enclosed in synovial membrane transmit blood vessels to the tendons within the digital synovial sheaths. The vincula brevia are triangular and pass to the tendons immediately proximal to their insertion. The vincula longa are more slender and lie nearer the root of the finger.

Flexor pollicis longus arises from the anterior surface of the radius between the attachments of flexor digitorum superficialis (radial head) and pronator quadratus, and from the interosseous membrane [Fig. 86]. The single tendon traverses the lateral part of the carpal tunnel, then the palmar surface of the thumb between the muscles of the thenar eminence and adductor pollicis [p. 91]. It enters the fibrous flexor sheath at the base of the proximal phalanx, and is inserted into the base of the terminal phalanx. **Nerve supply:** the anterior interosseous branch of the median nerve. **Action:** it flexes all the joints of the thumb (including the carpometacarpal joint) and the wrist.

Pronator quadratus [Figs. 81, 86] runs transversely between the anterior surfaces of the distal quarters of the ulna and radius. **Nerve supply:** the anterior interosseous branch of the median nerve. **Action:** pronation.

Dissection

Remove the deep fascia from the surfaces of the thenar and hypothenar eminences. Avoid damage to the branch of the median nerve and the deep branch of the ulnar nerve which supply their contained muscles.

In the **thenar eminence,** the most anterior muscle is **abductor pollicis brevis.** It hides the **opponens pollicis** and partly covers the **flexor pollicis brevis** which is incompletely fused with the medial margin of the opponens. Pass the handle of a scalpel behind the lateral border of the abductor and lift it from the underlying muscles. Define its attachments and cut across it to expose the opponens. Separate the flexor brevis from the opponens; the flexor brevis is inserted with the abductor brevis into the anterior aspect of the base of the first phalanx, the opponens to the anterior surface of the first metacarpal [Fig. 89]. *(The use of the terms anterior and posterior in the thumb may be misleading. It should be realized that the palmar surface of the thumb faces medially while the surfaces which correspond to the lateral and medial surfaces in a finger face anteriorly and posteriorly in the thumb.)* All three thenar muscles arise from the flexor retinaculum and the tubercle of the trapezium, but the flexor has a deep head from the trapezoid and capitate [Fig. 39].

Cut across the middle of flexor pollicis brevis and reflect its parts. This exposes the tendon of flexor pollicis longus and behind it the adductor pollicis passing to the posterior surface of the base of the proximal phalanx. Examine the synovial sheath of the long flexor tendon, then expose and divide the fibrous flexor sheath in the thumb to follow the tendon and its synovial sheath to the terminal phalanx.

In the **hypothenar eminence,** separate the **abductor digiti minimi** from the medial side of **flexor digiti minimi brevis.** Identify and follow the **deep branch of the ulnar nerve** and the deep palmar branch of the ulnar artery between these muscles. Define the attachments of these muscles and then cut through the middle of the abductor and reflect its parts to expose the **opponens digiti minimi.** Follow this muscle to its attachments.

Cut through the flexor digitorum profundus in the forearm and both ends of the superficial palmar arch in the hand. Turn the distal parts of the flexor digitorum superficialis and profundus towards the fingers. Note the nerves to the lumbricals as they are reflected with the tendons. This uncovers the remainder of the adductor pollicis, the deep palmar arterial arch, and deep branch of the ulnar nerve in the palm. Establish the continuity of the last two with the ulnar artery and nerve by tracing them over the medial surface of the hook of the hamate bone. Divide flexor digiti minimi brevis if necessary [Fig. 76]. Follow the artery and nerve laterally on the proximal parts of the bodies of the metacarpals deep to the long tendons. Find the branches of the nerve which pass to innervate the interosseous muscles between the metacarpals and trace its branch to the adductor pollicis.

Define the attachments of adductor pollicis [Fig. 89]. Cut across the muscle midway between its origins and insertion and follow the branch of the nerve and the artery between the two parts of the muscle. The nerve passes to the first dorsal interosseous muscle which is now exposed in the palm. The artery completes the arch by meeting the radial artery entering the palm between the two heads of the first dorsal interosseous muscle. Find the branch of the radial artery (**princeps pollicis**) which passes to the palmar surface of the thumb and the **radialis indicis artery** to the lateral side of the palmar surface of the index finger [Fig. 90]. Identify the three **palmar metacarpal arteries** which pass from the deep palmar arch to join the common palmar digital arteries close to their bifurcation into proper palmar digital arteries.

Fascial compartments of the palm

In the palm there is a central region enclosed in a fibrous sheath consisting of the palmar aponeurosis and the septa which pass posteriorly from its margins to become continuous with the fascia covering the palmar surfaces of the adductor pollicis and the medial two interosseous spaces. This sheath contains the long flexor tendons of the fingers, the lumbrical muscles, branches of the median and ulnar nerves, and the arteries in the palm. The space enclosed by the sheath is continuous proximally with the carpal tunnel and distally with the superficial tissues of the fingers through the apertures which transmit the lumbrical muscles [p. 77]. It is not directly continuous with the cavities of the fibrous flexor sheaths of the fingers for these are filled by the digital synovial sheaths. Distal to the common synovial sheath for the flexor tendons, several septa pass between the tendons from the palmar aponeurosis to the fascia covering the metacarpals. Posterior to the main structures in the sheath is a zone of loose connective tissue which may become distended with fluid in infections of the hand and thus form the '**midpalmar space**' of the surgeon. Such infections may spread to the space from the fingers along the lumbrical muscles or from the digital synovial sheaths.

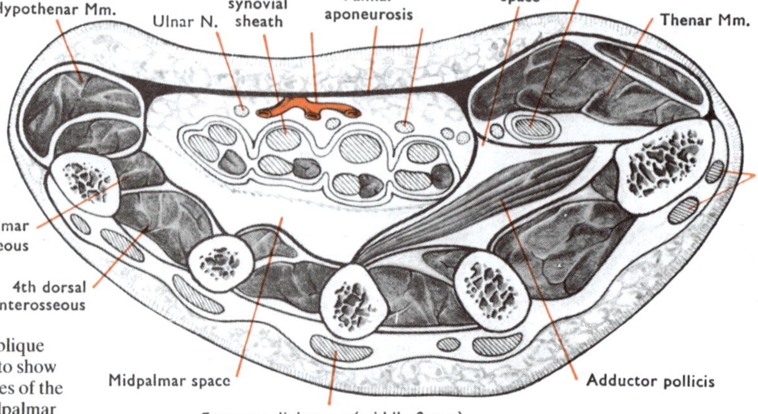

Fig. 88. Diagram of an oblique section through the hand to show the fascial layers and spaces of the palm. The thenar and midpalmar spaces are shown distended, and the thickness of the fascial layers is exaggerated.
A. Anterior.
P. Posterior.
M. Medial.
L. Lateral.

The adductor pollicis lies in a separate compartment posterior to the lateral part of the central sheath. This compartment may also be distended with fluid in infections which involve it, thus forming the **'thenar space'** [Fig. 88].

The thenar and hypothenar muscles lie in separate fascial compartments.

Infected puncture wounds of the palm may lead to a collection of fluid between the palmar aponeurosis and the tendons. This cannot escape to the

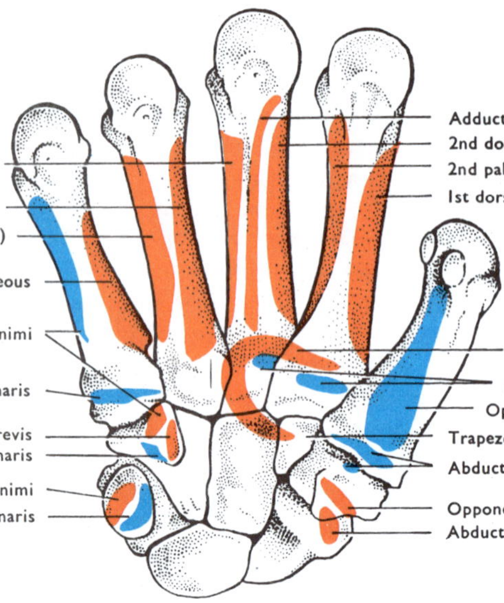

Fig. 89. Muscle attachments to palmar surfaces of carpus and metacarpus.

surface because of the aponeurosis and may involve the tendon sheaths if not allowed to drain by surgical incision. Minor injuries of the fingers may also become infected. These lead to considerable effusion of fluid with the development of pressure in the dense tissues of the finger. This may be in the pulp of the finger distal to the end of the fibrous flexor sheaths or within it in the synovial sheath. If untreated, the pressure may interfere with the blood supply of local tissues and lead to the death of the terminal phalanx if the pulp is involved, or of the flexor tendons if the flexor sheath is affected. Clearly, if pressure from such infections (whitlows) is allowed to develop, it must be relieved by opening the sheath and permitting drainage.

Short muscles of the thumb [Figs. 75, 76]

The **abductor brevis,** the **flexor brevis,** and the **opponens** form the thenar eminence and are normally supplied by the median nerve. Occasionally the flexor and rarely the abductor and opponens are supplied by the ulnar nerve. All three muscles arise from the lateral part of the flexor retinaculum and from the tubercles of the scaphoid and trapezium [Fig. 89].

The **opponens** fans out to be inserted along the anterior surface of the metacarpal of the thumb. It is covered anteriorly by the short abductor and medially by the short flexor. The **short abductor** and **flexor** are inserted together into the anteromedial surface of the base of the proximal phalanx through a tendon which contains a small sesamoid bone. The short abductor sends part of its tendon into the extensor (q.v.). Through this it is inserted into the dorsal surface of the base of the distal phalanx and thus can produce extension of the interphalangeal joint. The short flexor crosses the anteromedial surfaces of the carpometacarpal and metacarpophalangeal joints and so produces flexion at both. The short abductor crosses the anterior surfaces of the same two joints but produces abduction mainly at the carpometcarpal joint as this movement is very limited at the metacarpophalangeal joint of the thumb. The opponens acts only on the carpometacarpal joint. It moves the metacarpal towards the centre of the palm and rotates it medially so that the palmar surface of the thumb is turned to face the palmar surfaces of the fingers.

The **adductor pollicis** is supplied by the deep branch of the ulnar nerve. It lies deep in the palm. The oblique and transverse heads [Fig. 89] converge on the posteromedial surface of the base of the proximal phalanx as a common tendon containing a small sesamoid bone. This muscle draws the thumb posteriorly towards the palm moving the carpometacarpal joint, but it may also produce flexion at the metacarpophalangeal joint in the fully opposed thumb.

The **sesamoid bones** are small, ovoid bones buried in the tendons and capsule of the metacarpophalangeal joint. One flattened surface of each is covered with cartilage and slides directly on the cartilage of the palmar surface of the head of the metacarpal of the thumb. In a firm grip they prevent compression of the tendons against the bone and facilitate their movements on the bone.

Movements of the thumb [p. 119]

These are at right angles to the corresponding movements of the fingers and also differ from the fingers in the free movement at the **carpometacarpal joint**. This joint is saddle-shaped [pp. 12, 111] and permits flexion/extension and abduction/adduction. However, it is arranged on a curve so that flexion is associated with medial rotation of the metacarpal (action of opponens) and extension with lateral rotation. The range of these movements without rotation is very limited. The metacarpophalangeal and interphalangeal joints of the thumb allow little more than flexion and extension.

Opposition is a complex movement which brings the palmar surface of the distal segment of the thumb into contact with the corresponding surface of a finger. In the thumb this movement consists of abduction followed by combined flexion and medial rotation at the carpometacarpal joint with or without flexion of the other joints of the thumb. *Opposition of the thumb must not be confused with simple flexion of all of its joints* which can be produced by flexor pollicis longus acting alone. This brings the end of the thumb into contact with the lateral side of the terminal segment of any flexed finger and can still be carried out when true opposition is impossible because of paralysis of the short muscles of the thumb by injury to the median nerve distal to the origin of its anterior interosseous branch which supplies the long flexor of the thumb.

Short muscles of the little finger [Figs. 75, 89]

These muscles form the hypothenar eminence and all are supplied by the ulnar nerve. The **abductor digiti minimi** and **flexor digiti minimi brevis** lie side by side superficial to the **opponens digiti minimi**. They arise from the flexor retinaculum, the pisiform bone, and the hook of the hamate bone [Fig. 89]. The abductor and flexor brevis, partly fused, are inserted together into the anteromedial surface of the base of the proximal phalanx of the little finger. The opponens is inserted along the anteromedial surface of the metacarpal of the little finger [Fig. 89].

The little finger has the most mobile metacarpal of the four fingers. Even so, the degree of lateral rotation of the metacarpal which opponens can produce is very limited. This movement is supplemented by lateral rotation of the proximal phalanx by flexor digiti minimi brevis which also flexes the metacarpophalangeal joint with flexors digitorum superficialis and profundus.

Deep branch of the ulnar nerve [Fig. 85]

This branch arises from the ulnar nerve on the flexor retinaculum, supplies the short muscles of the hypothenar eminence, and then passes deeply between the abductor and the flexor digiti minimi brevis with the deep **palmar branch of the ulnar artery**. Both turn laterally on the hook of the hamate bone and cross the palm on the proximal parts of the bodies of the metacarpal bones, deep to the long flexor tendons. The nerve sends a branch to each of the medial three interosseous spaces to their interosseous muscles and the medial two lumbricals. It then supplies the adductor pollicis and the first dorsal interosseous muscle.

Thus the deep branch of the ulnar nerve supplies all the muscles in the palm medial to the tendon of flexor pollicis longus except the lateral two lumbricals which are supplied by the median nerve. The flexor pollicis brevis frequently receives a branch from the ulnar nerve in addition to that from the median; occasionally the ulnar nerve is its only source of supply.

Deep palmar arch

This is formed by the **radial artery** which enters the palm between the two heads of the first dorsal interosseous muscle in the first intermetacarpal space. It immediately gives off the **princeps pollicis** and **radialis indicis arteries** [Fig. 90] and, passing between the heads of adductor pollicis, unites

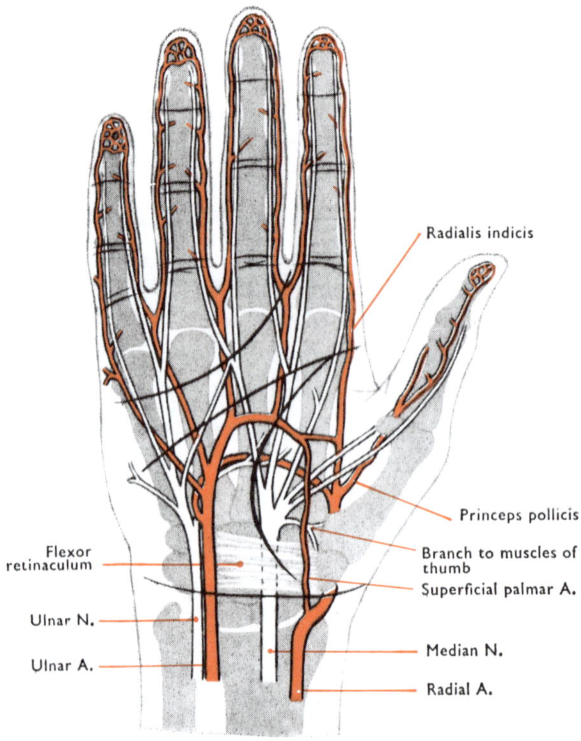

Fig. 90. Diagram of nerves and vessels of hand in relation to bones and skin markings.

with the deep palmar branch of the ulnar artery to complete the arch. This lies a finger's breadth proximal to the superficial palmar arch.

The arch gives a **palmar metacarpal artery** on each of the medial three interosseous spaces. These join the distal ends of the corresponding common palmar digital arteries and may sometimes replace them.

The **princeps pollicis artery** passes to the metacarpal of the thumb. Here it divides into the two palmar digital arteries of the thumb, one passing on each side of the tendon of flexor pollicis longus.

The **radialis indicis artery** passes distally between the first dorsal interosseous muscle and the adductor pollicis to become the lateral proper palmar digital artery of the index finger.

The extensor compartment of the forearm and hand

Begin by revising the surface anatomy [pp. 42–44] and cutaneous nerves [pp. 50–52] of the region.

The **posterior cutaneous nerve of the forearm** (a branch of the radial nerve) is the main cutaneous nerve in this region and extends at least as far as the wrist. The **medial** and **lateral cutaneous nerves of the forearm** also spread on to the posterior surface. In the hand, the main supply is usually from the **superficial branch of the radial nerve** and the **dorsal branch of the ulnar nerve,** often in almost equal proportions. These two nerves also form the **dorsal digital nerves** which usually do not extend beyond the proximal interphalangeal joint. The cutaneous supply of the dorsal surfaces of the hand and fingers shows considerable variation. Occasionally the lateral and/or the posterior cutaneous nerve of the forearm take part in this innervation, and the dorsal branch of the ulnar nerve regularly supplies a greater area than the branches of the ulnar nerve on the palmar aspect.

Dissection

Find the superficial branch of the radial nerve and the dorsal branch of the ulnar nerve on the front of the forearm. Trace both to their distribution on the dorsal surfaces of the hand and fingers if this has not been done already. Remove the deep fascia from the back of the forearm but leave intact its thickened part (**extensor retinaculum**) on the posterior aspect of the wrist [Fig. 91]. As the proximal edge of the retinaculum is defined, try to demonstrate the synovial sheaths of the tendons of the extensor muscles which pass deep to it [p. 97; Figs. 95, 96].

Separate the superficial muscles from each other starting with the tendons at the wrist. Because of their limited bony origin, these muscles arise mainly from extensive tendinous sheets between them, so that separation proximally is artificial but necessary if the deeper structures are to be seen. Completely separate the three anterolateral muscles (brachioradialis and the radial extensors of the carpus) from the extensor digitorum [Fig. 91] and expose the **supinator** muscle lying deep to them [Fig. 92]. Expose the **posterior interosseous nerve** emerging from supinator near its distal border. Follow the branches of this nerve to the extensor digitorum and the muscles medial and deep to it. Pull brachioradialis and the radial extensors of the carpus laterally to expose the radial nerve at the elbow. Complete the exposure of this nerve and its deep branch which gives branches to supinator and then pierces it. Find the branch to extensor carpi radialis brevis which arises here. Pull gently on the deep branch to establish its continuity with the posterior interosseous nerve by noting the movement of that nerve.

Find the posterior interosseous artery on the back of the forearm. It emerges from between the radius and ulna immediately distal to supinator and close to the posterior interosseous nerve. Trace the main branches of the artery.

Identify the remaining superficial muscles. Extensor digiti minimi is the separated medial part of extensor digitorum and leaves it at the extensor retinaculum to pass through a separate compartment medial to the extensor digitorum. Medial to this is the extensor carpi ulnaris. It is attached to the posterior border of the ulna by thick deep fascia

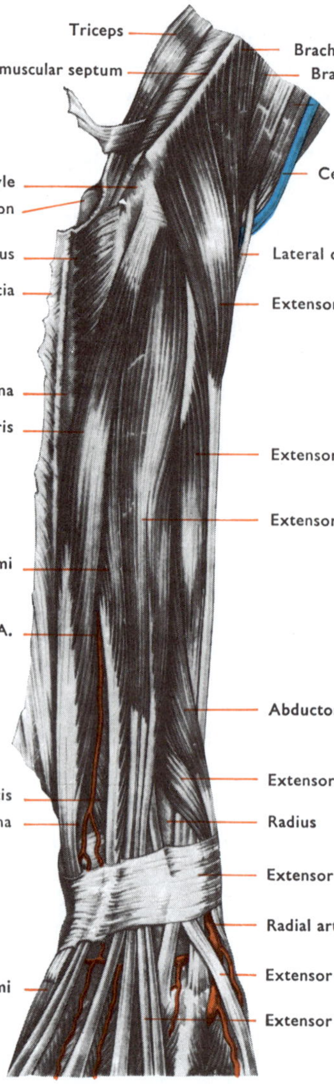

Fig. 91. Superficial dissection of back of forearm.

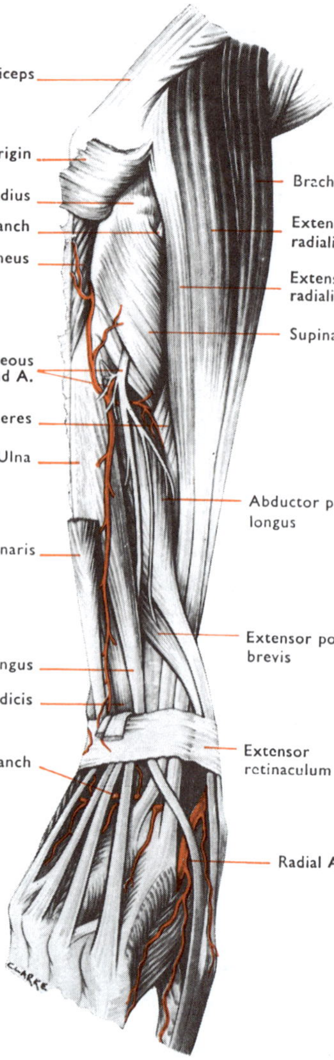

Fig. 92. Deep dissection of back of forearm.

which should be divided in the proximal third of the forearm to demonstrate anconeus [Fig. 91].

Lift extensor digitorum and expose the deep layer of extensor muscles. Immediately distal to supinator is abductor pollicis longus. The other three muscles (extensor pollicis brevis, extensor pollicis longus, and extensor indicis) arise distal to this [Fig. 93]. Trace the tendons of these muscles to the extensor retinaculum.

Expose the tendons on the back and lateral side of the hand, but do not follow them any further than is necessary to determine whether they enter the digits or end on the metacarpals. Note that the thumb and the index and little fingers each have two extensor tendons. Identify all these tendons at your own wrist and note which of them become taut in movements of the wrist with the fingers relaxed and in movements of the fingers and thumb. At the same time review the position of the flexor tendons on the anterior aspect of the distal part of your own forearm.

Muscles of the back of the forearm [Fig. 91]

These may be divided into three groups.

1. Superficial muscles which arise from the lateral supracondylar line and the lateral epicondyle of the humerus [Fig. 53] and pass to the bones of the forearm [Fig. 93], hand [Fig. 99], or digits.

(a) Centrally placed in this group are the **extensor digitorum** and **extensor digiti minimi** passing to the fingers.

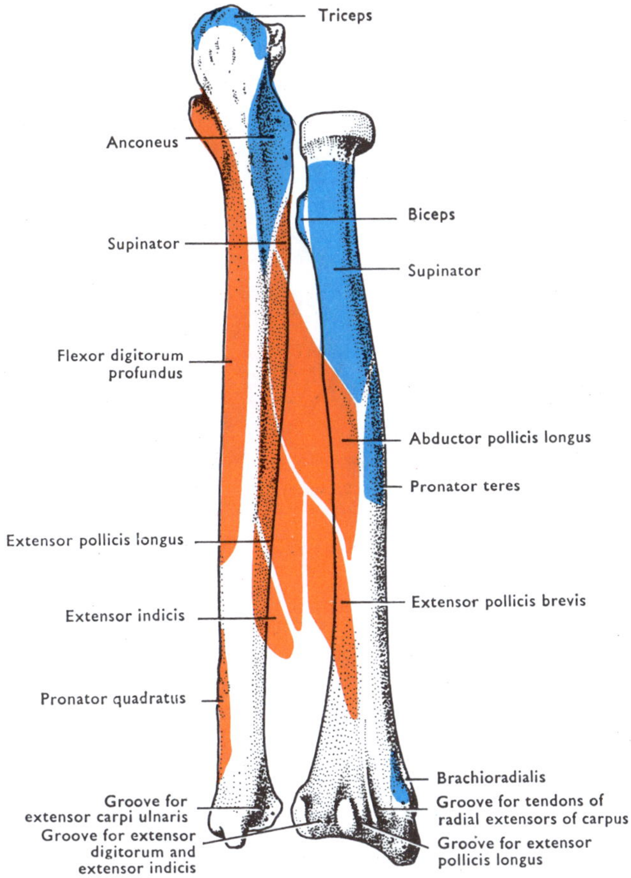

Fig. 93. Muscle attachments to posterior surface of right radius and ulna. The attachment of flexor carpi ulnaris to the posterior border of the ulna is not shown.

(b) On either side of the muscles in (a) are the corresponding extensors of the carpus which pass to metacarpal bones—laterally, **extensor carpi radialis longus** and **brevis** to the second and third metacarpals; medially, **extensor carpi ulnaris** to the fifth [Fig. 99].

(c) At each margin of this superficial group of muscles, a single muscle passes to the corresponding forearm bone. Anterolaterally, **brachioradialis** passes to the radius; posteromedially, **anconeus** fans out from the lateral epicondyle to the proximal third of the lateral surface of the ulna, posterior to the radial notch [Fig. 93].

2. Four deep muscles arise from the forearm bones and interosseous membrane [Fig. 93]. They pass only to the thumb and index finger. Laterally **abductor pollicis longus** and **extensor pollicis brevis** curve over the posterior surface of the radius and the tendons of the lateral three muscles of the superficial group to reach the lateral aspect of the base of the first metacarpal. Immediately medial to these is the **extensor pollicis longus**, the tendon of which curves round the medial side of the **dorsal tubercle of the radius**. The most medial muscle, **extensor indicis**, passes medial to the tendons of extensor digitorum.

3. A single deep muscle (**supinator**) passes between the two forearm bones. It arises from the lateral surfaces of the fibrous capsule of the elbow and superior radio-ulnar joints and of the ulna distal to the radial notch. It curves round the posterior and lateral surfaces of the radius [Fig. 92]. Anteriorly, its attachment to the radius reaches to the origin of the radial head of flexor digitorum superficialis [Fig. 86] and distally to the insertion of pronator teres.

The **nerve supply** to all these muscles is from the radial nerve and its branches. Brachioradialis, the two radial extensors of the carpus, and supinator are supplied by branches which arise from the radial nerve anteriorly. The remaining muscles, except anconeus, are supplied by the posterior interosseous nerve which is the continuation of the deep branch of

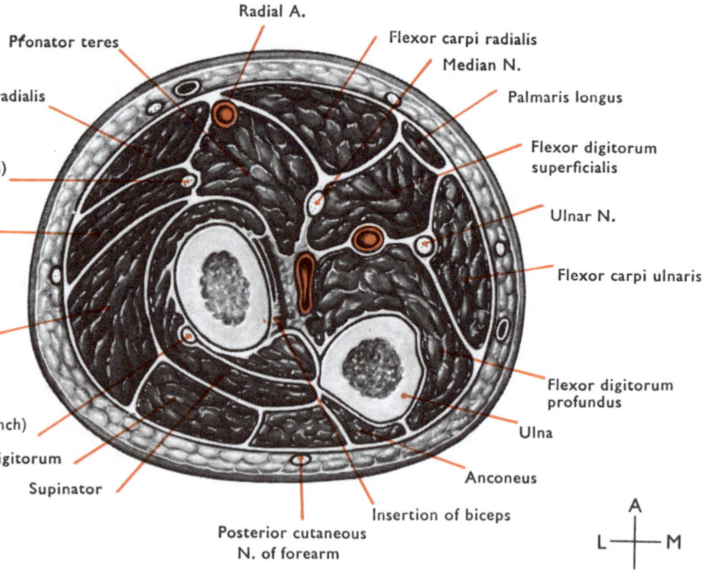

Fig. 94. Section through upper third of left forearm.
A. Anterior.
P. Posterior.
M. Medial.
L. Lateral.

the radial nerve. Thus injury to the deep branch of the radial nerve in the supinator paralyses only these muscles. Anconeus is supplied by the nerve to the medial head of triceps from the radial nerve.

Actions of extensor muscles of forearm

The actions of the extensor muscles of the fingers and thumb will be dealt with later when the muscles which act with them have been dissected [p. 102]. Brachioradialis is dealt with on page 86.

Extensor carpi radialis longus and **brevis** and **extensor carpi ulnaris** act together to extend the wrist. They also prevent flexion of the wrist by the flexor muscles of the fingers so that these muscles can apply the full range of their contraction to the fingers. When the wrist is flexed, the fist cannot be clenched because the flexor muscles of the fingers are unable to contract sufficiently and extensor muscles of the fingers cannot stretch adequately to allow this movement. The radial extensors of the wrist act with the radial flexor to produce *abduction of the wrist*. This is an important movement, e.g. in raising a hammer prior to striking with it—an action which requires the strength of two radial extensors even though the range of movement is less than that of adduction. The **extensor** and **flexor carpi ulnaris** act in a similar fashion to produce *adduction of the wrist*. The flexors and extensors of the wrist act together to fix the wrist so that fine movements of the fingers can take place on a stable hand.

Anconeus holds the ulna firmly against the humerus. It also contracts strongly when *pronation* is carried out around an axis passing through the radial side of the hand. In this movement the distal end of the ulna is displaced laterally by slight lateral rotation of the humerus, anconeus assisting. This occurs in many movements, e.g. in using a screwdriver in the right hand to remove a screw.

Supinator is a powerful lateral rotator of the radius which acts with biceps brachii and may be slightly assisted by abductor pollicis longus which arises in part from the ulna and runs parallel to supinator.

Abductor pollicis longus is inserted into the anterolateral surface of the base of the first metacarpal. It abducts the thumb at the carpometacarpal joint and produces some extension. See also supinator above.

Extensor retinaculum and synovial sheaths of extensor tendons

[Figs. 79, 95, 96]

The extensor retinaculum is a thickened strip of deep fascia, 2–3 cm wide, which passes across the extensor tendons from the triquetrum and styloid process of the ulna to the sharp anterolateral margin of the distal part of the radius. It produces a tunnel for each separate group of tendons and their sheaths by sending septa between them to the head of the ulna and to each of the ridges on the distal end of the radius [Fig. 93].

The tendons of extensor digitorum and extensor indicis lie in a common, central sheath. Each of the other tendons usually has its own separate sheath

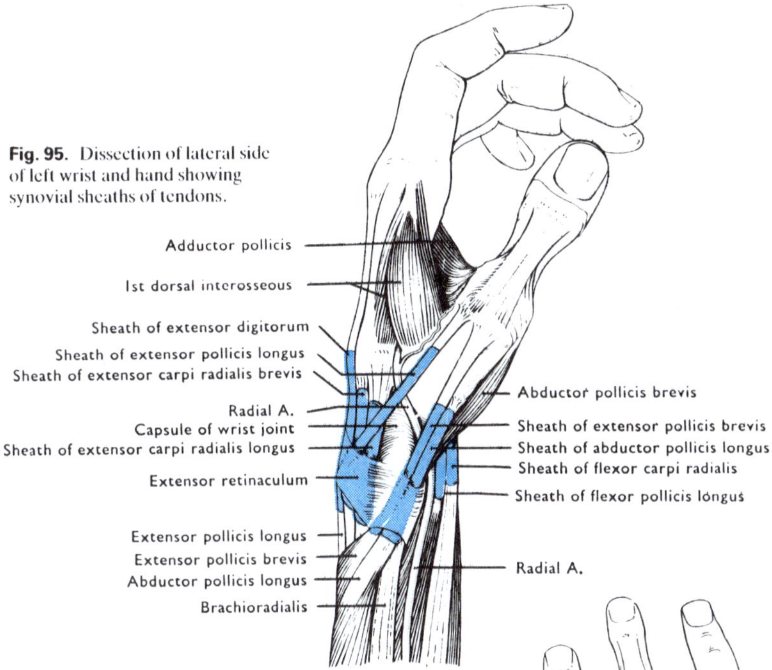

Fig. 95. Dissection of lateral side of left wrist and hand showing synovial sheaths of tendons.

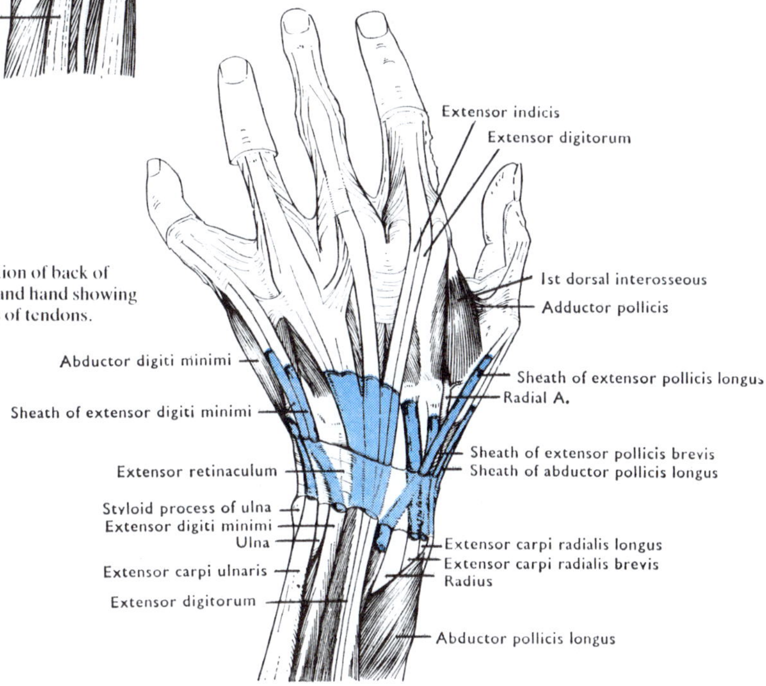

Fig. 96. Dissection of back of forearm, wrist, and hand showing synovial sheaths of tendons.

Positions of extensor tendons

Action	Muscles	Tendon palpable
Extension of wrist	Extensor carpi radialis longus and brevis	Between distal end of radius and bases of 2nd and 3rd metacarpals
	Extensor carpi ulnaris	Between distal end of ulna and base of 5th metacarpal
Extension of fingers	Extensor digitorum	Centrally over carpus and bases of 3rd and 4th metacarpals
	Extensor indicis	
	Extensor digiti minimi	On 5th metacarpal
Extension of thumb	Extensor pollicis longus	From dorsal tubercle of radius along posterior margin of anatomical snuff-box
	Extensor pollicis brevis	From styloid process of radius along anterior margin of snuff-box
Abduction of thumb	Abductor pollicis longus	Between styloid process of radius and base of 1st metacarpal

with the exception of abductor pollicis longus which lies in the same sheath as extensor pollicis brevis on the lateral surface of the distal end of the radius. The sheaths begin near the proximal edge of the extensor retinaculum and extend for a variable distance on to the corresponding metacarpal except in the case of the extensors of the carpus and the long abductor of the thumb which end near the base of the metacarpal to which each is attached.

Deep branch of radial nerve and posterior interosseous nerve
[Figs. 84, 92]

The deep branch of the radial nerve arises at the level of the lateral epicondyle of the humerus. The nerve descends between the elbow joint and brachioradialis and gives branches to extensor carpi radialis brevis and supinator. It then enters the supinator muscle and winds obliquely round the lateral and posterior surfaces of the radius within that muscle. It emerges a short distance proximal to the distal border of supinator as the posterior interosseous nerve. It gives branches to the surrounding muscles and descends between extensor digitorum and abductor pollicis longus, then deep to extensor pollicis longus to accompany the terminal part of the anterior interosseous artery on the posterior surface of the interosseous membrane. It ends on the back of the wrist joint by sending branches to that joint and the intercarpal joints.

Dissection

Trace the radial artery distally from its position on the anterior surface of the distal end of the radius. It passes through the anatomical snuff-box, deep to the tendons which form the margins of the box, and enters the proximal end of the first intermetacarpal space. Find its dorsal and palmar carpal branches and the dorsal digital arteries which it gives to the thumb and the lateral side of the index finger. Trace the dorsal carpal branch deep to the extensor tendons, dividing the extensor retinaculum where necessary to follow it into continuity with the corresponding branch of the ulnar artery through the dorsal carpal rete. Trace the dorsal metacarpal arteries distally from the rete on the medial three intermetacarpal spaces to their dorsal digital branches on the adjacent sides of the corresponding fingers. Note the dorsal digital artery to the medial side of the little finger arising from the medial end of the rete.

The arteries of the back of the forearm and hand
[Figs. 80, 92]

The **posterior interosseous artery** supplies the muscles on the back of the forearm, takes part in the anastomosis around the elbow joint, and ends in the dorsal carpal rete. The artery passes backwards from the common interosseous artery between the radius and ulna, immediately proximal to the interosseous membrane. It appears posteriorly between the supinator and abductor pollicis longus muscles, close to the posterior interosseous nerve. Here it gives muscular branches and sends the interosseous recurrent artery, deep to anconeus, to the elbow joint anastomosis. The tenuous remainder of the artery descends between the deep and superficial muscles to the dorsal carpal rete.

The terminal part of the **anterior interosseous artery** pierces the interosseous membrane 5–6 cm proximal to the distal end of the radius. It descends on the membrane to the dorsal carpal rete with the terminal branch of the posterior interosseous nerve.

The **dorsal carpal rete**—a mesh of anastomosing arteries on the dorsal surfaces of the carpal bones—is formed by the **dorsal carpal branches** of the radial and ulnar arteries and the anterior and posterior interosseous arteries. It supplies the dorsal surfaces of the wrist, carpal, and carpometacarpal joints, and of the hand and fingers. The rete gives rise to a **dorsal digital artery** to the medial side of the little finger and three **dorsal metacarpal arteries** which lie on the medial three intermetacarpal spaces. Each dorsal metacarpal artery receives **perforating branches** through the space from the deep palmar arch and the corresponding palmar metacarpal artery, and divides into a dorsal digital artery to each of the adjacent fingers.

The **radial artery** leaves the anterior surface of the radius and, passing deep to the tendons of abductor pollicis longus and extensor pollicis brevis, lies in the 'anatomical snuff-box' on the scaphoid and trapezium against which it can be palpated. Here it gives off its **palmar** and **dorsal carpal arteries**. The palmar artery anastomoses with the corresponding branch of the ulnar artery on the anterior surface of the carpus and communicates with the deep palmar arch. The dorsal branch passes to the dorsal carpal rete. The radial artery then passes deep to the tendon of extensor pollicis longus and gives off **dorsal digital arteries** to both sides of the thumb and the lateral side of the index finger. The artery then turns medially into the palm through the proximal end of the first intermetacarpal space, between the two heads of the first dorsal interosseous muscle.

Dissection

Follow the extensor tendons into the fingers and thumb. In each finger the tendon expands into a sheet as it passes towards the metacarpophalangeal joint. This **extensor expansion** is widest at the level of the metacarpophalangeal joint where the margins turn anteriorly on each side of the metacarpal head to be attached to the deep transverse metacarpal ligament immediately anterior to the head. This attachment cannot be seen at present. Distal to the joint, the expansion narrows to the dorsal surface of the proximal interphalangeal joint, passing over it to reach the middle and distal phalanges. Identify the thickened margins and central portion of the expansion over the proximal phalanx and follow the fibre bundles of both parts as they pass distally.

Follow the tendon of the **lumbrical muscles** on the palmar surface of the deep transverse metacarpal ligament into the lateral margin of the expansion.

Remove any fat and fascia covering the dorsal surfaces of the intermetacarpal spaces and expose a **dorsal interosseous muscle** in each. Trace the muscle distally to its tendon. Divide the dense fibrous tissue which lies between the dorsal parts of the metacarpal heads and trace part of the tendon into the corresponding margin of the extensor expansion distal to the metacarpophalangeal joint. A deeper part of the tendon may be traced into the base of the proximal phalanx. Identify the deep transverse metacarpal ligament lying between the palmar surfaces of the medial four metacarpal heads. Define the ligament in one space and then divide it. Now force the adjacent metacarpal heads apart and follow the proximal edge of the extensor expansion to the deep transverse metacarpal ligament and the tendon of the interosseous muscle to the proximal phalanx and the extensor expansion.

Separate the dorsal interosseous muscle from the two adjacent metacarpal bones from which it arises. Turn the muscle distally and expose the **palmar interosseous muscle** which arises only from the

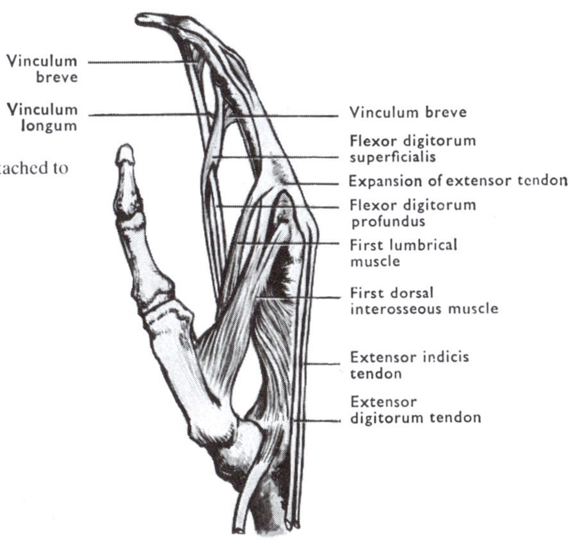

Fig. 97. The tendons attached to the index finger.

metacarpal of the finger to which it passes. In the first intermetacarpal space the first palmar interosseous muscle is only a slender slip. Trace the tendon of the palmar interosseous to the extensor expansion and sometimes to the base of the proximal phalanx. A dorsal interosseous muscle is present on the lateral side of the index and middle fingers and on the medial side of the middle and ring fingers. A palmar interosseous muscle is present on the medial side of the (thumb and) index finger and on the lateral side of the ring and little fingers. The tendons of the interossei in the medial three spaces lie posterior to the deep transverse metacarpal ligament—in the first space the ligament is absent.

Extensor tendons of the fingers

Four separate tendons of **extensor digitorum** pass on to the dorsum of the hand but are linked together by oblique strips of tendinous material, the **conexus intertendineus**, proximal to the metacarpophalangeal joints. These connections force the tendons of this muscle to work together. The index and little fingers each have an additional extensor tendon—**extensor indicis** and **extensor digiti minimi**, respectively. These fuse with the corresponding tendon of extensor digitorum distal to the conexus and so are able to extend the metacarpophalangeal joints of these fingers when the corresponding joints of the middle and ring fingers are flexed. The converse cannot happen because the middle and ring fingers receive only a tendon from extensor digitorum.

Extensor expansion

[Figs. 97, 98]

Just proximal to the metacarpophalangeal joint, each tendon joins a triangular extensor expansion which forms a hood over the joint and a considerable part of the proximal phalanx. The base of the triangle passes anteriorly on each side of the metacarpal head to the deep transverse metacarpal ligament in a plane immediately anterior to the metacarpal head. Distal to this, each margin of the expansion is thickened by the insertion into it of part of the tendon of the corresponding **interosseous muscle** and all of the tendon of the **lumbrical** (lateral margin only). These thickened margins pass obliquely backwards on the sides of the proximal phalanx towards the posterior surface of the proximal interphalangeal joint. As they do so they send tendinous bundles towards the tendon of the long extensor in the midline of the extensor expansion on the posterior surface of the phalanx. The main bulk of the long extensor tendon courses through the midline of the extensor expansion but is held in position by strong, transverse, tendinous bundles at the metacarpophalangeal joint. Distal to this joint, the tendon splits into three bundles in the expansion. The central part, joined by bundles

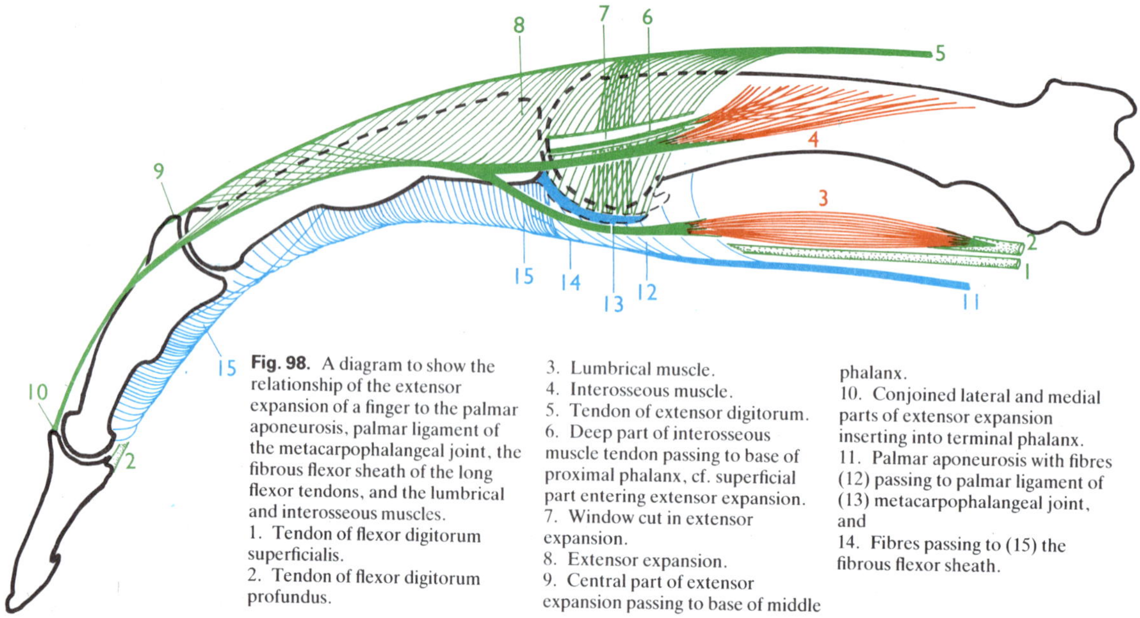

Fig. 98. A diagram to show the relationship of the extensor expansion of a finger to the palmar aponeurosis, palmar ligament of the metacarpophalangeal joint, the fibrous flexor sheath of the long flexor tendons, and the lumbrical and interosseous muscles.
1. Tendon of flexor digitorum superficialis.
2. Tendon of flexor digitorum profundus.
3. Lumbrical muscle.
4. Interosseous muscle.
5. Tendon of extensor digitorum.
6. Deep part of interosseous muscle tendon passing to base of proximal phalanx, cf. superficial part entering extensor expansion.
7. Window cut in extensor expansion.
8. Extensor expansion.
9. Central part of extensor expansion passing to base of middle phalanx.
10. Conjoined lateral and medial parts of extensor expansion inserting into terminal phalanx.
11. Palmar aponeurosis with fibres (12) passing to palmar ligament of (13) metacarpophalangeal joint, and
14. Fibres passing to (15) the fibrous flexor sheath.

from the thick margins of the expansion, crosses the proximal interphalangeal joint and is inserted into the base of the middle phalanx. The other two parts diverge, fuse with the remaining parts of the thickened margins, and pass over the posterior surface of the proximal interphalangeal joint on either side of the central part. These lateral and medial parts converge and fuse on the dorsal surface of the middle phalanx and then cross the posterior surface of the distal interphalangeal joint to be inserted into the base of the distal phalanx.

At the **metacarpophalangeal** and **interphalangeal joints**, the extensor expansion forms the dorsal part of the **fibrous capsule** of the joint. Thus it is continuous laterally with the remainder of the fibrous capsule and is held in position by it.

Deep transverse metacarpal ligament

This is a strong band which passes between the palmar ligaments of the metacarpophalangeal joints of the fingers but does not extend to the thumb. These **palmar ligaments** are thick, semi-rigid structures which are firmly attached to the base of the proximal phalanx of each finger. They are only loosely attached to the metacarpal. When the metacarpophalangeal joint is flexed the palmar ligament slides proximally on the palmar surface of the metacarpal; when the joint is extended, the ligament moves distally on the metacarpal head. In each case the attachment of the extensor expansion to the ligament moves with the ligament.

Muscles inserted into the extensor expansion

In addition to the long extensors, the lumbrical and interosseous muscles join the extensor expansion.

Lumbrical muscles

These four muscles arise from the tendons of flexor digitorum profundus in the palm of the hand—the first from the lateral side of the tendon to the index finger, the remainder often from the adjacent sides of two tendons. Each passes to the radial side of the corresponding finger, anterior to the metacarpophalangeal joint and the deep transverse metacarpal ligament (except the first) to join the lateral edge of the extensor expansion. Thus these muscles flex the metacarpophalangeal joints of the fingers and extend the interphalangeal joints—the position of the fingers in writing. **Nerve supply:** the lateral two are innervated by the median nerve, the medial two by the ulnar nerve.

Interosseous muscles

These muscles arise from the metacarpal bones [Figs. 89, 99]—the larger dorsal interossei from two adjacent metacarpals, the smaller palmar interossei from the metacarpal of the finger to which each passes. They enter the digits at the sides of the metacarpophalangeal joints posterior to the deep transverse metacarpal ligament (except those in the first intermetacarpal space). **Dorsal interossei** pass to the lateral sides of the index and middle fingers and to the medial sides of the middle and ring fingers. Part of the tendon passes deep to the extensor expansion (or pierces it) into the base of the proximal phalanx; the remainder joins the corresponding margin of the extensor expansion. They abduct these fingers from the line of the middle

Fig. 99. Muscle attachments to dorsal aspect of right metacarpus.

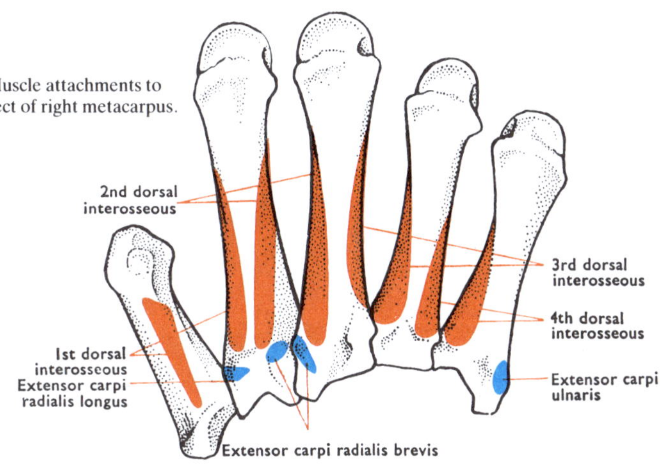

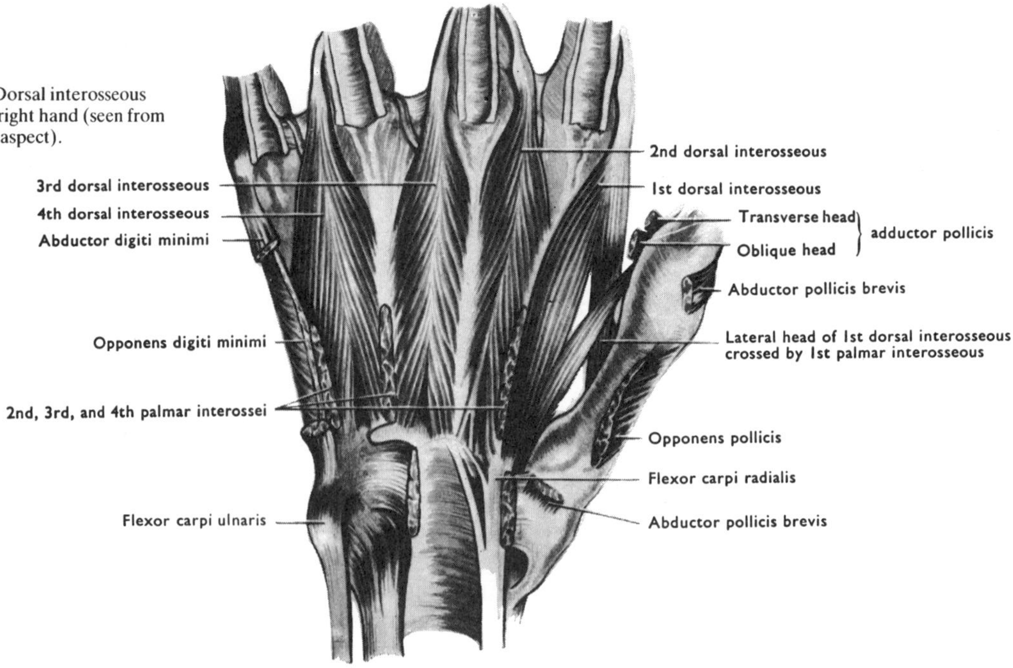

Fig. 100. Dorsal interosseous muscles of right hand (seen from the palmar aspect).

finger, extend the interphalangeal joints, and play a part in flexion of the metacarpophalangeal joints (especially the first dorsal interosseous).

Palmar interossei pass to the medial sides of the (thumb and) index finger and to the lateral sides of the ring and little fingers. They are inserted into the corresponding margin of the extensor expansion and some also into the base of the proximal phalanx. They adduct these fingers and the thumb to the line of the middle finger, extend the interphalangeal joints, and play a part in flexion of the metacarpophalangeal joints.

Abduction and adduction at the metacarpophalangeal joints is markedly reduced when these joints are flexed. This is because of tightening of the collateral ligaments and the reduced mechanical advantage of the interossei in the flexed position. **Nerve supply:** all the interossei are supplied by the deep branch of the ulnar nerve.

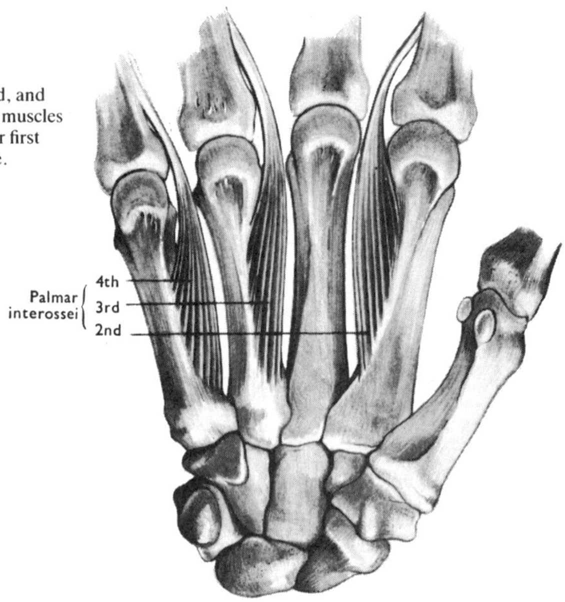

Fig. 101. The second, third, and fourth palmar interosseous muscles (right side). See Fig. 100 for first palmar interosseous muscle.

Movements of the fingers

[Table 6; p. 118]

The *fingers are flexed* at all joints by the flexor digitorum profundus, at the proximal two joints by flexor digitorum superficialis, at the metacarpophalangeal joints by the lumbricals and interossei. Inability to flex the distal interphalangeal joints occurs in paralysis of flexor digitorum profundus—a condition which is evident in the ring and little fingers in damage to the ulnar nerve above the elbow.

The *fingers are extended* together at all joints by the extensor digitorum. The index and little fingers are extended independently at all joints by extensor indicis and extensor digiti minimi. Extension of the interphalangeal joints is assisted by the lumbricals and interossei. *When the metacarpophalangeal joints are fully extended*, the transverse metacarpal ligament is pulled distally on the metacarpal head, making this the only effective insertion of the long extensor tendons. Their distal parts in the extensor expansion are slackened so that extension of the interphalangeal joints can only be produced by the **lumbricals** and **interossei**. When these muscles are paralysed and the metacarpophalangeal joints are fully extended, the interphalangeal joints are flexed by the unopposed action of the long flexors—a condition known as *'claw hand'*. It is best seen when both ulnar and median nerves are damaged at the wrist but occurs in the ring and little fingers when the ulnar nerve alone is damaged there (lumbricals of index and middle fingers are still innervated). Claw hand can be demonstrated in yourself. Fully extend your fingers and note the taut extensor tendons on the back of your hand. Keeping the metacarpophalangeal joints fully extended, flex your interphalangeal joints and note that this can be done without any movement of the extensor tendons.

Flexion of one finger at the metacarpophalangeal and proximal interphalangeal joints when the other fingers are extended, leaves the distal phalanx of that finger quite lax—it cannot be either extended or flexed. This arises because the flexor digitorum profundus cannot act on a single finger (insufficient separation of the parts of the muscle) and the extensor expansion can only extend the distal interphalangeal joint when the proximal interphalangeal joint is extended. A finger in which the extensor expansion has been ruptured from the base of the distal phalanx is set in this position to allow repair of the expansion to take place without it being exposed to traction either from the extensors or the flexors.

Abduction and adduction of the fingers (but not the thumb) occurs at the metacarpophalangeal joints. The interossei and abductor digiti minimi produce these movements which have a considerable range when the joints are extended but are limited when they are flexed [see movements of metacarpophalangeal joints]. Adduction also occurs in flexion of the fingers and abduction in extension. This is because the axes of the interphalangeal joints do not lie in a straight line but on an arc of a circle which is concave towards the palm. Confirm this movement in your own hand.

The little finger has the most mobile metacarpal of all the fingers. It can be rotated laterally to a small degree by opponens digiti minimi assisted by the short flexor and the abductor. This brings the pulp of the little finger into direct opposition with that of the thumb. Compare this with opposition of the thumb and index finger in your own hand.

Extensors of the thumb

Extensor pollicis longus arises from the middle third of the posterior surface of the ulna and adjacent interosseous membrane [Fig. 93]. Its tendon passes deep to the extensor retinaculum and bends laterally around the dorsal tubercle of the radius. It then crosses the tendons of the radial extensors of the carpus to the posterior margin of the dorsum of the first metacarpal along which it runs to the metacarpophalangeal joint. Here it is joined by the first palmar interosseous muscle and an extension from abductor pollicis brevis to form a limited **extensor expansion** which extends to the distal phalanx.

Extensor pollicis brevis and **abductor pollicis longus** arise together—the abductor from the posterior surfaces of the ulna, radius, and interosseous membrane distal to supinator; the extensor brevis from the posterior surfaces of the radius and interosseous membrane immediately distal to the abductor [Fig. 93]. Together the tendons of both muscles cross those of the radial extensors of the carpus and brachioradialis to reach the lateral side of the distal end of the radius [Fig. 92]. Thence they pass to the dorsum of the first metacarpal and form the anterior margin of the 'anatomical snuff-box'. Here the abductor pollicis longus is inserted while the extensor pollicis brevis continues to the base of the proximal (or distal) phalanx of the thumb.

These three muscles of the thumb are supplied by the posterior interosseous nerve from the radial nerve.

Movements of the thumb
[Table 7; p. 119]

Functionally the thumb is one-half of the hand for it acts in the opposite direction to the fingers in grasping any object.

The principal movements of the thumb take place at the **carpometacarpal joint**. This is a curved, saddle-shaped joint which allows abduction and adduction and also flexion and extension. However, its flexion and extension, when limited to movement at right angles to abduction and adduction, is very slight in any position of the joint unless accompanied by medial rotation in flexion and lateral rotation in extension—movements which can only occur freely when the thumb is abducted. This rotation, due to the curvature of the saddle joint, is permitted by the flatter surfaces of the joint which are in contact in abduction and cannot be avoided if the full range of movement is to occur. Flexion with medial rotation of the abducted thumb is known as **opposition** because it brings the palmar surface of the thumb to face that of one or other fingers.

At the **metacarpophalangeal joint** of the thumb there is flexion and extension (flexor pollicis longus and brevis and extensor pollicis longus and brevis) with a small amount of abduction and adduction produced respectively by the abductor pollicis brevis and the adductor pollicis assisted by the first palmar interosseous muscle.

At the **interphalangeal joint** only flexion and extension occur—flexion by flexor pollicis longus. Extension occurs by extensor pollicis longus and sometimes extensor pollicis brevis which may extend to the terminal phalanx, and abductor pollicis brevis.

Opposition is produced by the combined action of abductor pollicis longus and brevis followed by contraction of opponens pollicis (medial rotation) synchronously with flexor pollicis brevis and/or longus (flexion at the carpometacarpal joint with or without flexion at the other two joints of the thumb). Flexor pollicis longus is used principally when the tip of the thumb is opposed to the tip of a finger or when power is required; flexor brevis when the main flexion is at the carpometacarpal and metacarpophalangeal joints. Abductor pollicis brevis is used principally when the thumb is opposed to the little finger; abductor longus is continuously active during opposition and the reverse movement. In this reverse movement, extension is first produced by extensor pollicis brevis, which helps to maintain abduction at the carpometacarpal joint. Extensor pollicis longus comes more and more into play as the movement progresses helping to produce lateral rotation of the thumb. Extensor pollicis longus may also act as an adductor of the fully abducted thumb thus assisting adductor pollicis or mimicking its activity when paralysed.

Confirm these movements in your own hand and check the contraction of the muscles by noting, as far as possible, their tendons or the hardening of the muscles themselves.

The joints of the upper limb

Elbow joint

Dissection

If the joint is to be dissected, separate the muscles from the epicondyles and reflect them distally. Divide biceps, brachialis, and triceps a short distance proximal to the elbow and turn all three distally. Separate all the muscles from the fibrous capsule of the elbow joint and remove the loose connective tissue from its external surface so as to define its parts. Retain the median, ulnar, and radial nerves and the brachial artery.

This joint is formed by the articulation of the **trochlea** and **capitulum** of the

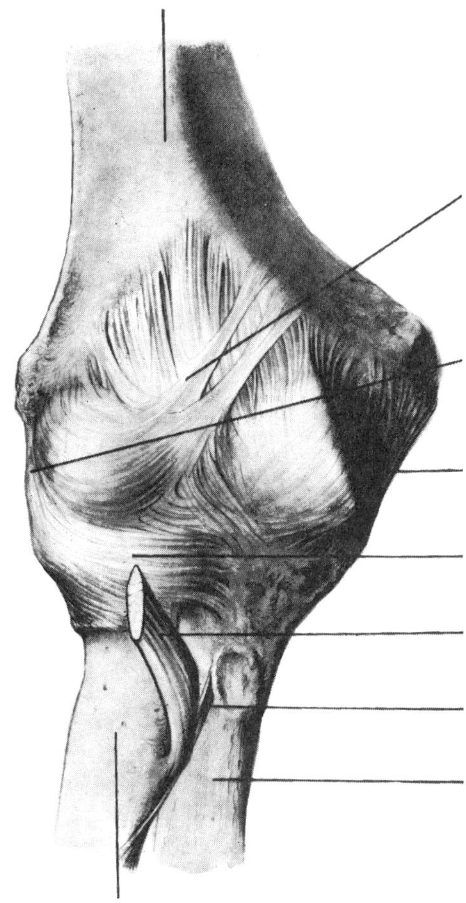

Fig. 102. Front of elbow joint.

humerus [Fig. 229] with the **trochlear notch** of the ulna [Fig. 233] and the proximal surface of the **head of the radius**, respectively. Its fibrous capsule and joint cavity are continuous with that of the proximal radio-ulnar joint. The elbow joint is essentially a hinge joint with strong radial and ulnar collateral ligaments, while the anterior and posterior parts of the fibrous capsule are weak and contain many oblique fibres which permit the full range of movement.

The **anterior ligament** passes from the epicondyles and the upper margins of the radial and coronoid fossae of the humerus to the coronoid process of the ulna and the anular ligament of the radius.

The **posterior ligament** is weak. It stretches from a line joining the epicondyles across the floor of the olecranon fossa to the articular margin of the olecranon.

The **radial collateral ligament** is strong. It passes from the distal surface of

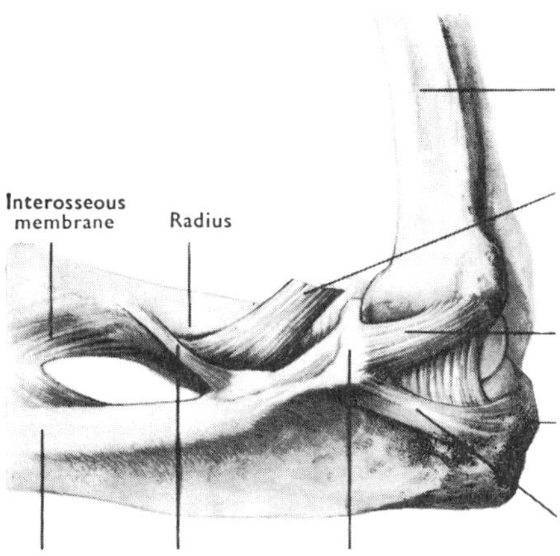

Fig. 103. Medial aspect of elbow joint. The anterior and posterior parts of the articular capsule were removed.

the lateral epicondyle to the lateral and posterior parts of the anular ligament of the radius [Fig. 102].

The **ulnar collateral ligament** radiates from the distal border of the medial epicondyle. Its thick borders pass to the medial edges of the coronoid process and olecranon. The thinner, central part is attached to a transverse band that bridges across the interval between these edges [Fig. 103]. The ulnar nerve lies on the posterior and middle parts of the ligament and has the posterior ulnar recurrent artery ascending close to it.

Dissection

Make transverse incisions through the anterior and posterior parts of the fibrous capsule and examine the synovial membrane.

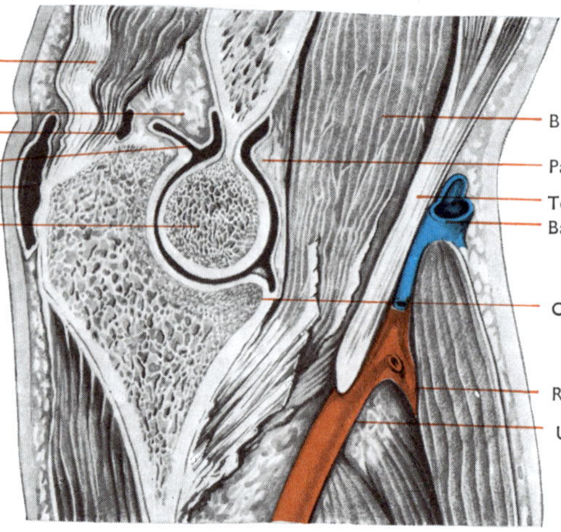

Fig. 104. Sagittal section of right elbow.

Synovial membrane

As in all synovial joints, the synovial membrane lines the deep surface of the fibrous capsule and the adjacent non-articular parts of the bones within the fibrous capsule. It is separated from the fibrous capsule over the olecranon, coronoid, and radial fossae by pads of fat which slide into the fossae when the bony processes are withdrawn [Fig. 104]. It is continuous with the synovial membrane of the proximal radio-ulnar joint on the lateral side.

The **nerve supply** of the joint is derived from all the adjacent nerves—median, ulnar, radial, posterior interosseous, and musculocutaneous.

Movements at the elbow joint [Table 3; p. 116]

The movements at the elbow joint are distinct from those which take place at the proximal radio-ulnar joint, though the head of the radius rotates on the capitulum of the humerus during movements at the radio-ulnar joint. The elbow joint is essentially a hinge joint, but the humero-ulnar part is a modified saddle joint [p. 12] which also allows some slight abduction and adduction of the ulna. The main movements are flexion and extension but these movements are not exactly in a sagittal plane. Thus the forearm bones lie parallel to the humerus in full flexion. In full extension the ulna is angled laterally so that the supinated forearm bones make an angle ('*carrying angle*') of approximately 165 degrees laterally with the humerus. This angulation of the ulna is obscured in pronation when the arm and forearm lie in the same straight line, the radius and ulna lying along the diagonals of the forearm. Table 3 summarizes the muscles which move the elbow joint.

Dissection

Remove the remains of the thenar and hypothenar muscles from their proximal attachments and separate the flexor and extensor retinacula from the bones. Reflect the flexor and extensor tendons distally.

Wrist joint

This **radiocarpal joint** consists of the articulation between the convex proximal surface of the carpus (formed by the scaphoid, lunate, and triquetrum bones and their interosseous ligaments) and the concave socket formed by the distal surfaces of the radius and the **triangular articular disc** [p. 109]. The disc joins the medial edge of the articular surface of the radius to the styloid process of the ulna. It separates the ulna from the joint. In the resting

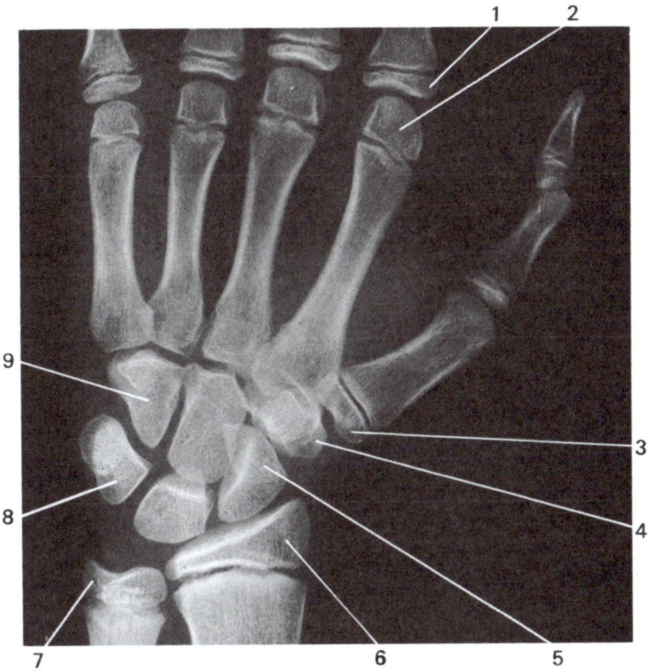

Fig. 105. Anteroposterior radiograph of hand. Age 12 years.
1. Epiphysis of proximal phalanx.
2. Epiphysis of metacarpal.
3. Epiphysis of metacarpal thumb.
4. Trapezium.
5. Scaphoid.
6. Distal epiphysis of radius.
7. Distal epiphysis of ulna.
8. Triquetrum.
9. Hamate.

Cf. Fig. 8.

position of the hand only the scaphoid and lateral part of the lunate articulate with the two shallow fossae on the distal surface of the radius [Fig. 106]. The remainder of the lunate is in contact with the articular disc while the triquetrum is applied to the medial part of the capsule of the joint. The direction of the radiocarpal joint is oblique—the lateral and dorsal margins of the radius extend further distally than its other margins. This reduces the likelihood of posterior dislocation of any of the carpal bones.

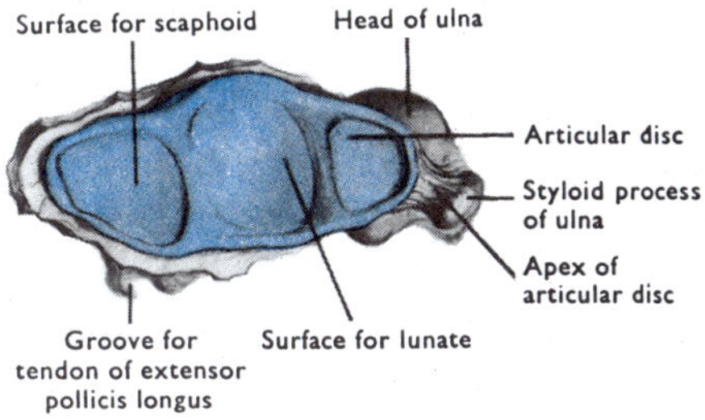

Fig. 106. Proximal articular surface of wrist joint.

Fibrous capsule

This passes from the margins of the distal ends of the radius and ulna and from the margins of the articular disc to the proximal row of carpal bones, excluding the pisiform. Slightly thickened portions attached to the styloid processes of the radius and ulna (**radial** and **ulnar collateral ligaments**) pass respectively to the scaphoid and triquetrum. The anterior and posterior parts of the fibrous capsule contain fibres which pass obliquely downwards and medially. The **synovial membrane** which lines the fibrous capsule and covers the interosseous ligaments of the carpus may be continuous with that of the distal radio-ulnar joint through a defect in the triangular disc. The **nerve supply** is through the anterior and posterior interosseous nerves and the dorsal branch of the ulnar nerve.

Movements at the wrist joint [Table 5; p. 117]

This ellipsoid joint [p. 12] has a long radius of curvature transversely which permits abduction and adduction and a short radius anteroposteriorly which permits flexion and extension. All these movements are supplemented by similar movements at the **intercarpal joints** [Fig. 107] which are principally responsible for abduction and greatly increase the range of flexion. At the radiocarpal joint, extension and adduction have the greatest range. In adduction, the carpal bones slide laterally, the lunate passing further on to the radius while the triquetrum comes into contact with the triangular disc.

Because of the two different curvatures of the joint at right angles to one another, rotation is not possible at this joint. As a result the carpal bones

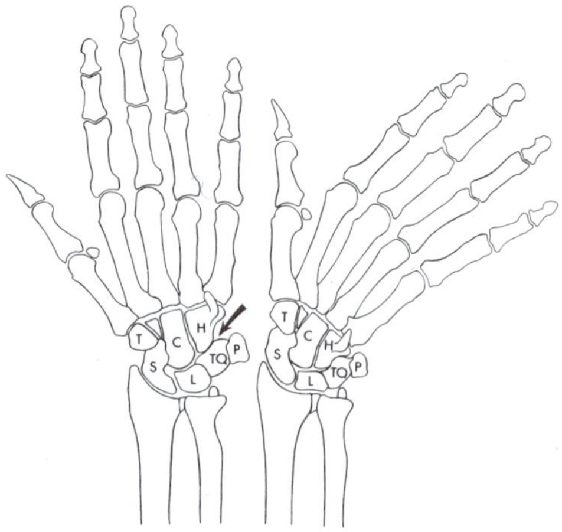

Fig. 107. Outline tracings of the bones of the hand taken from radiographs of the same individual in abducted and fully adducted positions of the wrist. Note how, in adduction, the proximal row of carpal bones slides laterally on the radius to bring the lunate into contact with the distal end of the radius, and the triquetrum against the disc on the distal end of the ulna. The distal row of carpal bones slides in the concavity of the proximal row, so as to bring the hamate into contact with the lunate, and the whole of its medial aspect against the triquetrum; the capitate sliding laterally off the lunate on to the scaphoid, and the trapezium gliding medially on the distal surface of the scaphoid.
C. Capitate
H. Hamate
L. Lunate
P. Pisiform
S. Scaphoid
T. Trapezium
TQ. Triquetrum

move with the radius in pronation and supination at the radio-ulnar joints. Thus the movement of adduction when the hand is pronated deviates the hand laterally but still towards the ulna which is now lateral to the radius in the distal forearm. For this reason, adduction is commonly called 'ulnar deviation' and abduction 'radial deviation'.

Dissection

Divide the anterior, medial, and lateral ligaments by a transverse incision across the front of the joint. Bend the hand backwards and expose the articular surfaces.

Radio-ulnar joints

Proximal radio-ulnar joint

This joint is between the side of the cylindrical head of the radius and the radial notch of the ulna. The ligaments are the anular and the quadrate.

Anular ligament of the radius

This strong, fibrous collar is attached to the anterior and posterior margins of the radial notch of the ulna. With that notch the ligament encircles the head of the radius and retains it in contact with the notch. The anular ligament is slightly conical and fits closely but is only loosely attached to the neck of the radius. Thus the head of the radius is free to turn within the ligament but

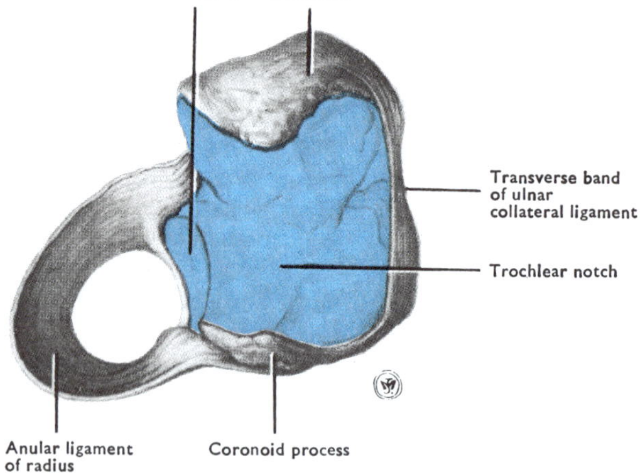

Fig. 108. Anular ligament of radius and proximal articular surfaces of ulna.

cannot be pulled downwards out of it. Proximally the anular ligament is continuous with and strengthened by the lateral and anterior ligaments of the elbow joint.

The **quadrate ligament** is a weak sheet of fibres which passes between the neck of the radius and the lower margin of the radial notch of the ulna.

Synovial membrane

This is continuous with the synovial membrane of the elbow joint. It lines the deep surface of the anular ligament and is reflected upwards from its distal margin to surround the intracapsular part of the neck of the radius.

Distal radio-ulnar joint

In this joint the side of the head of the ulna articulates with the ulnar notch of the radius. The articular disc, the interosseous membrane, and a weak fibrous capsule hold the bones together.

Articular disc

This triangular, fibrocartilaginous disc is the main structure holding the distal ends of the radius and ulna together. The disc is attached by its base to the distal margin of the ulnar notch of the radius and by its apex to a depression at the root of the ulnar styloid process. Thus it covers the distal end of the ulna, separating it and the distal radio-ulnar joint from the wrist joint and hence from the lunate and triquetrum. Occasionally the disc is perforated. Then the cavities of the two joints are continuous.

Fibrous capsule

This consists of lax fibres passing between the anterior and posterior borders of the disc and the adjacent surfaces of the radius and ulna. Between these bones it extends proximally to the distal border of the interosseous membrane enclosing a prolongation of the joint cavity, the **recessus sacciformis**.

Synovial membrane

This lines the fibrous capsule and the proximal surface of the articular disc.

Dissection

Expose the interosseous membrane by removing the muscles from the back or front of the forearm.

Interosseous membrane of the forearm

This fibrous sheet stretches between the interosseous borders of the radius and ulna and holds these bones together without preventing the movements which take place between them. It begins 2–3 cm distal to the tuberosity of the radius and blends distally with the capsule of the distal radio-ulnar joint. The fibres of the membrane run downwards and medially and thus transmit to the ulna compression forces applied to the radius from the hand. Such forces are then transferred to the humerus through its stable articulation with the ulna at the elbow joint, in addition to their transmission through the articulation of the head of the radius with the capitulum.

The posterior interosseous vessels pass backwards between the radius and ulna proximal to the interosseous membrane; the anterior interosseous vessels pierce it 5 cm from its distal end. The membrane increases the area of origin for the deep flexor and extensor muscles of the forearm.

Dissection

Cut through the anular ligament and divide the interosseous membrane from above downwards. Open the capsule of the distal radio-ulnar joint and draw the radius laterally to expose the connexions of the articular capsule and disc.

Movements at the radio-ulnar joints
[Table 4; p. 117]

These are **supination** and **pronation**. When the limb is supine, the thumb is directed laterally and the radius and ulna lie parallel to each other; when prone, the thumb and styloid process of the radius lie on the medial side and the posterior surfaces of the radius and hand face anteriorly. The body of the radius lies obliquely across the anterior surface of the ulna. In pronation, the radius describes a segment of a cone with its apex at the centre of the head of the radius and the centre of its base in the head of the ulna—the head of the radius rotating in the anular ligament, while the distal end turns around the stationary ulna carrying the hand and articular disc with it. As described above, the ulna remains stationary and the little finger rotates around its own axis. However, pronation and supination can be carried out around the axis of any one of the fingers. This shift of the axis is produced by *deviation of the distal end of the ulna* which moves laterally as the radius rotates into pronation and medially as it moves into supination. The lateral deviation can be produced by rotation of the humerus or contraction of anconeus.

Pronation

This is produced by muscles on the anterior surface of the forearm which run from the medial to the lateral side—pronator teres, pronator quadratus, and flexor carpi radialis. Pronator teres has the maximum mechanical advantage

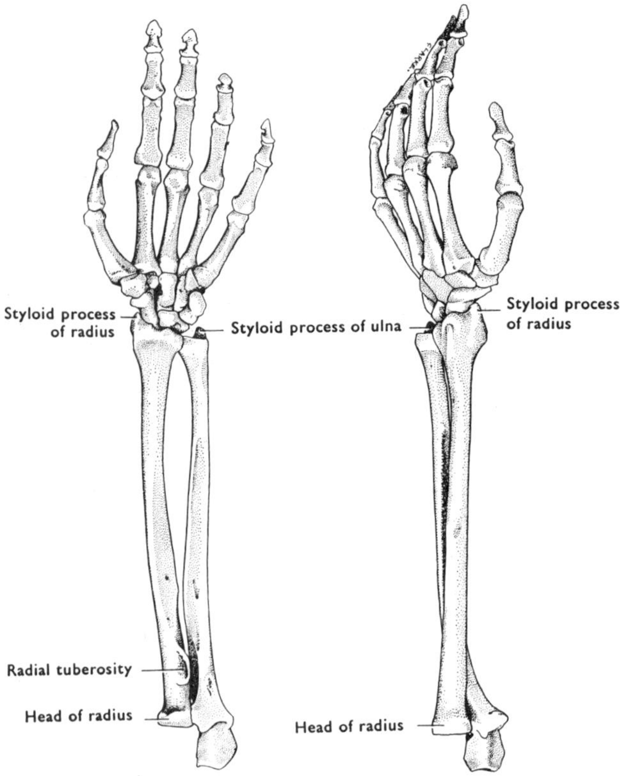

Fig. 109. Outline drawing of the left forearm and hand bones in the supine (left) and semiprone (right) positions. Note that the ulna remains stationary and that the distal end of the radius rotates around it carrying the hand. The head of the radius rotates in the radial notch of the ulna.

because it is inserted into the point of maximum lateral curvature of the radius.

Supination

Biceps is a powerful supinator. Its tendon turns round the medial side of the radius into the posterior aspect of the radial tuberosity. Thus it rotates the radius laterally on contraction. Muscles which pass from medial to lateral on the posterior aspect of the forearm also produce supination—supinator and abductor pollicis longus. Brachioradialis can help to start supination of the fully pronated forearm.

With the elbow extended, the range of pronation and supination is apparently increased by the added *rotation of the humerus*. For this reason, clinical tests for the range of movement at the radio-ulnar joints are always carried out with the elbow flexed to a right angle—the position in which biceps has its maximum supinating power.

Intercarpal, carpometacarpal, and intermetacarpal joints

[Fig. 110]

There are only three separate joint cavities within this complex of articulations: (1) the main joint complex; (2) the pisiform (intercarpal) joint; (3) the carpometacarpal joint of the thumb.

The main joint complex

The largest is a single, complex joint in which the cavity and synovial membrane are common to the articulations of the carpal bones with each other (intercarpal joints) and with the medial four metacarpals (carpometacarpal joint) and extend between the bases of these metacarpals (intermetacarpal joints) [Fig. 110]. The common fibrous capsule unites the exposed surfaces of all these bones. It is continuous proximally with the capsule of the wrist joint (though their cavities are separate) and it forms the three strong, intermetacarpal ligaments which limit the cavity distally. This fibrous capsule may be divided into palmar, dorsal, lateral, and medial ligaments of the joints it contains but these are simply parts of a continuous sheath and will not be dealt with further.

In addition to the intermetacarpal ligaments, **interosseous ligaments** unite each row of carpal bones. These ligaments between the proximal parts of the scaphoid, lunate, and triquetrum bones complete the distal articular surface of the wrist joint and separate its cavity from that of the intercarpal joints. Less regular ligaments unite the distal row of carpal bones and allow

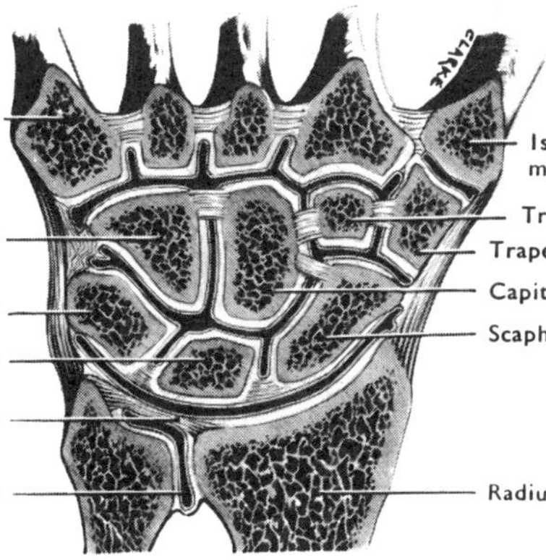

Fig. 110. Coronal section through radiocarpal, intercarpal, carpometacarpal, and intermetacarpal joints to show joint cavities and interosseous ligaments (diagrammatic).

continuity of the intercarpal and carpometacarpal joint cavities around them. The interosseous ligaments between the rows of bones are less well developed. The capitate is commonly attached to the scaphoid [Fig. 110] and to the base of the third metacarpal by a ligament which also arises from the hamate bone.

Articular surfaces and movements [Figs. 110, 239]

Intercarpal joints

In each row, the carpal bones articulate by flat surfaces which allow little movement but give some resilience to the carpus. The joint between the proximal and distal rows is deeply concavo-convex. The capitate and hamate fit into the concavity of the proximal row, while the concave surfaces of the trapezium and trapezoid fit the convex distal surface of the scaphoid.

The main movements are flexion and extension. The distal row also moves on the proximal row around an anteroposterior axis through the centre of the capitate producing some abduction and adduction [Fig. 107]. Thus the transverse intercarpal joint increases the range of movement at the wrist joint and the resilience of the region.

The pisiform joint

This is a small, flat area where the pisiform articulates with the palmar surface of the triquetrum. The pisiform is held in position against the pull of flexor carpi ulnaris by the **pisohamate** and **pisometacarpal ligaments** attached respectively to the hook of the hamate and the base of the fifth metacarpal bone. The joint allows the pisiform to maintain correct alignment during adduction and abduction of the hand.

Carpometacarpal joints—Medial four

The metacarpal of the index is fitted around the trapezoid bone, that of the middle finger has a flat joint with the capitate. Both metacarpals have very limited movements. Confirm this on your own hand and note that the metacarpal of the ring finger has considerably more movement while that of the little finger is the most mobile. The carpometacarpal joints of the ring and little fingers are flexed when the fist is clenched or the palm 'cupped' and the fifth has slight lateral rotation produced by the opponens digiti minimi.

The carpometacarpal joint of the thumb

This is separate from the remainder. This is a saddle-shaped joint with a loose capsule which permits the wide range of movement of the metacarpal of the thumb on the trapezium. The thumb lies anterior to the other digits and is rotated so that its nail faces laterally. Movements of the thumb are thus at right angles to those of the fingers and occur principally at this joint. The metacarpal may be moved laterally (extension) or medially (flexion) or anteriorly (abduction) or posteriorly (adduction). When the thumb is adducted the range of flexion and extension is small; when abducted the range is greatly increased. The metacarpal then moves on an arc of a circle so that it is medially rotated in flexion and laterally rotated in extension. This movement of flexion with medial rotation of the abducted metacarpal of the thumb is known as **opposition** for it opposes the palmar surface of the thumb to those of the fingers. It is essential in holding or grasping any object and makes the thumb functionally one-half of the hand.

Intermetacarpal joints

These permit slight movement between the bases of the metacarpals.

Nerve supply

The nerve supply of these joints is from the anterior and posterior interosseous nerves, and/or the dorsal and deep branches of the ulnar nerve, and/or the superficial branch of the radial nerve, depending on the position of each joint.

Metacarpo-phalangeal joints

These are condyloid joints in which the surface of the metacarpal is convex transversely and anteroposteriorly and fits the shallow, spherical fossa on the base of the proximal phalanx. In the thumb the metacarpal surface is flatter and less extensive than in the other metacarpals for the range of movement is smaller in the thumb.

Fibrous capsules

These are thickened anteriorly to form the palmar ligament and on each side to form a collateral ligament. On the dorsal surface they are replaced by the expansion of the extensor tendon [Fig. 97]—a mechanism which permits the full range of flexion with continuous support for the dorsal surfaces of the joints.

The **collateral ligaments** are strong, oblique bands which extend from the distal surfaces of the tubercles on the dorsal surface of the metacarpal heads to the sides of the base of the proximal phalanx anteriorly [Fig. 87].

The **palmar ligament** is a thick, fibrous plate attached firmly to the base of the proximal phalanx but loosely to the neck of the metacarpal. In full flexion of the joint the plate lies on the palmar surface of the body of the metacarpal. It passes on to the palmar surface of the head when the joint is straightened and on to its distal surface in full extension. In the medial four digits, the margins of the palmar plate give attachment (1) to the **deep transverse metacarpal ligaments;** (2) to the **fibrous flexor sheath;** (3) to the slips of the **palmar aponeurosis;** (4) to the **collateral ligaments;** (5) to the transverse fibres of the **extensor expansion**. Thus the palmar aponeurosis and the transverse fibres of the extensor expansion are tightened when the plate is drawn on to the distal aspect of the metacarpal head in full extension. This tethers the extensor digitorum tendon and prevents it from extending the interphalangeal joints when the metacarpophalangeal joint is in this position, though the extensor digitorum can extend the interphalangeal joints when the metacarpophalangeal joints are straight or flexed.

Sesamoid bones

A small, oval sesamoid bone is buried in each side of the palmar ligament of the metacarpophalangeal joint of the thumb where the tendons of adductor pollicis and flexor pollicis brevis fuse with the ligament. Each bone articulates with the corresponding surface of the head of the metacarpal and the tendon of flexor pollicis longus lies in the groove between them. Smaller sesamoid bones may be found in the palmar ligaments of the other joints, particularly in the index and little fingers.

Movements

On the basis of the shape of the joint surfaces, flexion, extension, abduction, adduction, and rotation could all take place. There is no provision for voluntary rotation but considerable passive rotatory movement is possible when the joint is extended and the collateral ligaments are relaxed—a situation in which abduction and adduction movements of the fingers are also possible. Both movements are restricted in flexion because of the tightening of the collateral ligaments. This occurs because the ligaments are excentrically attached near the dorsal surface of the metacarpal head and also because they are stretched over the wider palmar surface of the metacarpal as the phalanx moves on to that surface in flexion.

Because the metacarpals are arranged in an arc, convex dorsally, the phalanges converge on flexion and diverge on extension at the metacarpophalangeal joints. This occurs without the activity of the interossei which produce these movements when the joints are extended.

In **precision movements**, flexion of the metacarpophalangeal joints of the medial four digits is produced mainly by the interossei and lumbricals, the long flexor tendons acting in powerful movements. Extension of these joints is produced by extensor digitorum and by extensor indicis and extensor digiti minimi in the index and little fingers. These two muscles permit extension of the index and little fingers when the middle and ring fingers are flexed at the metacarpophalangeal joints.

In the thumb, the range of movement is much less in all directions at the metacarpophalangeal joint. Flexion is produced by flexor pollicis brevis and longus, abduction and adduction by the short abductor and adductor, and extension by the long and short extensor muscles.

Interphalangeal joints

These joints have the same arrangement as the metacarpophalangeal joints except that the articular surfaces only permit a hinge-like movement of flexion and extension. Two condyles, medial and lateral, on the head of one phalanx fit into concave facets on the base of the other, while the ridge between these facets slides in the groove between the condyles.

Flexor digitorum profundus flexes all the joints of the fingers. Flexor superficialis acts only on the proximal interphalangeal and metacarpophalangeal joints. Extension at the interphalangeal joints is produced by the long extensors of the digits and also by the interosseous and lumbrical muscles acting through the extensor expansion. When the metacarpophalangeal joints of the fingers are fully extended, the long extensors are unable to act on the interphalangeal joints (see above) which can then only be extended by the lumbricals and interossei. The **lumbricals** and **interossei** also flex the metacarpophalangeal joints, so paralysis of them permits the long extensor muscles to produce full extension at these joints, leaving the long flexor muscles of the fingers free to flex the interphalangeal joints and produce the *'claw hand'* which is so characteristic of this paralysis.

In the thumb, the single interphalangeal joint is operated by flexor and extensor pollicis longus and sometimes by extensor pollicis brevis. **Abductor pollicis brevis** (supplied by the median nerve) may be partly inserted into the extensor expansion. Thus some extension of the interphalangeal joint of the thumb may still be possible when all the extensor muscles of the thumb are paralysed by destruction of the radial nerve.

The movements of the fingers and thumb are summarized in Tables 6 and 7 [pp. 118, 119].

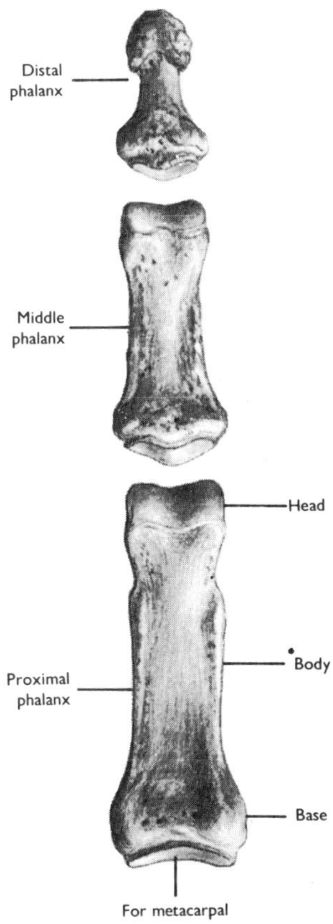

Fig. 111. Phalanges of a finger (palmar view). Comparison with the phalanges of a foot will show that in the foot the bases of the proximal phalanges are relatively large and the bodies are much thinner. The middle and distal phalanges are so short that they should not be mistaken. The bones of the big toe have special features.

Tables 1–8
The muscles, movements, and nerves of the upper limb

These Tables list the muscles in groups according to the joint or joint complex across which they act. The origin, insertion, and action of each muscle is given in the first part of Tables 1–7. In the second parts of these Tables, the muscles are grouped according to the actions which they produce on the particular joint or joint complex, and the nerve supply of each muscle is given. This allows an easy assessment of the degree of paralysis of a particular movement following destruction of a particular nerve. In Table 8, the total motor distribution of each nerve in the upper limb is shown, together with the paralysis which results from the destruction of that nerve at each level in the limb. The total cutaneous nerve supply of each of these nerves is shown in Fig. 48.

In the first parts of Tables 1–7, the numbers enclosed in square brackets, e.g. [24], refer to the Figures in which the attachments are shown.

The limitation of these Tables arises from the fact that they show only the actions of a particular muscle when it actively shortens. It should be remembered that muscles are also brought into action (1) to fix one part of the trunk or limb so that another part may have a stable base on which to act, e.g. movement of the free upper limb on a fixed scapula, or (2) to control the rate or strength of a movement which is in the direction opposite to that which the muscle would produce if it was shortening, e.g. the contraction of deltoid while the abducted arm is being lowered to the side.

Table 1

Trunk muscles acting on shoulder girdle
[Figs. 220–228]

Muscle	Origin	Insertion	Action on girdle
Trapezius	Superior nuchal line Ligamentum nuchae, 7th cervical and all thoracic vertebral spines	Clavicle, lat. ⅓ Acromion, medial edge Spine of scapula, superior margin	Elevates shoulder (a) Retracts scapula Depresses medial part of spine of scapula (b) (a)+(b) rotates scapula laterally
Serratus anterior	Upper 8 ribs anterolaterally	Scapula, medial border, entire length	Entire muscle protracts scapula and holds it against ribs Lower ⅝ rotates scapula laterally
Pectoralis minor	Ribs 3–5 anterolaterally	Coracoid process	Protracts scapula Depresses shoulder (medial rotation of scapula)
Rhomboid major	2nd–5th thoracic vertebral spines	Scapula, medial border inferior to spine	Retraction, medial rotation, elevation of scapula
minor	Lower lig. nuchae to 1st thoracic vertebral spine	Scapula, medial border at spine	Retraction and elevation of scapula
Levator scapulae	Cervical transverse processes 1–4	Scapula between superior angle and rhomboid minor	Elevation, medial rotation of scapula
Subclavius	1st costal cartilage	Clavicle, inferior surface	Holds clavicle to sternum

Trunk muscles acting on scapula when shoulder joint is fixed

Muscle	Origin	Insertion	Action on girdle
Pectoralis major, sternocostal	Sternum and costal cartilages 1–6	Humerus, crest of greater tubercle	Protracts scapula, depresses shoulder
Latissimus dorsi	Lower ribs, thoracolumbar fascia, iliac crest	Intertubercular sulcus of humerus	Depresses shoulder (medial rotation of scapula) Retracts scapula

Movements of shoulder girdle on trunk

Movement	Muscles	Nerve supply (motor)
Elevation	Levator scapulae	Dorsal scapular and C. 3 & 4
	Trapezius, upper part	Accessory
	Rhomboids	Dorsal scapular
Depression	Pectoralis minor	Medial pectoral
	Trapezius, lower part	Accessory
	Latissimus dorsi*	Thoracodorsal
	Pectoralis major, lower sternocostal part*	Medial pectoral
Protraction	Serratus anterior	Long thoracic
	Pectoralis minor	Medial pectoral
	Pectoralis major, sternocostal part*	Pectoral
Retraction	Rhomboid major and minor	Dorsal scapular
	Trapezius, middle part	Accessory
	Latissimus dorsi*	Thoracodorsal
Rotation: lateral, e.g. in abduction of arm	Serratus anterior, lower ⅝	Long thoracic
	Trapezius, upper and lower parts	Accessory
medial	Rhomboid major and minor	Dorsal scapular
	Levator scapulae	Dorsal scapular and C. 3 & 4
	Pectoralis minor	Medial pectoral
	Pectoralis major, lower sternocostal part*	Medial pectoral
	Latissimus dorsi*	Thoracodorsal

*These muscles can only act on the scapula through a fixed shoulder joint

---

Table **2**

Muscles acting on shoulder joint

[Figs. 221–236]

Muscle	Origin	Insertion	Action at shoulder
Pectoralis major	Clavicle, med. ⅔	Humerus, crest of greater tubercle	Flexion and medial rotation
	Sternum and costal cartilages 1–6		Adduction and medial rotation
Latissimus dorsi	Lower ribs, thoracolumbar fascia, iliac crest	Humerus, intertubercular groove	Adduction, medial rotation, extn. if flexed
Muscles passing from shoulder girdle to humerus			
Deltoid	Clavicle, lat. ⅓		Flexion and medial rotation
	Acromion	Humerus, deltoid tuberosity	Abduction
	Spine of scapula		Extension, lat. rotation
Biceps brachii			
short head	Coracoid process	Radius	Flexion
long head	Supraglenoid tubercle	Radius	Stabilization
Coracobrachialis	Coracoid process	Humerus, middle of body, medial	Flexion
Teres major	Inf. ⅓ lat. margin of scapula	Humerus, crest of lesser tubercle	Adduction, med. rotation
Supraspinatus	Scapula, supraspinous fossa	Humerus, gtr. tubercle superior surface	Abduction, stabilization
Infraspinatus	Scapula, infraspinous fossa	Humerus, gtr. tubercle post-sup. surface	Lat. rotation stabilization
Teres minor	Scapula, superior ⅔ lateral margin	Humerus, gtr., tubercle post. surface	Lat. rotation, stabilization*
Subscapularis	Scapula, subscapular fossa	Humerus, lesser tubercle	Med. rotation, stabilization*
Triceps, long head	Scapula, infraglenoid tubercle	Ulna	Stabilization

*Part of the stabilization which these muscles supply is in abduction at the shoulder. In this movement they prevent the head of the humerus from rising in the glenoid and abutting on the acromion when deltoid contracts.

Movements at the shoulder joint

Movement	Muscles	Nerve supply
Flexion	Pectoralis major, clavicular part	Pectoral nerves
	Deltoid, clavicular part	Axillary
	Biceps, short head	Musculocutaneous
	Coracobrachialis	Musculocutaneous
Extension	Deltoid, post. part	Axillary
	Latissimus dorsi (if shoulder flexed)	Thoracodorsal
	Teres major (if shoulder flexed)	Subscapular
Abduction	Deltoid, acromial part	Axillary
	Supraspinatus	Suprascapular
Adduction	Pectoralis major, sternocostal part	Pectoral
	Latissimus dorsi	Thoracodorsal
	Teres major	Subscapular
Lateral rotation of humerus	Deltoid, posterior part	Axillary
	Infraspinatus	Suprascapular
	Teres minor	Axillary
Medial rotation of humerus	Pectoralis major	Pectoral
	Latissimus dorsi	Thoracodorsal
	Deltoid, clavicular part	Axillary
	Teres major	Subscapular
	Subscapularis	Subscapular
Stabilization*	Subscapularis	Subscapular
	Supraspinatus	Suprascapular
	Infraspinatus	Suprascapular
	Teres minor	Axillary
	Triceps, long head	Radial
	Biceps, long head	Musculocutaneous

The actions of muscles shown in Table 2 presuppose a fixed scapula. If the arm is fixed, muscles passing from the shoulder girdle to the arm will move the girdle on the trunk. If the shoulder joint is fixed, muscles passing from the trunk to the humerus will move the girdle on the trunk at the sternoclavicular joint.

*All the muscles of stabilization are attached close to the shoulder joint, have a poor mechanical advantage over it, and are more effective in holding the joint than in moving it.

At the shoulder joint no movement is controlled by one nerve alone. However, some movements have their major muscle (or muscles) innervated by a single nerve and so are severely affected by damage to that nerve—e.g. the axillary nerve in abduction, extension, and lateral rotation. Thus destruction of the axillary nerve leads to the shoulder being held in a position of adduction, medial rotation, and flexion.

Table **3**

Muscles acting on the elbow joint

[Figs. 226, 230, 234, 236, 240]

Muscle	Origin	Insertion	Action at elbow
Brachialis	Humerus, ant. surface distal ½	Ulna, coronoid process	Flexion
Biceps brachii	Scapula, coracoid process Supraglenoid tubercle	Radius, tuberosity	Flexion
Brachioradialis	Humerus, lateral supracondylar line	Radius, base of styloid process	Flexion
Extensor carpi radialis longus	Humerus, lateral supracondylar line	2nd metacarpal	Flexion
Triceps	Scapula, infraglenoid tubercle. Humerus, post. surface—lat. head above groove for radial nerve, med. head below groove	Ulna, olecranon	Extension
Anconeus	Lateral epicondyle of humerus	Ulna, lat. surface, proximal ⅓	Holds ulna to humerus. Abduction of ulna
Pronator teres	Humerus, medial supracondylar line and		Minor role in elbow flexion
Flexor carpi radialis	medial epicondyle		

Movements at the elbow joint

Movement	Muscles	Nerve supply
Flexion	Biceps brachii	Musculocutaneous
	Brachialis	Musculocutaneous
	Brachioradialis	Radial
	Extensor carpi radialis longus	Radial
	Flexor carpi radialis	Median
	Pronator teres	Median
Extension	Triceps	Radial
Ulna, abduction	Anconeus	Radial

Table **4**

Muscles acting on the radio-ulnar joints
[Figs. 226, 230, 234, 236, 238]

Muscle	Origin	Insertion	Action on radio-ulnar joints
Pronator teres	Humerus, med. epicondyle and med. supracondylar line	Radius, lat. surface middle of body	Pronation
Pronator quadratus	Ulna, ant. surface, distal ¼	Radius, ant. surface, distal ¼	Pronation. Holds radius to ulna
Flexor carpi radialis	Humerus, med. epicondyle	2nd and 3rd metacarpal bases	Pronation
Supinator	Humerus, lat. epicondyle Ulna, supinator crest	Radius, post., lat., and ant. surfaces, proximal ⅓	Supination
Biceps brachii	Coracoid process Supraglenoid tubercle	Radius, tuberosity	Supination (with elbow flexion)
Brachioradialis	Humerus, lat. supracondylar line	Radius, distal end, lat. surface	Supination from pronation to midposition

Movements at radio-ulnar joints

Movement	Muscles	Nerve supply
Pronation	Pronator teres Pronator quadratus Flexor carpi radialis	Median Median* Median
Supination	Supinator Biceps brachii Brachioradialis	Radial Musculocutaneous Radial

*Ant. interosseous branch.
Pronation is seriously interfered with in destruction of the median nerve proximal to the elbow.

Table **5**

Muscles acting on the wrist joint
[Figs. 230, 234, 236, 238, 240]

Muscle	Origin	Insertion	Action at wrist
Flexor carpi radialis	Humerus medial epicondyle	2nd and 3rd metacarpal bases	Flexion, abduction
Flexor carpi ulnaris	Humerus medial epicondyle Ulna, subcutaneous border	Pisiform (hamate and 5th metacarpal)	Flexion, adduction
Extensor carpi radialis longus	Humerus, lateral supracondylar line	2nd metacarpal base	Extension, abduction
Extensor carpi radialis brevis	Humerus, lat. epicondyle	2nd and 3rd metacarpal bases	Extension, abduction
Extensor carpi ulnaris	Humerus, lat. epicondyle ulna, post. border	5th metacarpal base	Extension, adduction
Extensor digitorum	Humerus, lat. epicondyle	Extensor expansions of fingers [97]	} Extension, prevented by radial and ulnar flexor of carpus
Extensor digiti minimi	Humerus, lateral epicondyle	Extensor expansion 5th digit	}
Extensor pollicis longus	Ulna, middle ⅓ dorsal surface	Thumb, distal phalanx	}
Extensor indicis	Ulna distal to ext. pollicis longus	2nd digit, extensor expansion	}
Flexor digitorum profundus	Ulna, prox. ¾ ant. and med. surfaces	Fingers, terminal phalanges	} Flexion, prevented by radial and ulnar extensors of carpus
Flexor digitorum superficialis	Humerus, med. epicondyle Ulna, coronoid Radius, ant. border	Fingers, middle phalanges	}
Flexor pollicis longus	Radius, ant. surface middle 2 quarters	Thumb, distal phalanx	}

Movements at the wrist joint

Movement	Muscles	Nerve supply
Flexion	*Flexor carpi ulnaris* *Flexor carpi radialis* Flexor digitorum profundus Flexor digitorum superficialis	Ulnar Median Median* and ulnar Median

Movement	Muscles	Nerve supply
Flexion (cont)	Flexor pollicis longus	Median*
	Palmaris longus	Median
Extension	*Extensor carpi ulnaris*	Radial*
	Extensor carpi radialis longus and brevis	Radial
	Extensor digitorum	Radial*
	Extensor digiti minimi	Radial*
	Extensor pollicis longus	Radial*
	Extensor indicis	Radial*
Abduction	*Extensor carpi radialis longus and brevis*	Radial
	Flexor carpi radialis	Median
	Abductor pollicis longus	Radial*
Adduction	*Flexor carpi ulnaris*	Ulnar
	Extensor carpi ulnaris	Radial*

*Ant. or post. interosseous branch.
Terms in italic the principal muscles producing a given movement.

In the subsequent tables the following abbreviations are used. CM = carpometacarpal joint; MP = metacarpophalangeal joint; IP = interphalangeal joints; PIP = proximal interphalangeal joint; DIP = distal interphalangeal joint.

Table **6**

Muscles acting on the fingers
[Figs. 234, 236, 238, 240]

Muscle	Origin	Insertion	Action on fingers
Flx. digitorum superficialis	Humerus, med. epicond. Radius, ant. border	Middle phalanges [87]	Flexion, MP & PIP
Flx. digitorum profundus	Ulna, prox. ⅔ ant. and med. surfaces	Distal phalanges [87]	Flexion, all joints
Lumbricals	Tendons flx. digitm. profundus	Middle and distal phalanges *via* ext. expansion [97]	Flexion MP, extension IP
Extensor digitorum	Humerus, lat. epicondyle	Extensor expansion	Extends all joints all fingers. If MP fully extended, IP not extended
Interossei			
dorsal	Adjacent sides metacarpals 1–5	Corresponding side base of prox. phalanx Extensor expansion [97]	Abduction of MP of index, middle (2), and ring. Extension IP
palmar	Metacarpals, med. side 1 & 2, lat. side 4 & 5	Corresponding prox. phalanx base, exten. expansion	Adduction of MP of thumb, index, ring, and little Extension IP
Abductor digiti minimi	Pisiform, flexor retinaculum	Prox. phalanx, med. side of base (both)	Abduction MP (& CM) little finger
Flexor digiti minimi	Hamate, hook. Flexor retinaculum		Flexion CM & MP
Opponens digiti minimi	Hamate, hook	5th metacarpal, medial side	Rotates metacarpal laterally; flexion CM
Extensor indicis	Ulna, post. surface	Extensor expansion	Extension all jts. index (see ext. digitorum)
Extensor digiti minimi	Humerus, lateral epicondyle	Extensor expansion	As ext. indicis, for little finger and abduction MP

Movements of fingers

Movement	Muscles	Nerve supply
Flexion, all fingers		
All joints	Flexor digitorum profundus	Median* (index and middle) Ulnar (ring and little)
MP & PIP	Flexor digitorum superficialis	Median
MP only	Lumbricals	Median (index and middle) Ulnar (ring and little)
	Interossei	Ulnar
CM & MP, little finger	Flexor digiti minimi	Ulnar
CM only, little	Opponens digiti minimi	Ulnar
Extension		
All joints		
all fingers	Extensor digitorum	Radial*
index only	Extensor indicis	Radial*
little finger	Extensor digiti minimi	Radial*
MP only	Extensors digitorum, indicis, and digiti minimi if MP fully extended	Radial*

Movement	Muscles	Nerve supply
Extension (cont) IP only	Lumbricals	Median (index and middle) Ulnar (ring and little)
	Interossei	Ulnar
Abduction at MP		
all fingers except	Interossei, dorsal	Ulnar
little finger	Abductor digiti minimi	Ulnar
Adduction at MP		
all fingers except middle	Interossei, palmar	Ulnar
Opposition at CM of		
little finger only	Opponens digiti minimi	Ulnar

This table shows:

1. Little finger movements are seriously disturbed by destruction of ulnar nerve, but flexion at MP and PIP persists (flexor digitorum superficialis).
2. Extension at MP is lost if radial nerve destroyed, but IP extension is not (lumbricals and interossei).
3. Abduction and adduction at MP are lost when ulnar nerve is destroyed.
4. When median and ulnar nerves are destroyed, the extensors (radial*) acting against no resistance, pull MP into full extension. In this position the extensors cannot extend the IP and the lumbricals and interossei being paralysed, the IP are pulled into flexion by the passive insufficiency of the long flexor muscles (flexor digitorum profundus and superficialis) producing a 'claw hand'.

*Anterior or posterior interosseous branch.

Table **7**

Muscles acting on the thumb

[Figs. 234, 236, 238]

Muscle	Origin	Insertion	Action on thumb
Flexor pollicis longus	Radius, ant. surface middle 2 quarters	Distal phalanx	Flexion all joints
Flexor pollicis brevis	Tubercle of trapezium Flexor retinaculum	Prox. phalanx, base, ant. aspect	Flexion CM & MP
Abductor pollicis brevis	Scaphoid, tubercle Flexor retinaculum		Abduction CM & MP
Abductor pollicis longus	Radius and ulna, dorsal surfaces distal to supinator	Metacarpal base, ant. aspect	Abduction of CM some extension
Opponens pollicis	Trapezium, tubercle Flexor retinaculum	Metacarpal, ant. surface	Medial rotation and flexion of CM
1st palmar interosseous	1st metacarpal base	Prox. phalanx, base, post. aspect	Adduction of MP
Adductor pollicis	Metacarpals, bases of 2 & 3, body of 3		Adduction CM & MP
Extensor pollicis longus	Ulna, post. surface, middle ⅓	Distal phalanx	Extension all joints, esp. with CM lat. rotated
Ext. pollicis brevis	Radius, post. surface	Prox. (and distal) phalanx, base	Extension of CM, MP (& IP) esp, when thumb opposed

Movements of the thumb

Movement	Muscles	Nerve supply
Flexion		
All joints	Flexor pollicis longus	Median*
CM & MP	Flexor pollicis brevis	Median
CM only	Opponens pollicis	Median
Extension		
All joints	Extensor pollicis longus	Radial*
CM & MP (IP)	Extensor pollicis brevis	Radial*
CM only	Abductor pollicis longus	Radial*
IP only	Abductor pollicis brevis	Median
Abduction		
CM only	Abductor pollicis longus	Radial*
CM & MP	Abductor pollicis brevis	Median
Adduction		
CM & MP	Adductor pollicis	Ulnar
MP only	1st palmar interosseous	Ulnar
Opposition		
Abduction, see above		
Flexion, CM & MP, see above		
Extension, IP, see above		
Medial rotation, CM	Opponens pollicis	Median
Reverse of opposition		
Abduction at CM	Abductor pollicis longus	Radial*
Extension at CM & MP with lat. rotation		
initially	Extensor pollicis brevis	Radial*
later	Extensor pollicis longus	Radial*

*Anterior or posterior interosseous branch.

Table **8**

Motor distribution

In the following tables are shown the positions in the limb of the muscles innervated by the various nerves, the muscles, and the effects of paralysis of these muscles following injury to the nerves or their branches. Where a nerve innervates muscles in more than one segment of the limb (shoulder, arm, forearm, hand) the effects of injury to the nerve will depend on the level of injury. Thus when the median nerve is destroyed at the wrist, the muscles supplied by it in the forearm are not paralysed though those in the hand are. Since forearm and hand muscles may act together on the same joints, the degree of paralysis of some movements may be increased by the more proximal destruction in addition to the paralysis of different movements. An attempt has been made to show this by linking (with braces) those muscles which act together. In those cases where a number of muscles assist in an action and some are innervated by nerves other than those which are destroyed, those muscles which are still active are shown in brackets after the statement of the effect of the muscle paralysis.

Abbreviations.

Fingers are simply shown by their name—e.g 'index' for 'index finger'. CM = carpometacarpal joint. MP = metacarpophalangeal joint. IP = interphalangeal joints. PIP = proximal interphalangeal joint(s). DIP = distal interphalangeal joint(s).

Median nerve (For cutaneous supply, see Fig. 48)

Situation of innervated muscles	Muscles	Effects of paralysis by nerve destruction
Shoulder	Nil	
Arm	Nil	
Forearm	Flexor carpi radialis Pronator teres Pronator quadratus*	Weakened wrist flexion with ulnar deviation (flexor carpi ulnaris) *Pronation lost*
	Flexor pollicis longus*	Flexion of thumb lost at IP and weakened at CM & MP if only anterior interosseous nerve destroyed (flexor pollicis brevis, opponens pollicis). If total median nerve is destroyed above elbow, then thumb flexion is lost in all joints
	Flexor digitorum profundus, lateral half* Flexor digitorum superficialis	DIP flexion, lost, index and middle PIP flexion lost, index and middle PIP flexion weak, ring and little (flexor digitorum profundus) MP flexion weak all fingers: index and middle (interossei only); ring (flexor digitorum profundus, lumbrical, interossei); little (flexor digitorum profundus, flexor digiti minimi, interosseous)
Hand	Lumbricals, lateral two	IP extension weakened, index and middle (ext. digitorum and indicis, interossei)
	Abductor pollicis brevis Flexor pollicis brevis Opponens pollicis	CM & MP of thumb, weakened flexion (flexor pollicis longus) and abduction (abductor pollicis longus) *Opposition of thumb lost*

* = supplied by anterior or posterior interosseous branch.

Ulnar nerve (For cutaneous supply, see Fig. 48)

Situation of innervated muscles	Muscles	Effects of paralysis by nerve destruction
Shoulder	Nil	
Arm	Nil	
Forearm	Flexor carpi ulnaris	Weakened wrist flexion with radial deviation (flexor carpi radialis)
	Flexor digitorum profundus	*DIP loss of flexion* and MP & PIP weakness of flexion in ring and little (flx. digitorum superficialis)
Hand	Abductor digiti minimi	MP abduction lost in little finger
	Flexor digiti minimi brevis	MP flexion weakened (flx. digitorum superficialis [and profundus if ulnar nerve destroyed distal to branches to that muscle])
	Opponens digiti minimi	CM opposition of little finger lost
	All interossei	*MP abduction and adduction lost all fingers**
	Third and fourth lumbricals	IP extension weakened in all fingers (extensors digitorum, indicis, digiti minimi, and lumbricals of index and middle). No IP extension of ring and little if MP fully extended. These fingers then fixed in IP flexion—'claw'

Situation of innervated muscles	Muscles	Effects of paralysis by nerve destruction
	Adductor pollicis	Adduction of thumb lost, but long flexor and extensor of thumb acting together can mimic action of adductor

*Loss of abduction of little finger depends on the simultaneous paralysis of abductor digiti minimi, though extensor digiti minimi can mimic this action. Fingers are adducted in flexion and abducted in extension. This is due to the 'set' of the joints and is independent of the interossei. Hence interossei are tested with the fingers straight to overcome this and to avoid the restriction of the movement by tightening of the collateral ligaments in flexion.

Musculocutaneous nerve (For cutaneous supply, see Fig. 48)

Situation of innervated muscles	Muscles	Effects of paralysis by nerve destruction
Shoulder	Coracobrachialis Biceps brachii short head	Weakened shoulder flexion (deltoid; pectoralis major, clavicular part)
	long head	Some instability of shoulder joint in abduction (supraspinatus, subscapularis, deltoid)
Arm	Biceps brachii Brachialis	Weakened supination (supinator, brachioradialis) Severe weakening of elbow flexion (brachioradialis, ext. carpi. radialis longus, pronator teres, and flex. carpi radialis)

Axillary nerve (For cutaneous supply, see Fig. 48)

Situation of innervated muscles	Muscles	Effects of paralysis by nerve destruction
Shoulder	Teres minor Deltoid	Severe weakening of abduction (supraspinatus), extension (if not flexed), and lateral rotation of humerus (infraspinatus)

Subscapular nerves and thoracodorsal nerve

Situation of innervated muscles	Muscles	Effects of paralysis by nerve destruction
Shoulder	Subscapularis	Instability of shoulder joint with tendency to anterior dislocation
	Teres major	Weakened medial rotation of humerus (pectoralis major, deltoid clavicular part)
	Latissimus dorsi	Weakened adduction (pectoralis major). The paralysis of latissimus dorsi shows up in an inability to pull the body upwards with the upper limb

Radial nerve (For cutaneous supply, see Fig. 48)

Situation of innervated muscles	Muscles	Effects of paralysis by nerve destruction
Shoulder	Triceps, long head	Minor effect on shoulder stability in abduction. Downward dislocation in this position more likely
Arm	Triceps	*Loss of elbow extension*
Forearm	Supinator	Weakening of supination of prone hand (biceps brachii)
	Brachioradialis Extensor carpi radialis longus and brevis	Weakening of elbow flexion in midprone position (brachialis, biceps brachii, pronator teres)
	Extensor carpi radialis longus and brevis	Markedly weakened radial deviation of wrist (flexor carpi radlialis) *Loss of wrist extension—'wrist drop'*
	Extensor carpi ulnaris*	Weakened ulnar deviation of wrist (flexor carpi ulnaris)
	Extensor digitorum*	*Loss of extension at MP, all fingers* with weakened IP extension (interossei, lumbricals)
	Extensor indicis*	Loss of independent index extension
	Extensor digiti minimi*	Loss of independent little finger extension
	Extensor pollicis longus* Extensor pollicis brevis*	Loss of CM, MP, & IP extension of thumb (abd. pollicis brevis may act at IP as an extensor)
	Abductor pollicis longus*	Weakness of thumb abduction (abductor pollicis brevis)

*Posterior interosseous branch.

Suprascapular nerve

Situation of innervated muscles	Muscles	Effects of paralysis by nerve destruction
Shoulder	Supraspinatus	Difficulty with initiating abduction of humerus (deltoid [teres minor and subscapularis can assist deltoid by holding down humeral head])
	Infraspinatus	Slight weakness of lateral rotation of humerus (post. fibres deltoid, teres minor)

Long thoracic nerve

Situation of innervated muscles	Muscles	Effects of paralysis by nerve destruction
Shoulder girdle	Serratus anterior	Weakened protraction of scapula (pectoralis major and minor) Weakened lateral rotation of scapula (trapezius) and hence weakened and restricted abduction of upper limb on trunk Scapula not held against ribs—'winged scapula'

The lower limb

Introduction

The parts of the lower limb are the hip and buttock, the thigh, the leg, and the foot and toes.

The hip and buttock make up what is called the **gluteal region**. This overlies the side and back of the pelvis, extending from the waist down to the groove (**gluteal fold**) which limits the buttock inferiorly and to the hollow on the lateral side of the hip. The hip and buttock are not clearly distinguished from each other. The **hip** (*coxa*) is the upper part of the region in a lateral view; the **buttock** (*natis*) is the rounded bulge behind and below. The **natal cleft** is the groove between the buttocks. In it can be felt the lower part of the sacrum and coccyx (the end of the backbone). Anterior to this the perineum lies in the depths of the cleft and continues forwards between the thighs.

The skeleton of the hip and buttock is the **hip bone**. It consists of three parts which are fused together at the **acetabulum** [Fig. 114] where the head of the femur articulates with it. The **ilium** is the large, upper part with a crest [Fig. 114] which can be felt in the lower margin of the waist. The **ischium** is the postero-inferior part on which the body rests in a sitting position. The

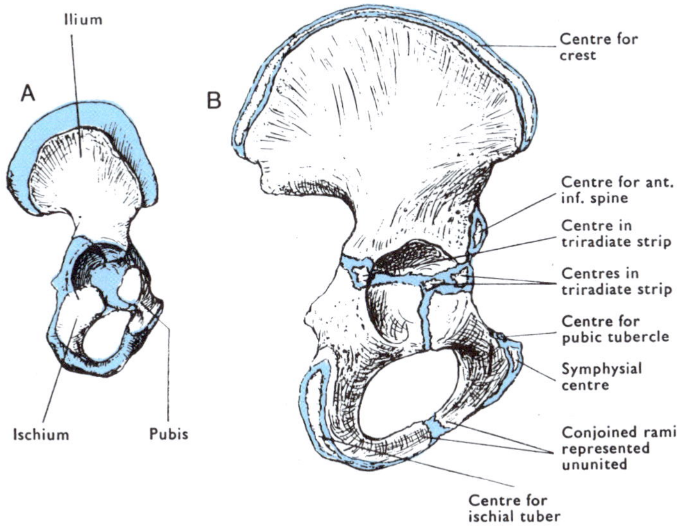

Fig. 112. Ossification of hip bone. The more anterior of the secondary centres in the acetabular cartilage may remain separate as an os acetabuli.

A. At birth
B. About 12 or 13 years

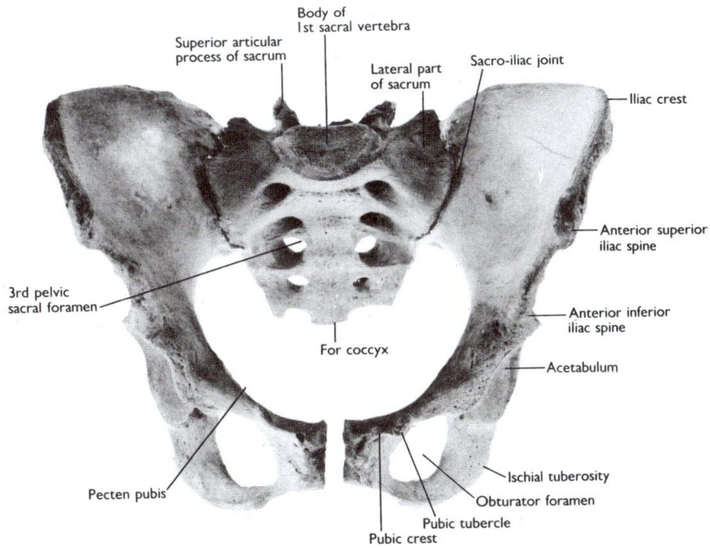

Fig. 113. The female pelvis seen from in front without the coccyx.

pubis is the anterior part. It can be felt in the lower part of the anterior abdominal wall where it meets its fellow in the **pubic symphysis** (*symphysis*= union) and separates that wall from the anterior part of the perineum.

The right and left hip bones, together with the sacrum and coccyx, make up the skeleton of the pelvis. The floor of the pelvic cavity is the **perineum**. The two hip bones together are sometimes called the **pelvic girdle**. Anteriorly, they articulate with each other at the pubic symphysis. Posteriorly they articulate with the sides of the sacrum at the **sacro-iliac joints**.

The **thigh** (*femur*) extends from the hip to the knee. Its bone is the **femur** which articulates at its upper end with the hip bone to form the hip joint. At the **knee joint**, the femur articulates with the **tibia** and with the **patella** (knee cap) which lies anterior to the knee joint.

The proximal extent of the thigh is at the gluteal fold posteriorly, at the groove of the groin (**inguinal region**) anteriorly, at the perineum medially, and at the hollow on the side of the hip laterally. The greater trochanter of the femur [Fig. 115] can be felt through the skin immediately anterior to the hollow. The ham (*poples*) is the lower part of the back of the thigh and the back of the knee where the hollow of the ham is the **popliteal fossa**.

The **leg** (*crus*) extends from the knee joint to the ankle joint. The term 'leg' is never used in anatomical descriptions to refer to the entire lower limb as it frequently is in colloquial speech. The soft, fleshy part of the back of the leg is the **calf** (*sura*).

The bones of the leg are the **tibia** or shin bone and the **fibula**. They lie side by side, with the slender fibula laterally, and articulate with each other (tibiofibular joints) only at their upper and lower ends. Elsewhere they are united by an **interosseous membrane**. The lower ends of the tibia and fibula form prominences at the sides of the ankle (**medial** and **lateral malleoli**) which are readily felt and which clasp the first bone of the foot (the **talus**) to form the **ankle joint**. The flattened superior surface of the expanded proximal end of the tibia (condyles of the tibia) articulates with the femur at the knee joint. The proximal end of the fibula (head) only reaches as far proximally as the inferolateral surface of the lateral tibial condyle and does not take part in the knee joint. A large part of the tibia is subcutaneous and readily felt. This includes the anterior [Fig. 250] and medial [Fig. 252] borders, the medial surface [Fig. 250] between these borders, and the parts of the condyles visible in [Fig. 250].

The fibula is mainly an attachment for muscles which cover it so that only its head and distal quarter [Fig. 250] are easily felt. Some of the muscles attached to the fibula are called **peroneal muscles** from *peroné*—the Greek equivalent of the Latin *fibula* (=a pin or skewer).

The **foot** extends from the point of the heel to the roots of the toes. Its superior surface is the **dorsum**, its inferior surface is the **sole** (*planta*). The foot is divided into tarsus and metatarsus. The **tarsus** is the posterior half formed by the tarsal bones. The **tarsal bones** are in two rows. The proximal row consists of two large bones set one (the **talus**) above the other (the **calcaneus**). The calcaneus is the largest bone of the tarsus and forms the skeleton of the heel. The talus articulates with the superior surface of the calcaneus and separates it from the ankle joint which the talus forms with the tibia and fibula. The distal row consists of the **cuboid bone** laterally and the three wedge-shaped **cuneiform bones** (*cuneus*=a wedge) set side by side, medially. The cuboid articulates proximally with the calcaneus and distally with the lateral two metatarsals. The cuneiforms articulate distally with the medial three metatarsals but are separated from the talus by the **navicular bone** which lies between the two rows. The navicular articulates proximally with the talus and distally with the three cuneiforms. Between the tarsal bones are the intertarsal joints [Figs. 254, 255].

The five **metatarsal bones** are set side by side. They are numbered 1–5 from the medial side. The proximal ends (**bases**) articulate with the tarsal bones (tarsometatarsal joints) and with each other (intermetatarsal joints—lateral four only). Each has a distal end (**head**) which articulates with the base of the proximal phalanx of the corresponding toe (metatarsophalangeal joint). The **toes** (digits) are numbered from the medial side. The first is the big toe or **hallux**, the fifth is the little toe or **digitus minimus**. The bones of the toes are the **phalanges**. The hallux has two phalanges, each of the other toes has three, though the middle and distal phalanges of the little toe may be fused together. The phalanges articulate at **interphalangeal joints**. The proximal end of the phalanx is its base, the distal end is its head.

There are several **sesamoid bones** in the lower limb. The largest is the patella. The remainder are small and inconstant except for two which are always present on the plantar surface of the metatarsophalangeal joint of the big toe. They produce grooves on the plantar surface of the head of the first metatarsal [Fig. 255].

The hip and thigh

Before starting to dissect, study the surface anatomy of the region on yourself or on another living subject and relate this to the appropriate dried bones.

Surface anatomy and bones

The **hip bone** [Fig. 114] has the appearance of a propeller with a large, sinuous blade (the **ilium**) directed upwards and a smaller blade, perforated by a large aperture (the **obturator foramen**) directed downwards. The two blades are almost at right angles to one another and meet at a narrow, thick hub where the fossa (**acetabulum**) for articulation with the head of the femur lies. The small blade consists of the **pubis** anteromedially and the **ischium** posterolaterally. These two are fused together (1) in the bar of bone inferior to the obturator foramen (**inferior ramus of the pubis** amd **ramus of the ischium**) and (2) at the **acetabular notch**. In the acetabulum they also fuse with the ilium, the superior ramus of the pubis at the **iliopubic eminence** [Fig. 244], and the ischium at the rough ridge on the posterior surface of the acetabulum.

The posterior margin of the ilium is deeply notched immediately above the acetabulum by the **greater sciatic notch**. The medial aspect of the ischium has a shallow **lesser sciatic notch** separated from the greater notch by the **spine of the ischium**. Immediately inferior to the lesser notch, the ischium expands posteriorly to form the **ischial tuberosity**.

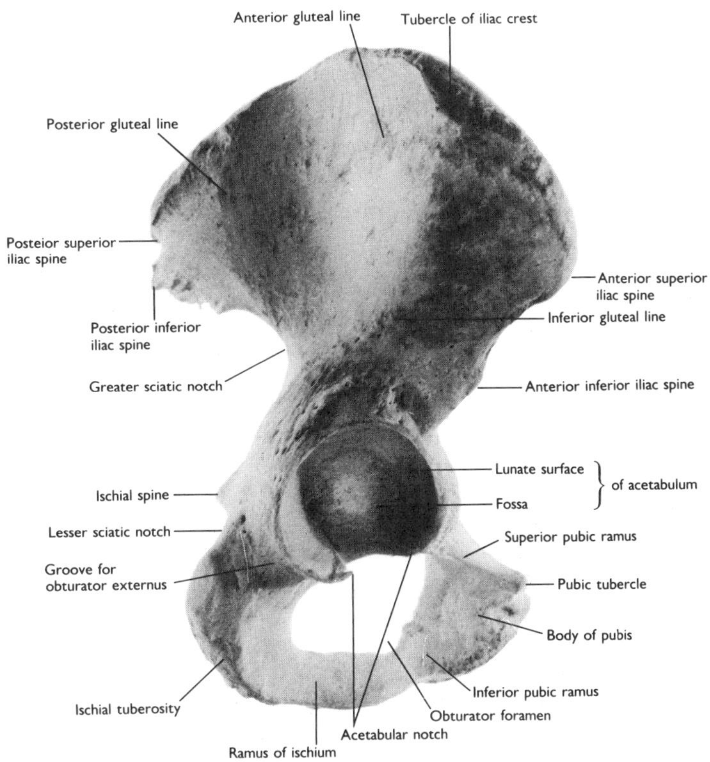

Fig. 114. Right hip bone seen from the lateral side.

The **body of the pubis** [Fig. 114] articulates with its fellow through a median fibrous pad. This is the **pubic symphysis** which may be felt at the inferior extremity of the abdominal wall in the median plane. Draw your finger laterally from the symphysis on the anterosuperior surface of the body of the pubis. The bone which is felt is the **pubic crest** which ends in a small, blunt prominence (the **pubic tubercle**) 2.5 cm laterally. The tubercle is less easily felt in the male because it is covered by the spermatic cord. Lateral to the pubic tubercle, a resilient band can be felt in the inguinal groove between the anterior surface of the thigh and the abdomen. This is the **inguinal ligament**. On the bone, note a sharp ridge which curves posterolaterally on the superior ramus of the pubis from the pubic tubercle to the iliopubic eminence. This is the **pecten pubis**. Deep fibres of the inguinal ligament turn posteriorly to be attached to the pecten and thus form the **lacunar ligament** [Fig. 128]. Below and behind the pubic symphysis, the **inferior pubic rami** diverge to form the **pubic arch**. Each inferior pubic ramus, with the corresponding **ramus of the ischium**, forms the boundary between the thigh and perineum and the entire length of the margins of these rami is palpable.

Find the **iliac crest** at the lower margin of the waist. Trace it forwards. It slopes downwards and slightly medially to end in a rounded knob, the **anterior superior iliac spine**. This may be grasped between finger and thumb in a thin individual. The inguinal ligament stretches from this spine to the pubic tubercle. On the bone, there is a notch on the anterior margin of the ilium inferior to the spine and below this the **anterior inferior iliac spine** lies immediately above the acetabulum. The inferior spine is in two parts. The upper for attachment of the tendon of the rectus femoris muscle, the lower for the strong **iliofemoral ligament** of the hip joint. Trace the outer lip of the iliac crest posteriorly until you feel a low prominence, the **tubercle of the iliac crest**. This is the widest part of the pelvis and the highest part seen from in front, though the highest point is further posteromedially at the level of the spine of the fourth lumbar vertebra. Further posteriorly the iliac crest turns steeply downwards to end in the **posterior superior iliac spine** at the level of the second sacral segment.

The superficial, **gluteal surface** of the ilium is marked by three ridges which curve upwards and forwards across it. These **gluteal lines** (posterior, anterior, and inferior [Fig. 114]) mark the attachment of aponeurotic layers between the **gluteal muscles**. Thus they mark the areas of attachment of these muscles to the ilium [Fig. 243].

The **greater trochanter of the femur** can be palpated indistinctly immediately in front of the hollow on the side of the hip. The top of the trochanter [Fig. 115] lies at the level of the pubic crest. The **head of the femur** can be felt indistinctly even though it is deeply buried in muscles. Place your finger just below the inguinal groove at the **mid-inguinal point**, that is *midway between the anterior superior iliac spine and the pubic symphysis*. Press firmly and rotate your limb medially and laterally. The head will be felt moving behind the muscles. With lighter pressure the **femoral artery** can be felt pulsating at the same spot.

Study the main features of the femur with reference to Figs. 115 and 116.

The spherical **head of the femur** fits into the acetabulum where it articulates with the C-shaped **lunate surface**. This is a broad strip extending inwards from the margin of the acetabulum to the edge of the non-articular **acetabular fossa** in the centre of the acetabulum. This fossa is continuous inferiorly with the floor of the **acetabular notch** between the ends of the lunate surface. The acetabular notch is converted into a foramen by the **transverse ligament of the acetabulum** which bridges the notch and thus completes the acetabular margin. The foramen and the acetabular fossa give rise to a sleeve of synovial membrane which contains some connective tissue and small blood vessels and converges on the non-articular **pit of the head of the femur**. This **'ligament' of the head of the femur** may transmit some small blood vessels to the head of the femur. They pass through foramina in the pit of the head.

The **neck of the femur** joins the head to the body and greater trochanter of the femur. It meets them posteriorly at a prominent, rounded ridge (the **intertrochanteric crest**) which extends from the **greater trochanter** above to

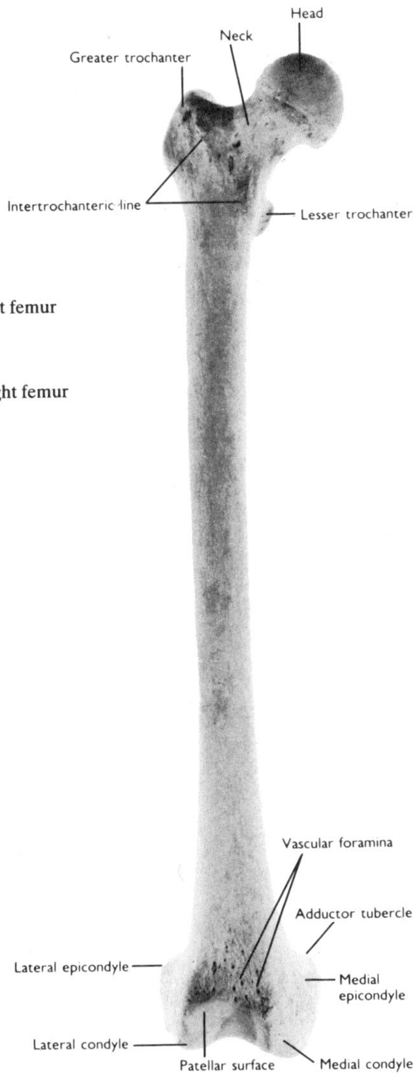

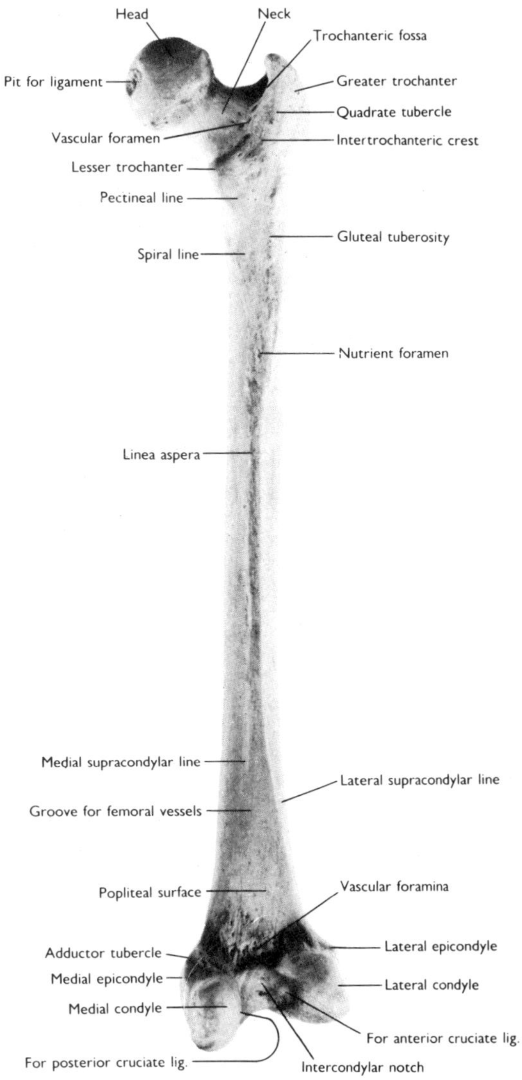

Fig. 115 (*left*) Right femur (anterior aspect).

Fig. 116 (*right*) Right femur (posterior aspect).

the **lesser trochanter** below. Anteriorly, the neck meets them in a rough **intertrochanteric line** which extends downwards from the greater trochanter and turns backwards on the inferior surface towards the posteriorly situated lesser trochanter. This line gives attachment to the powerful **iliofemoral ligament**—a thickening of the fibrous capsule.

The **neck** forms an angle of approximately 125 degrees with the body of the femur and deepens as it approaches the body. This is because of a thick bar of bone which is present in the lower part of the neck to carry the compressive forces applied to it by the weight of the body resting on the head of the femur. The neck is ridged longitudinally by bundles of fibres **(retinaculae)** which curve back along it from the fibrous capsule of the hip joint and transmit many blood vessels which pierce the neck. Note the foramina for these vessels, particularly on the superior surface of the neck and sometimes on a small, non-articular area of the superior margin of the head. These vessels form the main blood supply for the head and neck of the femur.

From the postero-inferior surface of the neck a slight groove can be traced upwards on the posterior surface of the neck of the femur towards the trochanteric fossa. This groove lies approximately midway between the head and intertrochanteric crest and marks the edge of the **tendon of obturator externus** [p. 150] and the attachment of the weak, posterior part of the **fibrous capsule of the hip joint**.

The greater trochanter overhangs the neck posteriorly and is excavated on its medial side by the **trochanteric fossa**.

The **body of the femur** is surrounded by muscles and cannot be felt easily. It is convex anteriorly, particularly in its proximal half. Most of its surface is smooth except for a keel-like ridge (the **linea aspera**) which projects posteriorly from its middle two quarters for the attachment of muscles. Superiorly and inferiorly the medial and lateral lips of the linea aspera diverge. Superiorly they pass on either side of the lesser trochanter and the **pectineal line** which descends from it, to form the **spiral line** anteriorly and the rough **gluteal tuberosity** posteriorly. The spiral line becomes continuous above with the intertrochanteric line and can be traced along the lower margin of the greater trochanter into continuity with the gluteal tuberosity posteriorly. Inferiorly the lips of the linea aspera form the medial and lateral **supracondylar lines** [Fig. 116]. These are the boundaries of the flattened **popliteal surface of the femur**. The lateral supracondylar line continues downwards to the lateral epicondyle. The medial line is interrupted where the femoral artery crosses it to become the popliteal artery. It reappears inferiorly and continues to the **adductor tubercle** on the medial epicondyle of the femur.

The distal end of the body of the femur widens into the two **condyles**. Posteriorly the condyles are separated by a wide **intercondylar fossa**. Anteriorly their articular surfaces unite in the grooved **patellar surface**. The lateral surface of this groove is more extensive and projects further fowards than the medial surface. The margin of the lateral surface may be felt proximal to the patella when the knee is flexed. Each condyle has a flattened, conical projection (**epicondyle**) from its superficial surface [Figs. 115, 116]. The lateral epicondyle has a fossa at its apex for the attachment of the lateral head of the muscle **gastrocnemius** [Fig. 249]. Below this is a fossa with a groove running posteriorly from it. The **tendon of popliteus** is attached to the fossa and lodges in the groove when the knee is flexed. The posterior surface of the medial epicondyle is marked by the attachment of the medial head of gastrocnemius; the adductor tubercle is on the superior surface of the epicondyle.

Identify the condyles of the femur and their epicondyles in your own knee. The condyles of the tibia and femur can be differentiated by the movement of the tibia when the knee is flexed and extended. Grasp the **patella** and try to move it. The patella is mobile when the knee is extended but becomes rigid when the knee is flexed. Feel the strong **ligamentum patellae** which stretches inferiorly from the patella to the **tibial tuberosity** (a blunt prominence on the front of the upper end of the tibia) and becomes taut when the knee is flexed. In this movement, the patella slides on to the distal end of the femur exposing the upper part of the patellar surface.

With your knee straight, a muscular strip with three tendons posterior to it

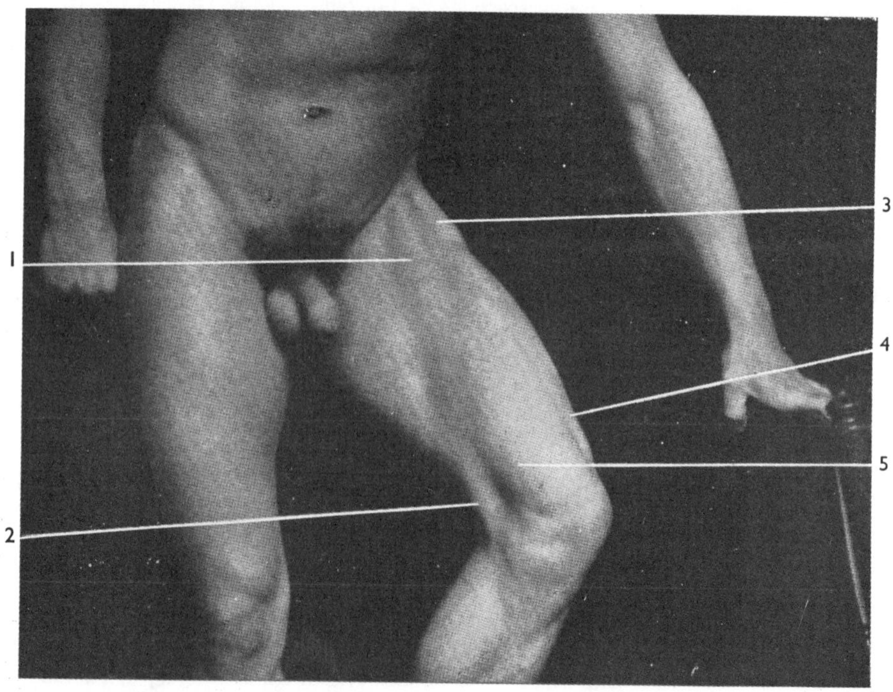

Fig. 117. (A) Sartorius in action.
1. Sartorius.
2. Semitendinosus applied to semimembranosus covered by sartorius and gracilis.
3. Tensor fasciae latae.
4. Vastus lateralis.
5. Vastus medialis.

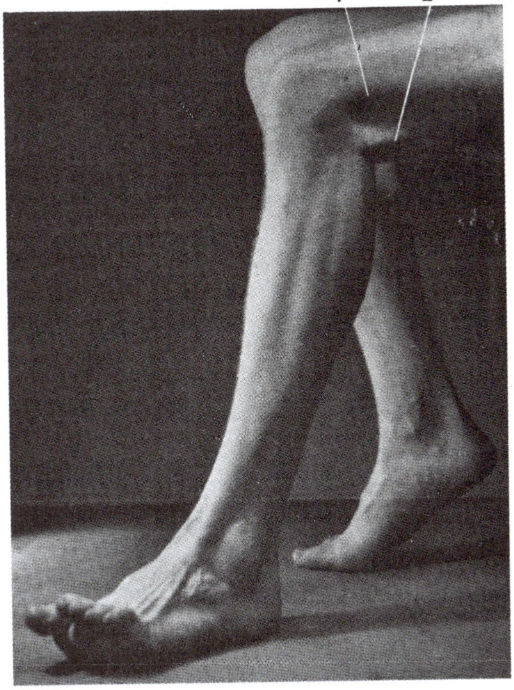

(B) Lateral rotation of leg upon thigh. Note the interval between the tendon of biceps femoris and the iliotibial tract covering vastus lateralis.
1. Iliotibial tract.
2. Biceps femoris.
(Both photographs courtesy of Professor R. D. Lockhart.)

can be felt on the medial side of the knee posterior to the medial epicondyle. As the knee flexes, these pass backwards to form a projecting medial border to the popliteal fossa, which is behind the knee. The muscle is **sartorius**, the two cord-like tendons are those of **gracilis** and **semitendinosus**. The third tendon, more deeply placed and less readily felt, is that of **semimembranosus**. On the lateral side, a single stout tendon can be felt posterior to the lateral epicondyle when the knee is bent. This is the tendon of **biceps femoris**. Trace it to the **head of the fibula**. Anterior to this tendon is a depression and then a broad, tendon-like structure which is best felt when standing with the knee slightly bent. This **iliotibial tract** is a thickened strip of deep fascia of the thigh through which gluteus maximus and tensor fasciae latae are inserted into the lateral condyle of the tibia.

Proximal to the medial epicondyle of the femur is a fleshy swelling. This is the lowest part of the **vastus medialis muscle** [Fig. 117]. When the knee is bent, a shallow groove appears posterior to this part of the muscle. Press your finger into the groove and feel the **tendon of the muscle adductor magnus**. Slide your finger distally on the tendon to the adductor tubercle where the tendon is attached.

Front of the thigh

Dissection

Make incisions 9 and 10 [Fig. 118] through the skin. Reflect the skin from the superficial fascia and turn it laterally. As there is very little superficial fascia at the knee, care must be taken not to destroy the patellar plexus of cutaneous nerves [Fig. 123].

Superficial fascia

In the thigh, the superficial fascia consists of a thick superficial layer and a deeper membranous layer which are continuous with the same layers in the anterior abdominal wall. The membranous abdominal layer is attached to the deep fascia of the thigh by a linear fusion which extends medially to the pubic tubercle [Fig. 119]. Thence the line of fusion extends downwards across the front of the body of the pubis to the superficial margin of the inferior pubic ramus along which it extends to the ischial tuberosity. This fusion separates the zone of loose fibrous tissue deep to the membranous layer in the anterior abdominal wall and perineum from the thigh [Fig. 119] but leaves communication between the abdominal wall and perineum anterior to the pubic bones. This is the route of descent of the testis into the scrotum and of

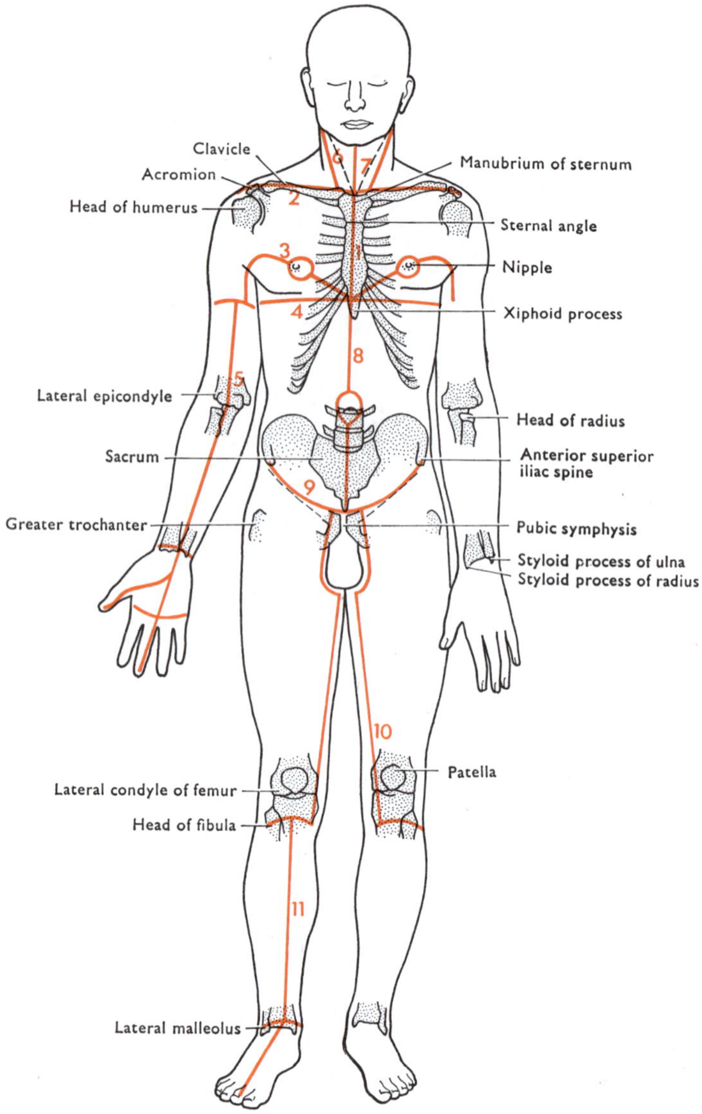

Fig. 118. Landmarks and incisions. For the bony landmarks of the lower limb, see illustrations of individual bones.

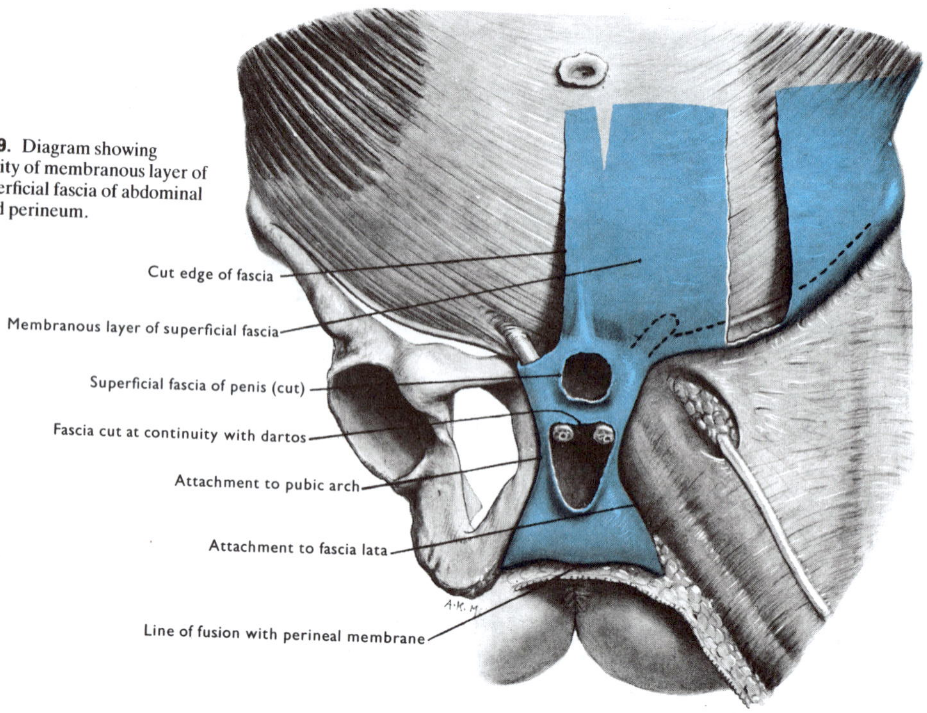

Fig. 119. Diagram showing continuity of membranous layer of the superficial fascia of abdominal wall and perineum.

fluid from the perineum into the abdominal wall, e.g. in rupture of the urethra in the male.

If the abdomen is being dissected at the same time as the lower limb, the following dissection should be carried out.

Dissection

If the abdomen has not been dissected, make a horizontal incision through the entire thickness of the superficial fascia of the anterior abdominal wall from the anterior superior iliac spine to the midline. Raise the superficial fascia inferior to the cut and pass the fingers downwards between the membranous layer of the fascia and the aponeurosis of the external oblique muscle [Fig. 119]. Little resistance to the passage of the fingers is felt till the line of fusion of the membranous layer with the deep fascia is reached at the fold of the groin. Pass the fingers medially along this line and find the opening into the perineum just medial to the pubic tubercle. Note that a finger can easily be passed into the perineum but cannot be carried laterally into the thigh because of the line of fusion. In the male, the finger passes beside the spermatic cord towards the scrotum; in the female, it passes into the base of the labium majus.

Dissectors of the lower limb should now find the **great saphenous vein** in the superficial fascia of the medial part of the anterior surface of the thigh. Trace the vein downwards to the knee and upwards to the point where it turns sharply backwards through the deep fascia to enter the femoral vein. As the upper part is exposed, note the lower group of **superficial inguinal lymph nodes** scattered along the vein and the delicate, thread-like lymph vessels which enter them.

At least three small veins enter the great saphenous vein at its upper end. Follow these and the small superficial inguinal branches of the femoral artery which pierce the deep fascia and accompany them to supply the adjacent skin and lymph nodes. The **superficial external pudendal vessels** pass medially to the external genital organs, the **superficial epigastric** run superiorly to the anterior abdominal wall, and the **superficial circumflex iliac** course in the lateral part of the groin [Fig. 121]. When tracing these vessels, note the upper group of superficial inguinal lymph nodes which lie scattered along the lower border of the inguinal ligament. They vary greatly in number and size.

Identify the **superficial inguinal ring.** This is an opening in the aponeurosis of the external oblique muscle of the abdomen immediately superolateral to the pubic tubercle. The **spermatic cord**

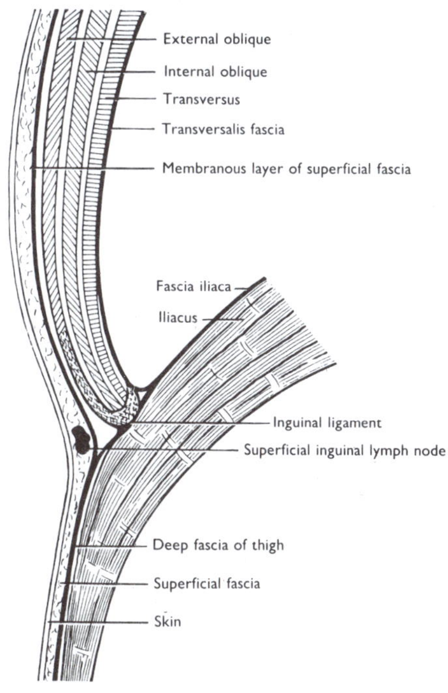

Fig. 120. Diagram of fasciae and muscles of inguinal and subinguinal regions lateral to femoral sheath. Cf. Fig. 130.

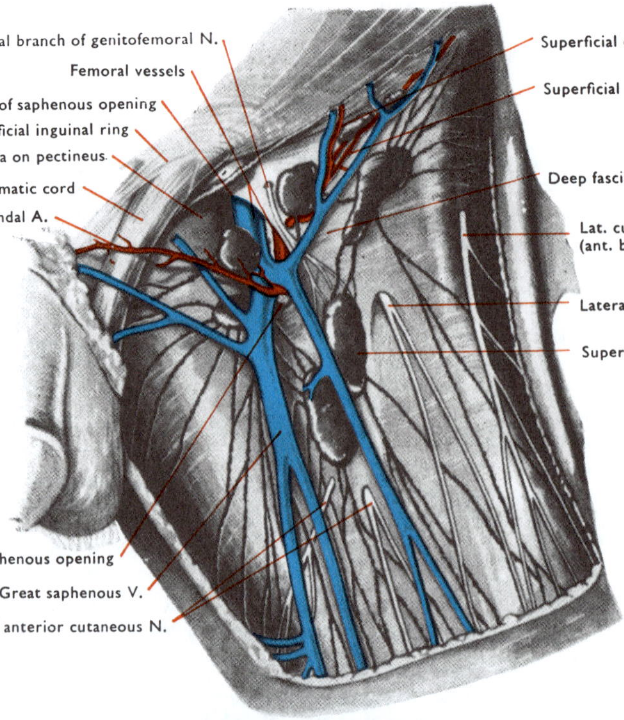

Fig. 121. Superficial dissection of proximal part of front of thigh. The saphenous opening and the superficial lymph nodes and lymph vessels of the groin are displayed. The lymph vessels may be recognized by their beaded appearance.

(round ligament of the uterus in the female) emerges through this ring with the **ilio-inguinal nerve** on its lateral side [Fig. 123]. Trace the branches of the ilio-inguinal nerve to the skin of the upper medial part of the thigh. It also sends branches to the external genital organs.

Lift the upper extremity of the great saphenous vein and note that it turns backwards over a sharp edge of the deep fascia. Follow this edge round the lateral side of the vein and upwards towards the inguinal ligament. This is the falciform margin of the **saphenous opening** [Fig. 121]. From this margin, the thin **cribriform fascia** passes in front of the opening and the femoral vessels in the femoral sheath and fuses with the deep fascia of the thigh medial to these vessels.

Remove the cribriform fascia to expose the femoral sheath. Take care not to damage the structures which pierce the cribriform fascia or lie posterior to it.

The **femoral sheath** is an extension of the fascial lining of the abdominal cavity which surrounds the upper 4 cm of the femoral artery and vein. The vein lies posterior to the saphenous opening, the artery is behind its lateral margin. Medial to the vein, the sheath surrounds the tubular **femoral canal** through which a femoral hernia [p. 139] may pass into the groin. Here the hernia lies posterior to the thin cribriform fascia and pushes it forwards producing a swelling beside the upper end of the great saphenous vein. This swelling may be mistaken for a distention of the upper end of the great saphenous vein especially as both types of swelling are made more obvious by raising the intra-abdominal pressure, e.g. by coughing, for both are connected with the abdomen.

Saphenous opening

In this area the deep fascia is the thin, perforated, **cribriform fascia** (*cribrum*=a sieve). It transmits the great saphenous vein, one or more of the superficial inguinal arteries, and efferent lymph vessels from the superficial inguinal lymph nodes. The area lies approximately 3–4 cm inferolateral to the pubic tubercle and is about 3 cm long and 1.5 cm wide. Except on the medial side it is limited by the sharp, **falciform margin** of the thicker deep fascia which surrounds it [Fig. 121]. The cribriform fascia lies anterior to the femoral sheath and becomes continuous medially with the fascia covering the pectineus muscle which slopes backwards and laterally behind the femoral sheath.

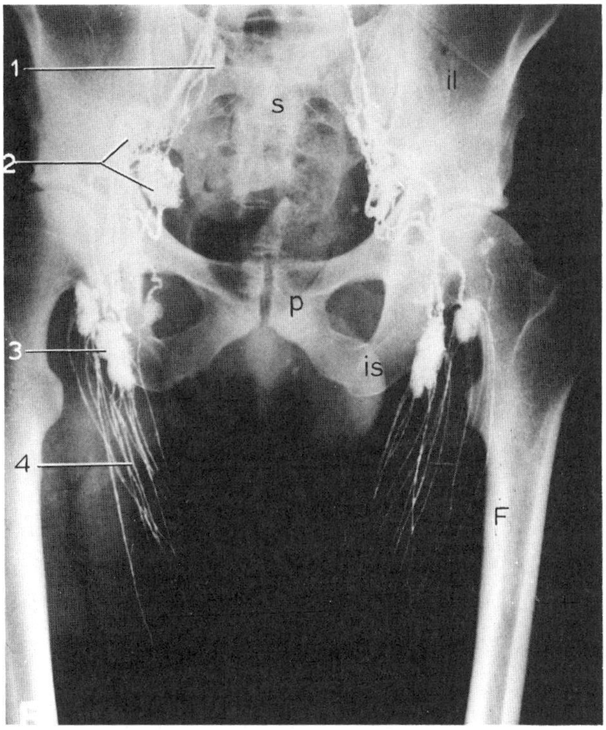

Fig. 122. Lymphangiogram of some of the lymph vessels and nodes draining the thigh. This is produced by the injection of some lymph vessels with X-ray-opaque dye followed by a radiograph after an interval to permit the dye to ascend in the vessels and through the nodes. Only the lymph vessels and nodes which drain lymph from the injected region are shown; the remainder are invisible.
F. Femur.
il. Ilium.
is. Ischium.
p. Pubis.
s. Sacrum.
1. Common iliac lymph node.
2. External iliac lymph nodes.
3. Inguinal lymph nodes.
4. Superficial lymph vessels of the anterior surface of the thigh.

Superficial inguinal lymph nodes

These lie in the superficial fascia and are arranged in the shape of a T. The upper nodes are below and more or less parallel to the inguinal ligament. The lower nodes are placed along the upper part of the great saphenous vein [Figs. 121, 179].

The nodes receive lymph from the skin and superficial fascia over a wide area. (1) *From the trunk* below the level of the umbilicus. This includes the perineum together with the anal canal, lower vagina and urethra, the external genitalia and scrotum. *It excludes (a) the testis from which lymph drains exclusively to the lumbar lymph nodes in the abdomen;* (b) the glans penis which drains principally to the deep inguinal lymph nodes. (2) *The lower limb*. This includes the gluteal region but *excludes the heel and lateral part of the foot from which lymph drains into the popliteal fossa* with the small saphenous vein [Figs. 179, 180]. (3) A few lymph vessels from the fundus and body of the uterus reach the superficial inguinal lymph nodes along the round ligament of the uterus.

The superficial inguinal lymph nodes are connected together by many lymph vessels. Their efferents pass through the cribriform fascia to the deep inguinal lymph nodes on the femoral vessels and the external iliac nodes on the external iliac vessels in the abdomen [see Vol. 2].

Great saphenous vein

This is the largest and thickest-walled superficial vein of the lower limb. It begins on the medial side of the dorsum of the foot and runs upwards and backwards anterior to the medial malleolus and then on the medial surface of the distal third of the tibia. It then ascends on the medial border of the tibia to the posteromedial surface of the knee and inclines anteriorly through the thigh to enter the femoral vein through the saphenous opening. In the leg, the great saphenous vein lies between two layers of membranous fascia and is crossed by a more superficial plexus of veins which tend to join it near the knee. The vein has several *communications* through the deep fascia with the deep veins. Most contain valves which only permit blood to flow from the great saphenous vein into deep veins after these have been emptied by compression from surrounding muscles. They include: (1) communications with the medial plantar veins on the medial surface of the foot; (2) communications with the anterior tibial veins anterior to the ankle; (3) communications with tributaries of the posterior tibial veins behind the medial margin of the tibia; (4) it is continuous with the femoral vein at the saphenous opening.

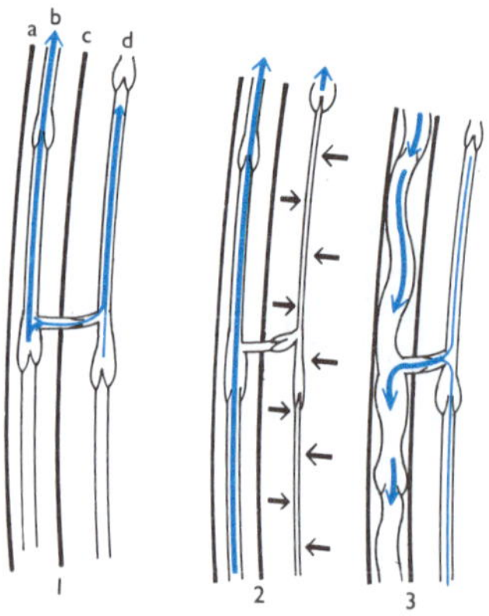

Fig. 124. Diagrams to show the flow of blood in the superficial and deep veins. In 1, blood flows from a superficial vein through a communicating vein into a deep vein which has previously been emptied by contraction of the surrounding muscles as shown in 2. Such segments of deep veins emptied by surrounding pressure can only be filled with blood either from lower parts of the same vein or from the superficial veins at a pressure which is independent of the pressure above the next superior competent valve. In 3, dilatation of the superficial and communicating veins makes their valves incompetent so that blood flows distally in the superficial veins and from the deep veins to the superficial veins when the muscles contract. This further distends and elongates the superficial veins which become tortuous and are continually subjected to the full head of venous pressure in the erect position. Clearly such varicose veins prevent proper venous return and dam back the entry of arterial blood to the region thus leading to poor nutrition and the non-healing of injuries. Also, small cuts into the vein wall can lead to rapid exsanguination unless elevated above the heart level.
a. Skin.
b. Superficial vein in the superficial fascia.
c. Deep fascia.
d. Deep vein.

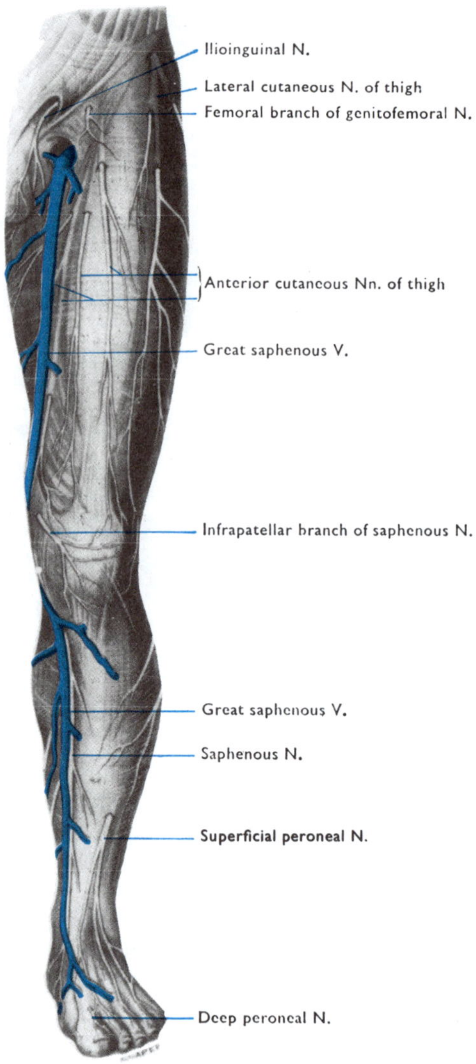

Fig. 123. Cutaneous nerves on front of lower limb. See also Fig. 140.

Valves in the great saphenous vein divide its column of blood into segments and so reduce the pressure on the distal parts of its walls in the upright position so long as blood from these segments is draining into emptied deep veins through communicating vessels. This system breaks down if there is no muscular contraction to empty the deep veins or if the valves in the communicating vessels become incompetent. When they do, muscular contraction forces blood into the superficial veins instead of pushing it upwards through the valves of the deep veins. This raises the pressure in the superficial veins which eventually dilate thus making their valves incompetent and worsening the position.

Superficial inguinal ring

This aperture in the aponeurosis of the external oblique muscle of the abdominal wall transmits the spermatic cord or the round ligament of the uterus. It lies above the medial end of the inguinal ligament immediately superolateral to the pubic tubercle.

Dissection

Strip the superficial fascia downwards from the front and lateral side of the thigh by blunt dissection. Leave the deep fascia in place. With the assistance of Figs. 121 and 123 find the points at which the cutaneous nerves pierce the deep fascia and follow them distally. Note how most of these nerves terminate in the patellar plexus anterior to the patella. Check for the presence of a prepatellar bursa between the skin and lower part of the patella.

Cutaneous nerves

From the lumbar plexus	Ilio-inguinal nerve Femoral branch of the genitofemoral nerve Lateral cutaneous nerve of the thigh
From the femoral nerve	Anterior cutaneous branches to the thigh Saphenous nerve
From obturator nerve	Occasional branch to medial side of thigh

The **ilio-inguinal nerve** (L. 1) emerges through the superficial inguinal ring. It is distributed to the scrotum or to the labium majus and the adjacent part of the thigh.

The **femoral branch of the genitofemoral nerve** (L. 1, 2) is small and difficult to find. It enters the thigh posterior to the inguinal ligament and pierces the deep fascia lateral to the saphenous opening. The nerve supplies an area of skin immediately below the inguinal ligament.

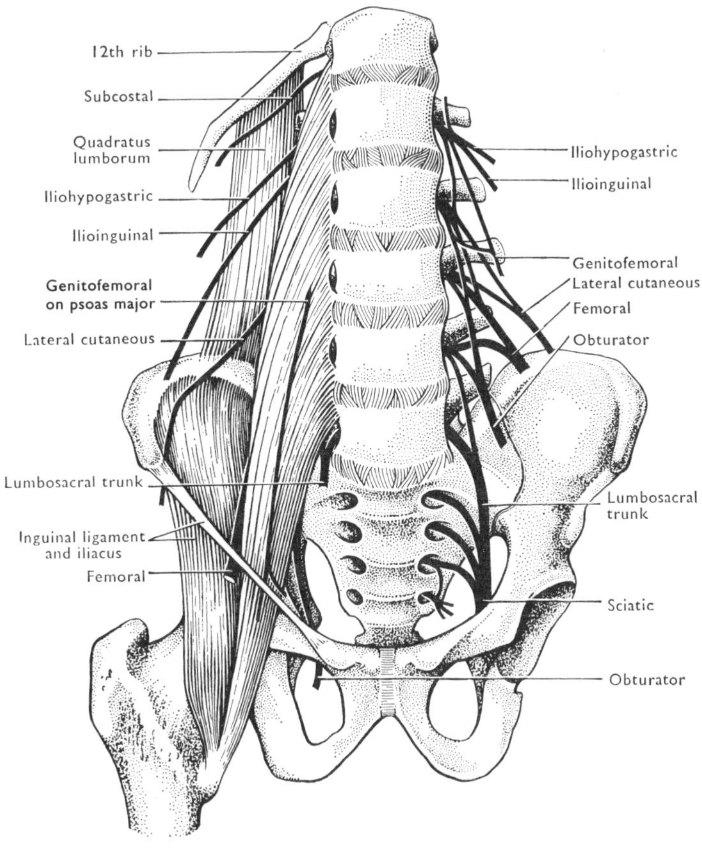

Fig. 125. Lumbar plexus (semi-diagrammatic) in relation to quadratus lumborum and iliopsoas muscles.

The **lateral cutaneous nerve of the thigh** (L. 2, 3) enters the thigh posterior to the lateral part of the inguinal ligament. A posterior branch pierces the deep fascia first and passes backwards to supply an area of skin over the greater trochanter [Fig. 140]. The remainder of the nerve pierces the deep fascia lower down. It descends to the lateral side of the patella sending branches to the skin of the lateral and anterior surface of the thigh.

There are commonly three **anterior cutaneous branches** of the femoral nerve (L. 2, 3) [Figs. 123, 140]. They supply the skin of the anterior and medial surfaces of the thigh and upper part of the medial surface of the leg. The more medial the branch, the more distal the point at which it pierces the deep fascia. (Occasionally the anterior branch of the obturator nerve supplies the distal two-thirds of the medial surfaces of the thigh.)

The **saphenous nerve** (L. 3, 4) descends with the femoral artery deep to the sartorius muscle [Fig. 132]. It sends an **infrapatellar branch** through that muscle [Fig. 123] to supply skin medial to the knee and distal to the patella. The main nerve pierces the deep fascia posterior to sartorius at the knee. It then descends with the great saphenous vein supplying branches to the skin of the medial surface of the leg. It ends in the skin of the medial surface of the foot.

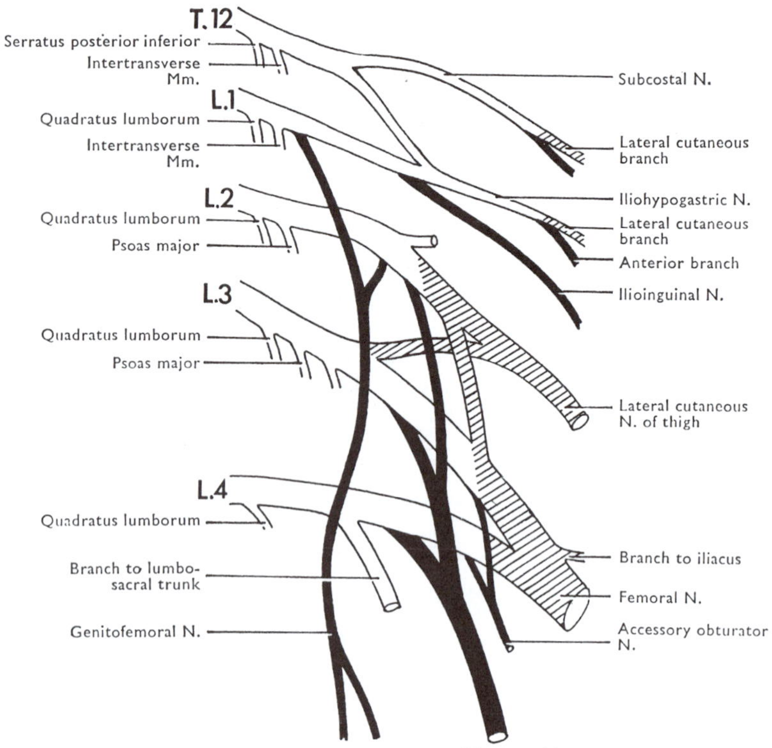

Fig. 126. Diagram of lumbar plexus. Ventral offsets, black: dorsal offsets, cross hatched. Cf. the arrangement of the brachial plexus [Fig. 24]. For the sacral part of the lumbosacral plexus see Fig. 145.

Patellar plexus

This is formed by branches from the lateral cutaneous nerve of the thigh, the lateral and intermediate anterior cutaneous branches of the femoral nerve, and the infrapatellar branch of the saphenous nerve. The nerve fibres which run through the plexus supply skin over the patella, the ligamentum patellae, and the proximal part of the tibia anteriorly. Here, as in other nerve plexuses, the individual nerve fibres entering the plexus do not anastomose but merely run in the same connective tissue sheath.

Dissection

Complete the exposure of the deep fascia of the front and lateral side of the thigh leaving at least the stumps of the cutaneous nerves as they pierce it so that they may be followed to their origins later. Trace the deep fascia upwards to the iliac crest, inguinal ligament, and the body of the pubis.

Fascia lata

This is the name given to the deep fascia of the thigh. Like deep fascia elsewhere in the body it is continuous with the periosteum of the underlying bones either directly where the bone is subcutaneous or indirectly through intermuscular septa where the bones are covered by muscles. Thus the stocking of fascia lata is attached around the root of the limb (a) to the iliac crest laterally, (b) to the inguinal ligament anteriorly, (c) to the body and inferior ramus of the pubis and to the ramus and tuberosity of the ischium medially, and (d) to the sacrotuberous ligament (q.v.) and sacrum posteriorly. At the knee it fuses with the patella, the femoral and tibial condyles, and the head of the fibula. Posteriorly it is continuous with the dense fascia covering the popliteal fossa.

The fascia lata is thin medially and where it forms the cribriform fascia. Laterally it forms a thick band from the iliac crest to the lateral tibial condyle,

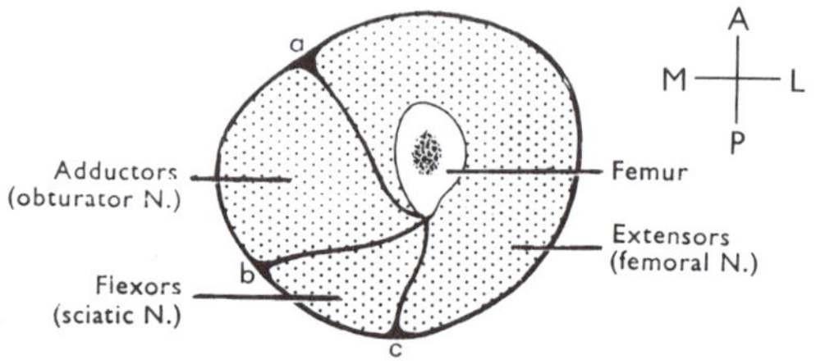

Fig. 127. Diagram to show the arrangement of the three intermuscular septa and the three osteofascial compartments of the right thigh seen from above.
a. Medial intermuscular septum
b. Posterior intermuscular septum
c. Lateral intermuscular septum
A. Anterior.
P. Posterior.
M. Medial.
L. Lateral.

the **iliotibial tract**. From the iliac crest the **gluteus maximus** posteriorly and the **tensor fasciae latae** anteriorly pass into the tract. Through it they help to stabilize the pelvis on the thigh and to maintain extension of the knee in standing.

Between its proximal and distal attachments the fascia lata sends intermuscular septa to the linea aspera of the femur. These (medial, posterior, and lateral [Fig. 127]) separate the thigh into three *compartments* each of which contains a group of muscles and the nerve which supplies them: (1) *anteriorly and laterally, the extensor muscles and the femoral nerve;* (2) *medially, the adductor muscles and the obturator nerve;* (3) *posteriorly, the flexor muscles (hamstrings) and the sciatic nerve*. The extensor group consists principally of four large muscles (quadriceps femoris) which are inserted together into the patella. Their tendinous fibres also continue over the anterior surface of the patella into the patellar ligament which anchors the patella to the tibial tuberosity and represents the continuation of the tendon of quadriceps.

Patellar bursae
[Fig. 200]

A number of bursae are present in the region of the knee. These allow free movement of the skin on the underlying tissues, e.g. in kneeling, and of the deep tissues on each other. There are two or three subcutaneous bursae in front of the patella and of the lower part of the ligamentum patellae and the tibial tuberosity.

Deep bursae

(1) A large **suprapatellar bursa** separates the tendon of quadriceps femoris from the front of the femur. It extends a hand's breadth proximal to the patella and is usually continuous with the cavity of the knee joint. (2) A **deep infrapatellar bursa** lies between the tibia and the ligamentum patellae immediately proximal to the tuberosity.

Deep dissection of the front of the thigh

Inguinal ligament

The free lower border of the aponeurosis of the external oblique muscle of the abdomen forms the inguinal ligament. It extends from the anterior superior iliac spine to the pubic tubercle and its edge is curved back on itself to form a groove on the abdominal aspect. The fascia lata is attached to the rounded external surface of the entire length of the ligament making it convex inferiorly by the tension which that fascia applies to it.

Lateral to the pubic tubercle, the deep surface of the inguinal ligament extends posteriorly to be attached to the pecten pubis. This triangular **lacunar ligament** [Fig. 128] has its apex at the pubic tubercle while its base

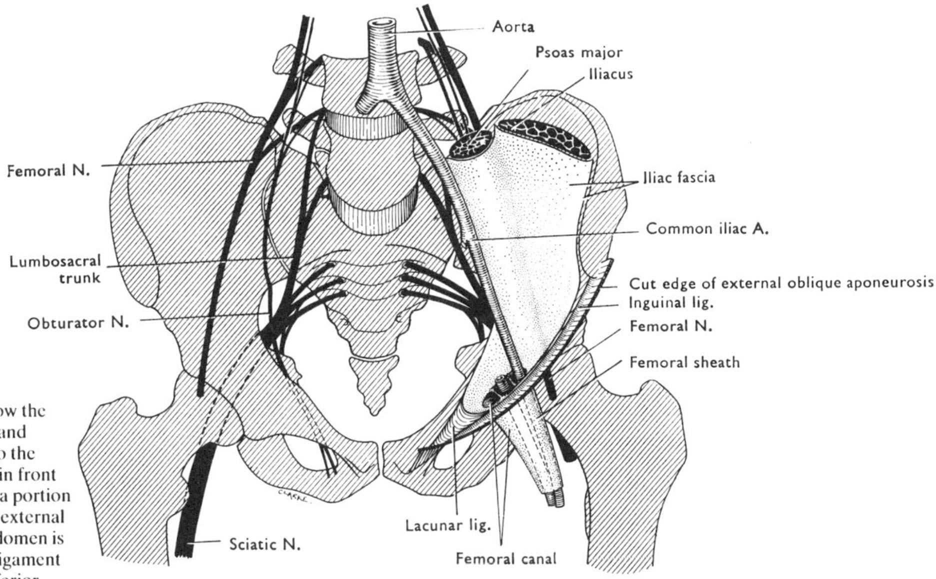

Fig. 128. Diagram to show the routes of entry of nerves and femoral blood vessels into the lower limb, viewed from in front and above. On the right, a portion of the aponeurosis of the external oblique muscle of the abdomen is shown with the inguinal ligament formed from its rolled inferior margin. The lacunar ligament passes posteriorly from this to be attached to the pubis and encircle the medial border of a funnel of fascia, the femoral sheath, which encloses the femoral vessels and femoral canal, and passes into the femoral triangle. The fascia of this sheath is continuous above with the fascia iliaca, which covers the psoas and iliacus muscles on the posterior abdominal wall, and anteriorly with the transversalis fascia, which lines the deep surface of the anterior abdominal wall. Note that the femoral nerve lies posterior to the fascia iliaca and hence is outside the femoral sheath as it enters the thigh. On the left, note how the sciatic and femoral nerves are packed close to the plane of the hip joint, thus minimizing tension on them during movements of the limb.

Fig. 129. Dissection to show femoral sheath and structures which pass between inguinal ligament and hip bone. Seen from below and in front.

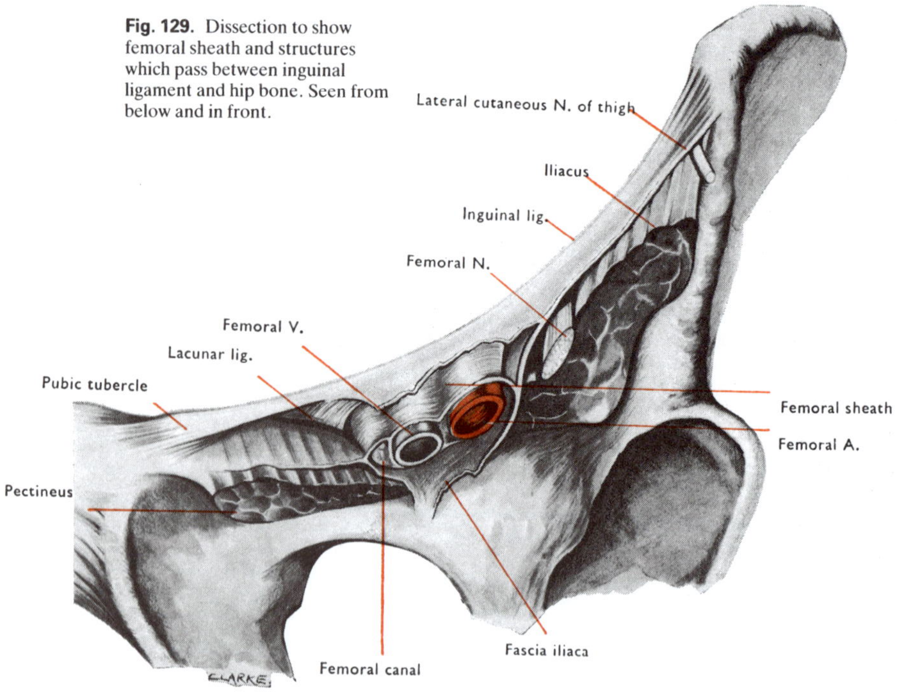

forms a sharp, crescentic margin medial to the aperture through which the femoral vessels enter the thigh enclosed in the femoral sheath.

Femoral sheath

To understand this region, the dissector should appreciate certain general points. (1) The anterior and posterior abdominal walls and the thigh meet at the inguinal ligament. (2) The inguinal ligament bridges a gap between it and the hip bone through which structures pass from the abdomen into the thigh. (3) The abdominal and pelvic walls are lined by a complete fascial sac inside which are the peritoneum, the abdominal viscera, and the major blood vessels. Thus the part of the sac lining the deep surface of the anterior abdominal wall (**transversalis fascia**) meets the part of it covering the lower part of the posterior abdominal wall (**iliac fascia**) at the inguinal ligament [Fig. 120]. Here muscles (psoas and iliacus) and nerves (femoral and lateral cutaneous of thigh) in the posterior abdominal wall escape into the thigh behind the iliac fascia and the lateral part of the inguinal ligament. The external iliac vessels in the abdomen become the femoral vessels as they pass behind the medial part of the inguinal ligament carrying with them a funnel-shaped sheath of the fascial lining of the abdomen, transversalis fascia anteriorly and iliac fascia posteriorly [Fig. 130]. This **femoral sheath** lies

Fig. 130. Diagram of fasciae and muscles of inguinal and subinguinal regions in the line of the femoral vein. Cf. Fig. 120.

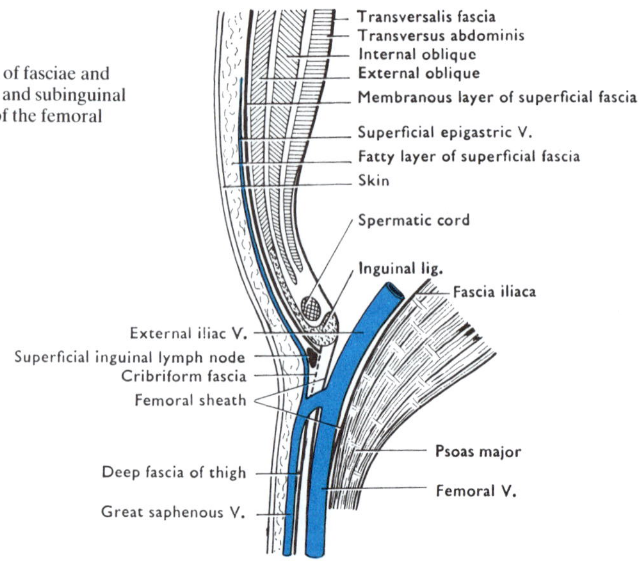

immediately lateral to the lacunar ligament [Figs. 128, 129] and encloses the femoral artery and the **femoral branch of the genitofemoral nerve** laterally, the femoral vein, and medial to that a space, the **femoral canal**. This canal, which allows for the expansion of the femoral vein within the sheath, narrows inferiorly and disappears where the sheath fuses with the adventitia of the vessels at the lower margin of the saphenous opening. The canal contains a little loose fatty tissue (the femoral septum), a small lymph node, and some lymph vessels.

Dissection

Follow the great saphenous vein through the anterior wall of the femoral sheath and expose the femoral vein which it enters. Split the femoral sheath lateral and medial to this to expose the femoral artery and the femoral canal, respectively. Note the septa of the sheath which separate the compartments in which the artery, vein, and canal lie and that the canal is much shorter than the spaces which contain the vessels. Introduce your little finger into the canal and push it upwards. It is possible to enter the abdomen through the canal but the tip of your finger is separated from the peritoneal cavity by the peritoneum which covers the abdominal opening of the canal. At the abdominal opening of the canal (the **femoral ring**) feel the edge of the lacunar ligament medially, the inguinal ligament anteriorly, and the pecten pubis posteriorly.

Femoral canal

This short fascial tube rapidly diminishes in width from above downwards and is closed inferiorly by fusion of its walls. The wide upper end (femoral ring) faces into the abdomen and is separated from the abdominal cavity only by the peritoneum—the smooth, innermost lining of the abdominal walls. The **boundaries of the femoral ring** are: the inguinal ligament, anteriorly; the sharp edge of the lacunar ligament medially; the pecten of the pubic bone, posteriorly; the femoral vein, laterally. Below the inguinal ligament, the canal lies posterior to the saphenous opening and the thin cribriform fascia and anterior to the fascia covering the pectineus muscle [Fig. 131].

Femoral hernia

This is the name given to the protrusion of some of the abdominal contents through the femoral canal into the thigh. With the assumption of the erect posture in man, the weight of the abdominal contents presses on the inguinal region where the femoral ring forms a point of weakness inviting the entry of a loop of intestine. The size of the femoral ring is limited anteriorly by the inguinal ligament. Thus anything which stretches the inguinal ligament and draws it forwards away from the pubic bone allows the femoral ring to enlarge. This is common in abdominal distention with weakening of the abdominal muscles and is frequently the result of childbearing—a situation which is aggravated by the larger space which is normally present posterior to the inguinal ligament in the female because of the wider female pelvis. For these reasons, femoral hernia is commoner in the female. It is obvious also that any condition which raises the intra-abdominal pressure, e.g. repeated coughing or straining, will predispose to the development of such a hernia.

If a loop of intestine is forced into the femoral ring, it carries the peritoneum covering the abdominal opening of the canal in front of it. This forms a hernial sac which descends in the femoral canal posterior to the weak cribriform fascia and bulges forwards through it into the superficial fascia of the thigh close to the saphenous vein. If the sac continues to enlarge, it expands superolaterally in the superficial fascia so that the entire hernia comes to be U-shaped. Because of this, any attempt to return the hernial sac and its contents to the abdomen by external pressure requires that the sac should first be pushed towards and through the cribriform fascia before an attempt is made to return it through the distended femoral canal.

However much the hernial sac may expand in the subcutaneous tissue, the margins of the femoral ring form a constricting neck to the sac, especially the sharp edge of the **lacunar ligament**. This tends to obstruct the passage of the contents of any loop of gut in the sac and may even occlude the blood vessels passing to it (strangulation of the hernia) so that the loop becomes gangrenous and may rupture. Surgical reduction of the hernia commonly requires division of the lacunar ligament to make room for the return of the sac and its contents to the abdomen. Care has to be exercised in dividing the lacunar ligament because of the presence of an abnormal obturator artery in 30 per cent of individuals. This abnormal artery arises from the inferior epigastric artery instead of the internal iliac artery and commonly crosses the abdominal aspect of the lacunar ligament [Vol. 2].

Femoral triangle

This triangle is bounded by [Fig. 131]: the inguinal ligament (base) superiorly; the medial border of sartorius laterally; the medial border of adductor longus medially. Inferiorly, the apex of the triangle is continuous with a narrow intermuscular space, the **adductor canal**, through which the femoral vessels travel down to the popliteal fossa.

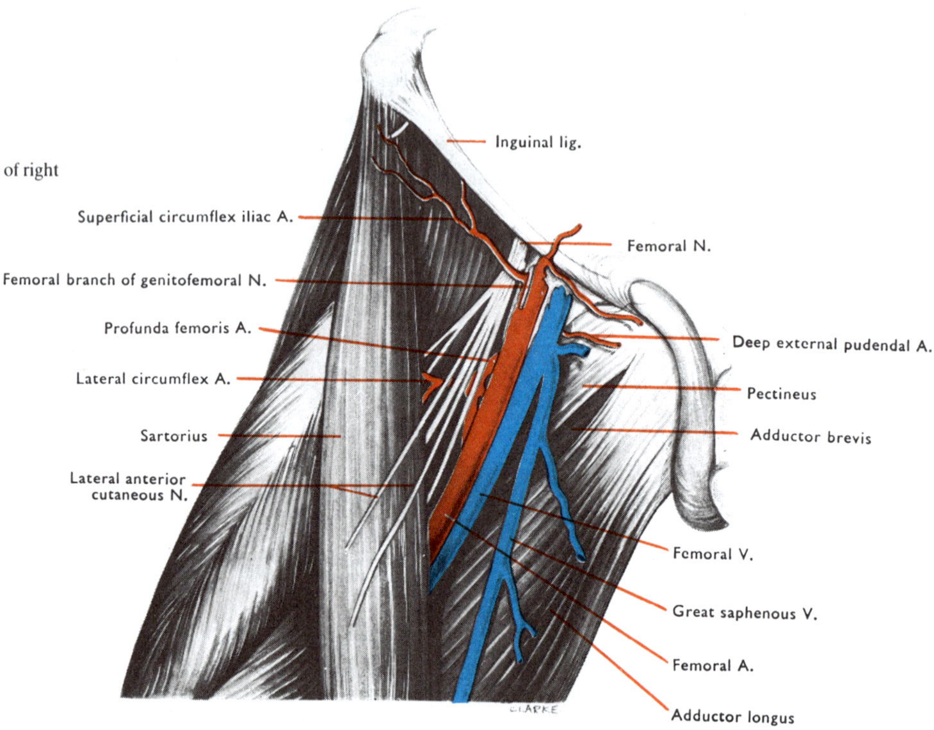

Fig. 131. Dissection of right femoral triangle.

The superficial fascia of the *anterior wall* of the triangle contains the superficial inguinal lymph nodes and lymph vessels, the upper part of the great saphenous vein, the femoral branch of the genitofemoral nerve, branches of the ilio-inguinal nerve, and the superficial branches and tributaries of the femoral vessels. Most of these structures pierce the cribriform fascia of this wall.

The *posterior wall* consists of adductor longus, pectineus, psoas major, and iliacus, from medial to lateral side. The posterior wall is concave anteriorly with its central hollow occupied by the femoral vessels with the profunda and medial circumflex vessels posteriorly.

Dissection

Expose the sartorius and adductor longus muscles down to the apex of the triangle where they meet. Preserve the nerves in the vicinity of the sartorius [Fig. 131].

Place a block under the knee to flex the hip joint and relax the structures in the triangle.

Find the femoral nerve lateral to the artery in the groove between the psoas and iliacus muscles and note that it rapidly divides into a number of cutaneous and muscular branches. Find the nerve to pectineus passing medially behind the femoral artery. Follow the other branches of the femoral nerve till they leave the triangle. Avoid injury to the lateral circumflex artery which passes laterally among these nerves near their origin.

Trace the vessels. Retain the large venous trunks but remove the venae comitantes of the smaller arteries to get a clear picture of the arrangement of the vessels. Find the deep external pudendal artery which arises from the upper part of the femoral artery and runs medially. Identify the root of the large profunda femoris artery which arises from the posterolateral surface of the femoral artery about 5 cm below the inguinal ligament. Follow it downwards with the profunda vein behind the femoral vessels till it leaves the triangle. Find the lateral and medial circumflex arteries which stem from the profunda near its origin or from the adjacent femoral artery. Trace the lateral artery as far as sartorius and the medial one backwards as far as possible behind the femoral vessels. Preserve the proximal parts of the circumflex veins which enter the femoral vein.

Trace the nerve to pectineus behind the femoral vein. Remove the fascia from the pectineus and find the anterior branch of the obturator nerve behind the interval between it and adductor longus. The nerve descends behind both muscles in front of the adductor brevis.

Strip the fascia from the surface of iliacus and psoas major. Place your finger on the anterior surface of the tendon of psoas and push it downwards and backwards following the line of the tendon. It is usually possible to reach the lesser trochanter of the femur to which the tendon is attached. The medial circumflex artery passes backwards between the psoas and pectineus muscles parallel to your finger. Expose it as far as possible.

Contents of the femoral triangle

1. The **femoral vessels** traverse the triangle from base to apex. The vein is medial to the artery at the base but behind it at the apex.

2. The **profunda femoris artery** [p. 168] is the main artery supplying the thigh. It arises from the posterolateral side of the femoral artery, curves downwards behind it, and passes posterior to the adductor longus close to the femur. The profunda vein is anterior to its artery and ends in the femoral vein.

3. The **lateral** and **medial circumflex arteries** usually spring from the profunda near its origin. The lateral artery runs among the branches of the femoral nerve and leaves the triangle posterior to sartorius. The medial artery passes backwards between the psoas and pectineus muscles. The circumflex veins end in the femoral vein.

4. The **deep external pudendal** is a small artery which arises from the medial side of the femoral artery near the base of the triangle. It runs medially to the scrotum in the male and to the labium majus in the female.

5. Three or four **deep inguinal lymph nodes** lie along the medial side of the femoral vein. Afferent lymph vessels reach them from the superficial inguinal and popliteal lymph nodes and from the deep structures of the limb. Efferent lymph vessels pass from the deep inguinal nodes along the femoral vessels to the external iliac nodes on the external iliac vessels in the abdomen.

6. The **femoral branch of the genitofemoral nerve** [p. 135] is distributed to the skin over the femoral triangle.

7. The **lateral cutaneous nerve of the thigh** crosses the lateral angle of the triangle.

8. The **femoral nerve** [p. 143].

Dissection

Expose the sartorius down to its insertion into the tibia.

Make a vertical incision through the fascia lata from the tubercle of the iliac crest to the lateral margin of the patella. Remove the fascia lata between the incision and sartorius. This uncovers the tensor fasciae latae and parts of the four elements of the quadriceps muscle, while leaving the greater part of the iliotibial tract in position.

Find: (1) the rectus femoris in the middle of the front of the thigh; (2) part of the vastus lateralis lateral to rectus femoris; (3) a small part of the vastus intermedius which appears to be the lower part of the vastus lateralis; (4) part of the vastus medialis between the lower parts of rectus femoris and sartorius. Raise the rectus femoris and follow it to its origin on the hip bone [Fig. 133].

Trace the lateral circumflex artery behind the sartorius and the rectus femoris. Follow its three branches: (1) The descending branch follows the anterior border of the vastus lateralis; (2) The ascending branch runs between sartorius and tensor fasciae latae on a deeper plane. Remove the fat and fascia from this interval; (3) A small transverse branch enters vastus lateralis.

Lift the middle third of sartorius laterally. This exposes a narrow strip of fascia, the roof of the adductor canal, between the vastus medialis and the adductor muscles. Divide the fascia longitudinally and find the femoral vessels, the saphenous nerve, and the nerve to vastus medialis in the canal [Fig. 132].

Sartorius
[Figs. 133, 141, 157, 161]

This long, strap-like muscle arises from the anterior superior iliac spine and runs a spiral course across the front of the thigh to reach the posterior part of the medial side of the knee. Inferior to this, it curves forwards as a thin tendinous sheet to the upper part of the medial surface of the tibia [Fig. 171]. This tendon is separated by a bursa (**bursa anserina**) from the tendons of gracilis and semitendinosus which are inserted posterior to it.

The sartorius forms the lateral boundary of the femoral triangle, covers the roof of the adductor canal, and produces a vertical, fleshy ridge far back on the medial side of the extended knee. When the knee is flexed, the muscle slips backwards into the medial boundary of the popliteal fossa. **Nerve supply:** the femoral nerve. **Action:** it flexes both the hip joint and the knee joint and rotates the thigh laterally to bring the limb into the position adopted by a cross-legged tailor (*sartor*=a tailor). When the knee is flexed, it medially rotates the tibia on the femur.

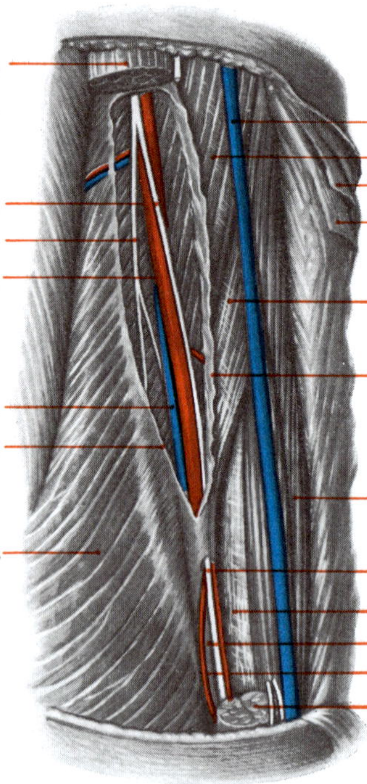

Fig. 132. Dissection of adductor canal in the right thigh. A portion of the sartorius has been removed.

Adductor canal

The femoral vessels, the **saphenous nerve**, and the nerve to vastus medialis lie in this canal. It is a deep furrow on the medial side of the thigh between vastus medialis anteriorly and the adductor longus and magnus muscles posteriorly. The furrow is converted into the canal by a strong fascial layer stretched across it on which the sartorius muscle lies. This fascial layer is pierced inferiorly by the saphenous nerve and then fuses with the tendon of adductor magnus. At this level, there is an aperture in the adductor magnus muscle, the tendinous (adductor) opening, through which the femoral vessels pass from the canal into the popliteal fossa.

The **nerve to vastus medialis** descends for some distance in the canal before all its branches enter that muscle.

Femoral artery
[Figs. 129, 131, 158, 161]

This is the main artery of the lower limb and is directly continuous with the external iliac artery of the abdomen behind the inguinal ligament at the mid-inguinal point [p. 126]. Here it is medial to the femoral nerve and lateral to the femoral vein and lies on psoas major anterior to the hip bone against which it may be compressed to control bleeding from a more distal point. The artery enters the femoral triangle anterior to the head of the femur and is covered only by skin and fasciae in the triangle. It leaves the triangle at its apex and traverses the adductor canal with the femoral vein, the saphenous nerve, and the nerve to vastus medialis. Here it lies close to the posteromedial surface of the shaft of the femur, anterior to adductor longus and then adductor magnus, and receives a branch from the obturator nerve. It becomes the **popliteal artery** by passing through the tendinous opening in adductor magnus.

The *course* of the femoral artery may be indicated on the skin by the upper two-thirds of a line drawn from the mid-inguinal point to the adductor tubercle with the thigh in a position of slight flexion, abduction, and lateral rotation.

Branches

The main branch and the principal artery of the thigh is the **profunda femoris,** though one or both circumflex arteries may arise directly from the femoral artery. Three small superficial arteries of the groin [p. 131] and the deep external pudendal artery also arise in the femoral triangle. Muscular twigs are given off in the adductor canal, and the **descending genicular artery** arises a short distance above the opening in the adductor magnus. This branch supplies adjacent muscles and the knee joint, and sends a branch with the saphenous nerve to the medial side of the knee and leg [Fig. 153].

Femoral vein
[Figs. 131, 132, 158, 161]

This is the direct continuation of the popliteal vein. It begins at the opening in the adductor magnus and accompanies the femoral artery to the inguinal ligament behind which it becomes the external iliac vein. The vein is mainly posterior to the artery but is posterolateral inferiorly and medial in the upper part of the femoral triangle.

The femoral vein contains several **valves.** One is constantly present proximal to the entry of the profunda vein. Open the vein and examine the valves.

Tributaries

The veins in the thigh correspond to the branches of the arteries. However, the *superficial veins of the groin end in the great saphenous vein* and the circumflex veins enter the femoral vein, though the corresponding arteries are usually branches of the profunda artery.

Femoral nerve

It arises from the lumbar plexus in the abdomen [Figs. 125, 126], descends in the grove between iliacus and psoas major, behind the iliac fascia, and enters the thigh posterior to the inguinal ligament and lateral to the femoral sheath [Fig. 129]. It ends by dividing into a number of branches 2 cm below the inguinal ligament.

Muscular branches to:
- Pectineus.
- Sartorius.
- Quadriceps femoris, with articular branches.

Cutaneous branches:
- Anterior cutaneous nerves of the thigh (medial and lateral).

Saphenous nerve.

The supply to quadriceps femoris is by separate nerves to each of its four parts—rectus femoris and the three vasti. **Articular branches**. The nerve to rectus femoris sends a branch to the hip joint; the nerves to the vasti send branches to the knee joint. Thus the nerves to the parts of the quadriceps which act only on the knee joint (vasti) send branches to that joint; the nerve to the part that acts also on the hip joint sends a branch to that joint.

The **lateral anterior cutaneous nerve** (L. 2, 3) may pierce the medial border of sartorius. For distribution see Fig. 218.

The **medial anterior cutaneous nerve** (L. 2, 3) runs along the medial margin of sartorius and crosses the femoral vessels at the apex of the femoral triangle [Fig. 123].

The **saphenous nerve** (L. 3, 4) is the longest branch of the femoral nerve and the only one that has its main distribution in the leg and foot. It accompanies the femoral vessels in the adductor canal, pierces the fibrous roof of the distal part of the canal, and appears at the posterior border of the sartorius medial to the knee [p. 191].

The **nerve to pectineus** arises a short distance below the inguinal ligament. It runs medially and downwards behind the femoral vessels to pectineus.

Two or three **nerves to sartorius** usually arise in common with the lateral anterior cutaneous nerve.

The **nerves to rectus femoris** (usually two) enter the deep surface of the muscle. The upper one supplies a twig to the hip joint.

The **nerve to vastus medialis** enters the adductor canal and divides into branches which enter the muscle at different levels. It sends a branch to the knee joint.

The **nerve to vastus lateralis** passes deep to rectus femoris and accompanies the descending branch of the lateral circumflex artery to the anterior border of the muscle. It usually gives a branch to the knee joint.

Two or three **nerves to the vastus intermedius** enter its anterior surface. The most medial nerve is a long slender branch which runs along the medial edge of vastus intermedius to the articularis genus muscle [p. 146]. Its terminal filaments pass to the knee joint.

Lateral circumflex artery
[Figs. 131, 160]

This is the largest branch of the profunda femoris artery. It supplies structures on the lateral side of the hip and thigh from iliac crest to knee joint. It arises from the profunda near its origin and runs laterally among the branches of the femoral nerve and then deep to rectus femoris. Here it divides into ascending, transverse, and descending branches.

The **ascending branch** passes along the intertrochanteric line of the femur under cover of tensor fasciae latae to the gluteal surface of the ilium. It supplies the surrounding muscles and the hip joint, and anastomoses with the **superior gluteal artery**. The small **transverse branch** passes backwards through the vastus lateralis. It anastomoses with other arteries posterior to the femur [p. 158]. The **descending branch** runs along the anterior border of vastus lateralis. It supplies a large part of the quadriceps and sends a long branch through vastus lateralis to the anastomosis at the knee joint.

Tensor fasciae latae
[Figs. 133, 158, 160]

This thick, short muscle lies at the junction of the gluteal region and the upper part of the front of the thigh. It is enclosed between layers of the iliotibial tract. The muscle arises from the anterior part of the iliac crest and is inserted into the iliotibial tract 3–5 cm below the level of the greater trochanter. **Nerve supply:** superior gluteal nerve. **Actions:** it flexes and medially rotates the hip joint, and extends the knee through the iliotibial tract.

Iliotibial tract
[Figs. 158, 159]

This thick band of fascia lata runs vertically on the lateral side of the thigh from the iliac crest to the lateral condyle of the tibia.

Inserted into it are the greater part of gluteus maximus behind and the tensor fasciae latae in front. These muscles help to steady the pelvis on the thigh and, through the tract, keep the knee joint firmly extended in the erect posture. Then the tensed tract is readily felt on the lateral side of the thigh immediately proximal to the lateral condyle of the femur. By comparison the flaccid quadriceps and mobile patella indicate that quadriceps is not responsible for maintaining knee extension in standing.

Superiorly most of the posterior part of the tract passes deep to gluteus maximus while its anterior part splits to enclose tensor fasciae latae, the intermediate part passing directly to the iliac crest. Inferiorly the tract is

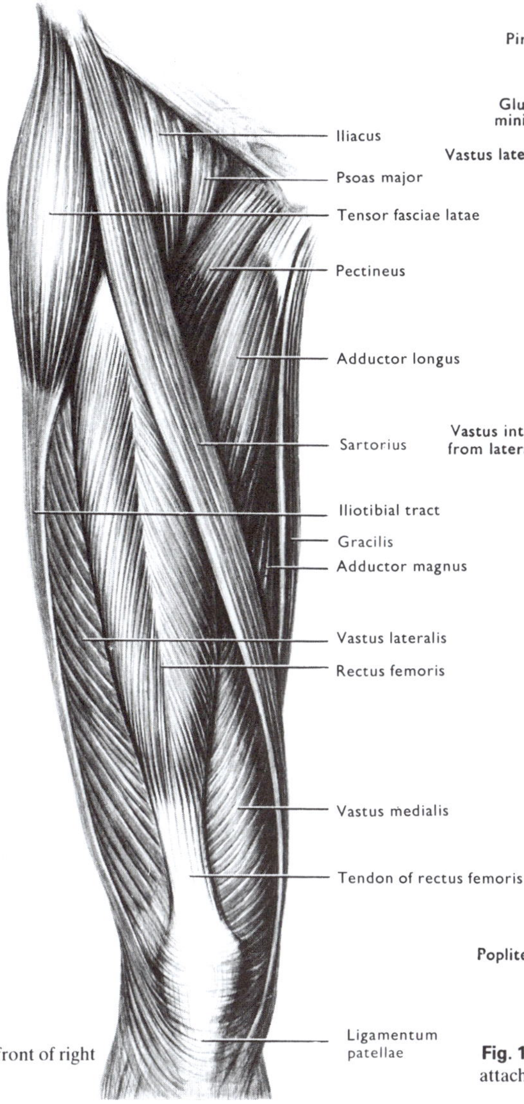

Fig. 133. Muscles of front of right thigh.

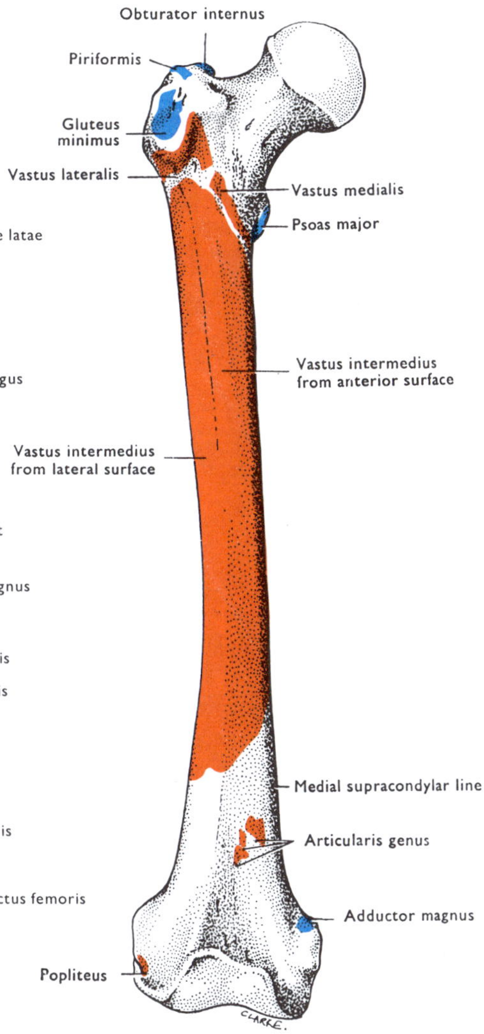

Fig. 134. Right femur (anterior aspect) to show muscle attachments.

continuous with the rest of the fascia lata and the lateral intermuscular septum.

Dissection

To expose the lateral intermuscular septum, detach vastus lateralis from it and reflect the muscle forwards.

Intermuscular septa

In the thigh there are lateral, medial, and posterior intermuscular septa [Fig. 127]. The lateral is strong; the others are thin fascial layers on the front and back of the adductor muscles. All three pass to the linea aspera (rough line) and the corresponding supracondylar line. All muscles attached to the body of the femur pass only to these lines except vastus intermedius [Figs. 134, 136]. The order of attachment of these muscles to the linea aspera is that of their position in the thigh, i.e. from medial to lateral, vastus medialis, the adductors, the short head of biceps (the only representative of the flexor muscles of the thigh attached to the femur), and vastus lateralis.

The fibrous **lateral intermuscular septum** passes from the deep surface of the iliotibial tract to the lateral supracondylar line and the linea aspera between vastus lateralis and the short head of biceps femoris which arise from it.

Quadriceps femoris
[Figs. 133, 158, 160]

This is the powerful extensor of the knee joint. All its four parts are inserted into the patella and act together *on the tibial tuberosity through the patella and the patellar ligament*. Vastus medialis, intermedius, and lateralis arise from the femur and, acting solely on the knee joint, are more or less fused together. The rectus femoris arises from the hip bone and is also a flexor of the hip joint. It is more separate than the vasti and only fuses with them as it approaches insertion into the patella. Because of the wide range of movement which is possible at the knee joint, the tendon of quadriceps, the patella, and the patellar ligament form the anterior part of the fibrous capsule of that joint and of the suprapatellar bursa [p. 12].

Rectus femoris

This muscle arises from the anterior inferior iliac spine (straight head) and from a long groove immediately above the acetabulum (**reflected head**) [Figs. 135, 141]. In varying degrees of flexion of the hip joint, one or other of these heads takes the major part of the strain. The muscle runs vertically down the front of the thigh in a groove between iliopsoas and tensor fasciae latae, superiorly, and vastus lateralis and vastus medialis, inferiorly. It overlies the anterior part of vastus intermedius.

Vastus lateralis

Together with vastus intermedius with which it is partly fused, this muscle covers the lateral aspect of the femur. It has a long linear origin from the root of the greater trochanter to the lateral supracondylar line [Figs. 134, 136]. The muscle fibres run downwards and forwards to the patella and the anterolateral part of the fibrous capsule of the knee joint. The lowest fibres lie 3–4 cm proximal to the patella.

Vastus medialis

This muscle has a long linear origin from the intertrochanteric and spiral lines, the linea aspera, the medial supracondylar line [Figs. 116, 136], the medial intermuscular septum, and the tendons of adductors longus and magnus. Most of its muscle bundles are directed downwards and forwards except the lowest which run horizontally into the medial aspect of the upper half of the patella. These help to hold the patella medially and form a prominent bulge just proximal to the medial condyle of the femur. Some of the fibres of vastus medialis run into the anteromedial part of the fibrous capsule of the knee joint.

Vastus intermedius

It arises from the lateral and anterior surfaces of the body of the femur [Fig. 134]. Some of the lowest fibres which arise from the front of the body of the femur are inserted into the upper margin of the **suprapatellar bursa**—the **articularis genus muscle** which elevates the bursa during extension of the knee joint. The remainder of vastus intermedius passes to the common tendon of the quadriceps which is inserted into the proximal surface of the patella. **Actions** of quadriceps: extension of the knee and flexion of the hip (rectus femoris). **Nerve supply:** the femoral nerve.

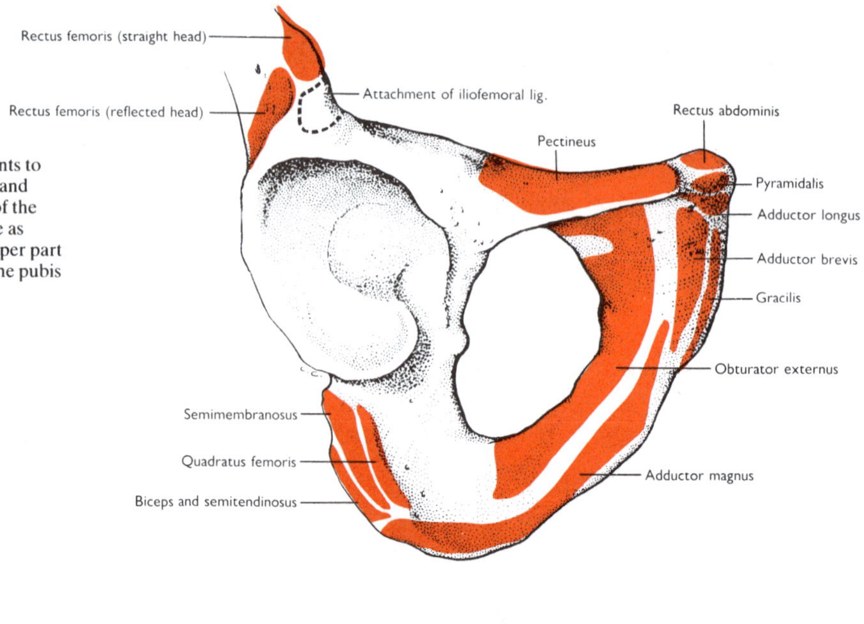

Fig. 135. Muscle attachments to outer surface of right pubis and ischium. The actual origin of the pectineus is not so extensive as shown; it arises from the upper part of the pectineal surface of the pubis and overlies the remainder.

The medial side of the thigh

The group of muscles on the medial side of the thigh is concerned with adduction at the hip joint. These **adductor muscles** are disposed in three layers. The anterior layer consists of pectineus and adductor longus which lie in the same plane. The middle layer is adductor brevis. The posterior layer is adductor magnus. All three pass from the hip bone to the back of the femur. Medial to these is the gracilis muscle. It is long and slender (*gracilis*=slender) and the only member of the group which is inserted into the tibia. As a result it acts on the knee joint in addition to the hip joint.

The two branches of the **obturator nerve** descend between the muscles and are separated by adductor brevis. The nerve supplies these muscles and obturator externus but not pectineus. The **profunda artery** descends posterior to adductor longus, close to the femur [Fig. 153].

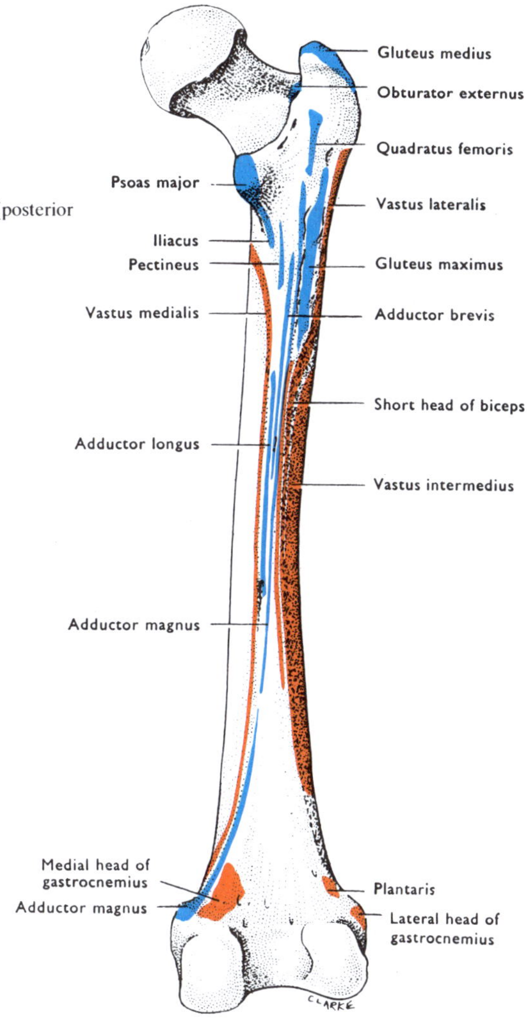

Fig. 136. Right femur (posterior aspect) to show muscle attachments.

Adductor longus

This triangular muscle arises by a narrow tendon from the front of the body of the pubis immediately below the pubic crest [Fig. 135]. It widens as it passes inferomedially, medial and edge to edge with pectineus. Its thin aponeurosis is inserted into the linea aspera of the femur, between vastus medialis and the other adductors [Fig. 136]. **Nerve supply:** anterior branch of the obturator nerve. **Action:** see below.

Dissection

Divide the adductor longus transversely 2–3 cm below its origin. Turn the distal part towards the femur, find its nerve supply and the anterior branch of the obturator nerve from which the supply comes. Follow the anterior branch of the obturator nerve inferiorly to gracilis, and find a twig entering the adductor canal inferior to adductor longus. Trace gracilis to its attachments.

Define the attachments of pectineus [Figs. 135, 136]. Avoid injury to the branches of the obturator nerve behind it and the medial circumflex artery superolateral to it. Detach pectineus from its origin and turn it laterally. Trace the anterior branch of the obturator nerve and the medial circumflex artery as far as possible. Identify the obturator externus. It lies superior to the medial circumflex artery and has the anterior branch of the obturator nerve passing anterosuperior to it [Fig. 137].

Pectineus [Figs. 133, 158, 160]

This muscle separates adductor longus from psoas major. It arises from the pecten and pectineal surface of the pubis [Fig. 135] and passes to the upper half of a line joining the lesser trochanter of the femur to the linea aspera [Fig. 136]. **Nerve supply:** the femoral nerve. **Action:** see below.

Accessory obturator nerve

This slender nerve, when present, arises from the lumbar plexus or from the obturator nerve near its origin. It descends along the medial side of psoas major and crosses the superior ramus of the pubis into the thigh. It may end in the hip joint or in pectineus, or it may pass between psoas and pectineus to replace part of the distribution of the obturator nerve [Fig. 126].

Medial circumflex artery [Fig. 137, 138, 160]

This vessel arises either from the profunda near its origin or occasionally direct from the femoral artery. It passes backwards superior to pectineus and the adductor muscles, and inferior to psoas, obturator externus, and quadratus femoris muscles. It gives branches to the adjacent muscles and a supply to the hip joint through the acetabular notch. The terminal branches take part in the formation of the **cruciate anastomosis** posterior to adductor magnus [p. 158].

Adductor brevis [Figs. 153, 161]

This muscle arises from the pubis inferior to adductor longus. It lies behind pectineus and adductor longus and is inserted into the femur in this position [Fig. 136]. **Nerve supply:** the obturator nerve. **Action:** see below.

Dissection

Divide the adductor brevis close to its origin. Turn it laterally preserving the anterior branch of the obturator nerve. Find and trace the posterior branch of the obturator nerve behind the muscle. Remove the fascia from the surface of obturator externus and adductor magnus without damaging the branches of the obturator nerve. Define the attachments of adductor magnus.

Gracilis [Figs.133, 161]

This muscle arises from the lower half of the body of the pubis, close to the symphysis, and from the anterior part of the inferior pubic ramus [Fig. 135]. It passes down the medial side of the thigh to the upper part of the medial surface of the tibia, posterior to sartorius [Fig. 171]. It is separated from sartorius and the tibial collateral ligament of the knee by a complex bursa anserina. **Nerve supply:** anterior branch of the obturator nerve. **Action:** see below.

Adductor magnus [Fig. 161]

This muscle arises from the ischiopubic ramus and the lower part of the ischial tuberosity [Fig. 135]. It passes posterior to the other adductor muscles, to the back of the femur from the medial side of the gluteal tuberosity to the adductor tubercle [Fig. 136]. At intervals the insertion is to tendinous slips which arch over the **perforating vessels** on the surface of the femur. The opening through which the femoral vessels pass is the largest of these arches. It lies at the medial supracondylar line about the junction of the middle and lower thirds of the thigh.

The muscle is fan-shaped [Fig. 153] with horizontal anterior fibres, oblique middle fibres, and nearly vertical posterior fibres. The last form the thick posteromedial border of the muscle and pass from the ischial tuberosity to the adductor tubercle. Here its cylindrical tendon is continuous with the medial intermuscular septum and, like it, gives attachment to the lower fibres of vastus medialis. **Nerve supply:** the part which arises from the ischiopubic

Fig. 137. Scheme of adductor group of muscles and obturator nerve.

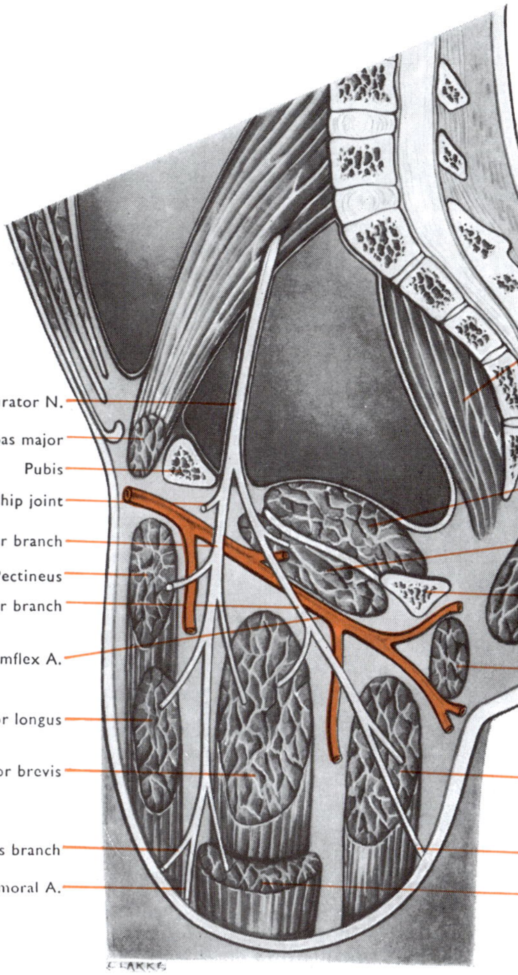

ramus is supplied by the posterior branch of the obturator nerve. (2) The part which arises with the hamstring muscles [p. 166] from the ischial tuberosity shares their nerve supply from the tibial part of the sciatic nerve.

Actions of the adductor muscles

The three adductor muscles, pectineus, and gracilis all adduct the thigh. In addition, **gracilis** is a flexor of the knee joint and a medial rotator of the leg when the knee is flexed. The ischial part of adductor magnus acts with the hamstring muscles to extend the hip joint, but unlike them it has no action on the knee joint. One of the principal actions of the adductor muscles is to stablize the hip bone on the femur. They prevent the hip bone from tilting laterally when standing on one leg. Hence they are active in the supporting limb during the whole period in which it performs this function in walking [see also gluteal muscles, p. 159]. From the position of the adductor muscles it might appear that they would produce lateral rotation of the thigh. Electromyographic evidence shows that they are only concerned with medial rotation of the thigh.

Obturator nerve
[L. 2, 3, 4]

This nerve arises from the lumbar plexus in the abdomen [Fig. 125]. It descends, medial to the psoas muscle, on to the lateral wall of the lesser pelvis where it lies lateral to the **ovary**. Here it joins the obturator vessels and enters the **obturator canal** [Fig. 128] where it divides into anterior and posterior branches. The **anterior branch** descends in the thigh anterior to obturator externus and adductor brevis. It sends branches to adductor longus, adductor brevis, gracilis, and the **hip joint** [Fig. 137]. Distal to adductor longus it enters the adductor canal. Here it gives a branch to the femoral artery and forms a plexus with twigs from the medial anterior cutaneous and saphenous branches of the femoral nerve. Through this plexus it may become cutaneous to the medial side of the thigh [Fig. 218].

The **posterior branch** supplies and pierces obturator externus and descends between adductors brevis and magnus supplying both. An **articular branch** passes through the lower part of adductor magnus to the back of the knee joint.

Obturator externus
[Fig. 159]

This fan-shaped muscle arises from the anterior half of the obturator membrane and from the anterior and inferior margins of the obturator foramen [Fig. 135]. It passes backwards and laterally curving upwards over the inferior and posterior surfaces of the neck of the femur to be inserted into the trochanteric fossa [Fig. 116]. **Nerve supply:** posterior branch of the obturator nerve. **Action:** it can flex and laterally rotate the thigh but its main function is to act as an extensile ligament [p. 10] of the hip joint.

Dissection

Carefully remove the obturator externus from its origin. This exposes the obturator artery and its branches.

Obturator artery
[Figs. 157, 158]

This branch of the internal iliac artery in the lesser pelvis accompanies the obturator nerve and divides into anterior and posterior branches which form an arterial circle on the obturator membrane deep to the obturator externus. It supplies the adjacent muscles, bone, and hip joint. Its **articular branch** traverses the acetabular notch and enters the ligament of the head of the femur, sometimes playing a minor role in the supply of the femoral head.

Psoas major and iliacus
[Figs. 133, 138, 158, 160]

These muscles arise within the abdomen and fuse as they enter the thigh posterior to the inguinal ligament, the femoral nerve, and the lateral part of the femoral sheath [Fig. 138]. Here they are only separated from the capsule of the hip joint by a **bursa** which may communicate with the joint cavity through the fibrous capsule [Fig. 155]. The muscles then pass backwards, inferior to the neck of the femur and the joint capsule to the lesser trochanter (psoas) and the surface of the femur below it (iliacus).

Nerve supply: the ventral rami of L. 2 and L. 3.

Action: the iliopsoas is the chief flexor of the hip joint. If the limb is fixed, it flexes the trunk on the thigh. It also produces slight medial rotation of the thigh because its insertion is lateral to the axis of rotation of the femur. This is important only because spasm of the psoas produces flexion and medial rotation of the hip joint—a position taken up by the right lower limb in appendicitis when the inflamed appendix is applied to the muscle. However, if the neck of the femur is broken, iliopsoas produces marked lateral rotation of the body of the femur and of the distal part of the limb with it. As a result, the toes of the affected limb point laterally in the recumbent patient.

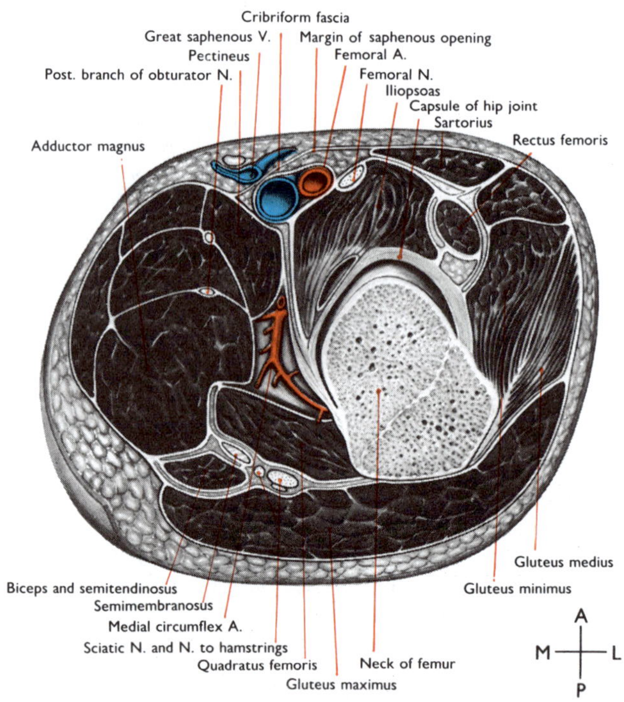

Fig. 138. Dissection of oblique section through upper part of thigh to show structures adjacent to the hip joint. The section is cut transversely to the neck of the femur.
A. Anterior.
P. Posterior.
M. Medial.
L. Lateral.

The gluteal region

Surface anatomy
[Figs. 139, 141]

The gluteal region extends from the iliac crest superiorly to the **gluteal fold** at the lower limit of the round **buttock** inferiorly, and from a line joining the anterior superior iliac spine to the front of the greater trochanter of the femur laterally to the **natal cleft** between the buttocks medially. The horizontal gluteal fold is caused by a linear adherence of the skin to the deep fascia obliquely across the inferior border of the large buttock muscle, gluteus maximus [Fig. 140]. Deep to the lower part of this muscle is the **ischial tuberosity** [Fig. 139]. This can be felt by pressing your fingers upwards into the medial part of the gluteal fold, but is most easily identified as the rounded bony mass on which you sit.

The natal cleft begins near the third spine of the sacrum. The lower part of the sacrum and coccyx are in its floor. Palpate your own sacrum and coccyx. The **coccyx** can be identified by its relative mobility. Between the lower part of the sacrum and the ischial tuberosity a deep resistance can be felt through the posterior part of the gluteus maximus. This is the **sacrotuberous ligament**. It holds down the lower part of the sacrum and prevents its anterosuperior part from tipping downwards under the weight transmitted to it through the vertebral column [Fig. 143].

Trace your iliac crest forwards to the anterior superior iliac spine and backwards to the **posterior superior iliac spine**. The latter lies in a skin dimple at the level of the second sacral spine and the middle of the sacro-iliac joint. The posterior surface of the sacrum lies between the two posterior superior iliac spines (right and left) and limits the gluteal region superomedially.

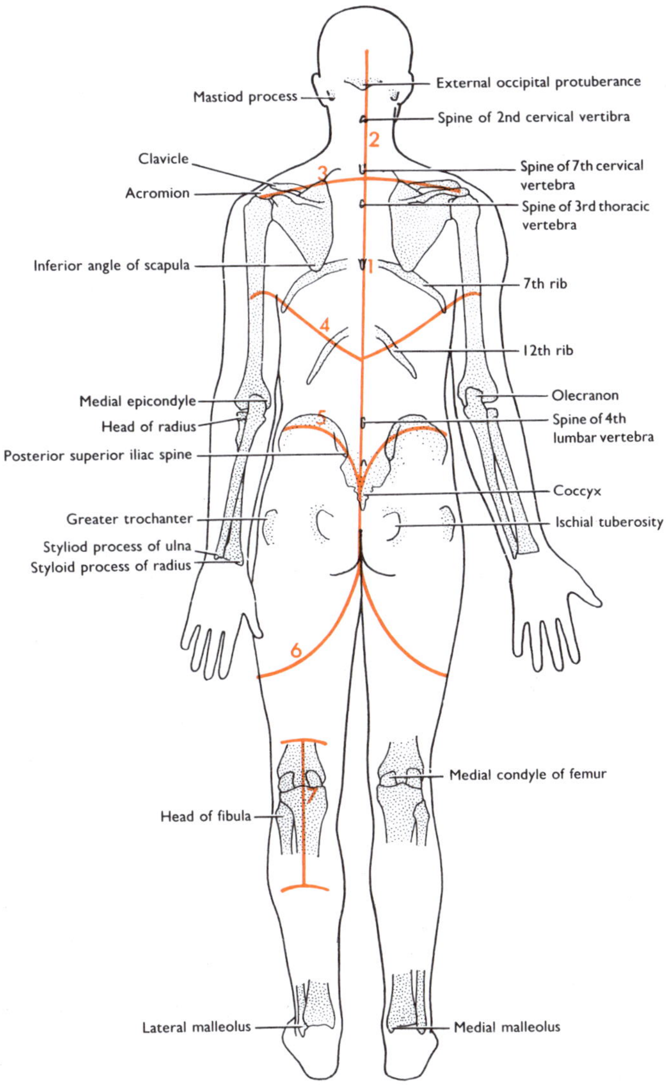

Fig. 139. Landmarks and incisions. For the bony landmarks of the lower limbs, see illustrations of individual bones.

Dissection

Make the skin incisions 5 and 6 [Fig. 139]. Reflect the flap of skin and superficial fascia laterally. Attempt to find the cutaneous nerves which enter the gluteal region from every direction. They are difficult to find because of the density of the superficial fascia, but it is usually possible to identify the branches of the lumbar nerves [Fig. 140].

Superficial fascia

This is dense and heavily laden with fat, especially at the upper and lower margins of gluteus maximus. It forms a tough, stringy cushion over the gluteal tuberosity.

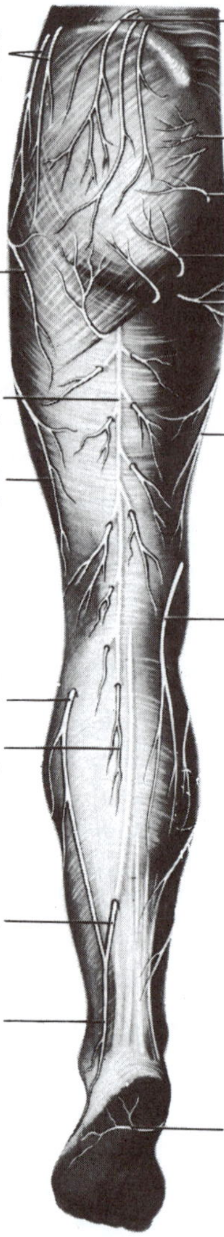

Fig. 140. Cutaneous nerves on back of lower limb. See also Fig. 123.

Cutaneous nerves [Fig. 140]

These converge on the gluteal region from all directions.

1. From above: the **lateral cutaneous branches** of the subcostal (T. 12) and **iliohypogastric** (L. 1) nerves pass downwards anterior and posterior to the tubercle of the iliac crest. They reach the level of the greater trochanter.

2. From in front: the posterior branch of the **lateral cutaneous nerve of the thigh** (L. 2, 3) supplies the antero-inferior region.

3. From below: branches of the **posterior cutaneous nerve of the thigh** curl over the lower border of gluteus maximus to the postero-inferior part.

4. From the medial side; cutaneous branches of the **dorsal rami** of L. 1–3 and S. 1–3 and the **perforating cutaneous nerve** (S. 2 and 3 ventral rami) supply the medial and intermediate regions. The long lumbar branches descend obliquely across the region almost to the gluteal fold. The sacral branches are short. The perforating cutaneous pierces the sacrotuberous

ligament and gluteus maximus midway between the coccyx and the ischial tuberosity.

Deep fascia

This is thick over the anterior border of gluteus maximus where the iliotibial tract splits to enclose the muscle. Elsewhere the fascia is thin over the muscle but forms a thick layer deep to it.

Dissection

If any branches of the posterior cutaneous nerve of the thigh have been found on the lower border of gluteus maximus, follow them back to the trunk of the nerve. Remove the thin deep fascia from gluteus maximus and define the attachments of the muscle. Leave the insertion of the muscle into the iliotibial tract intact.

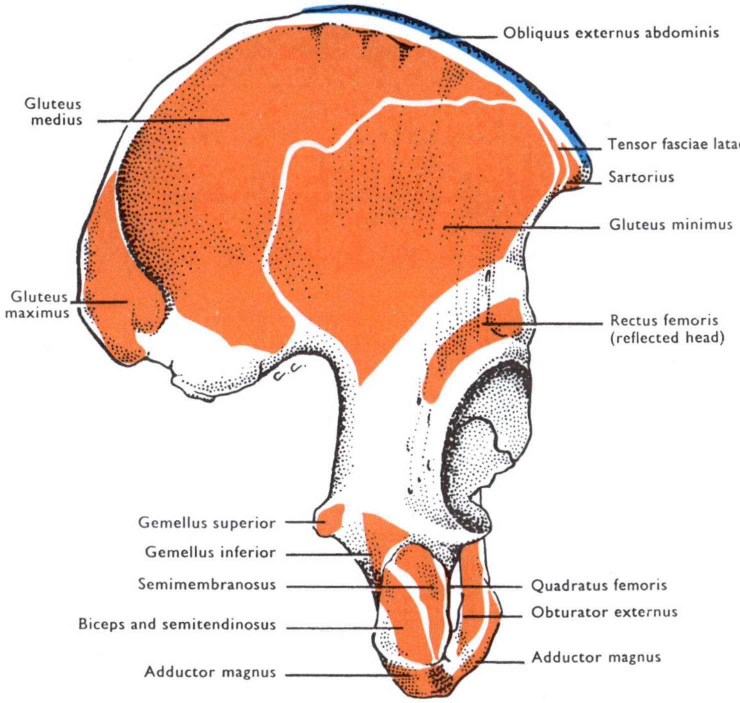

Fig. 141. Muscle attachments to outer surface of right hip bone.

Gluteus maximus
[Figs. 157, 161]

This powerful muscle arises from: (1) the external surface of the ilium behind the posterior gluteal line; (2) the back of the sacrum and coccyx; (3) the sacrotuberous ligament. Its fibres pass downwards and forwards and become suddenly aponeurotic. This abrupt thinning produces the hollow of the hip posterior to the greater trochanter of the femur. Only the lower, deep quarter is inserted into the **gluteal tuberosity** of the femur [Fig. 136]. The remainder passes to the iliotibial tract. This part of the aponeurosis runs superficial to the greater trochanter and the upper part of vastus lateralis, while the lower part of the muscle crosses the ischial tuberosity. It is separated from all three by large **bursae**.

Nerve supply: the inferior gluteal nerve. **Actions:** it is a powerful extensor of the hip joint used principally when strength is required, e.g. in lifting heavy weights from the floor. It is also used in running and climbing, more especially in full extension of the hip joint, e.g. when raising the foot from the ground prior to swinging it forwards when walking. It acts reciprocally with the tensor fasciae latae to stabilize the pelvis on the thigh in an anteroposterior plane, and acts with it to extend the knee through the iliotibial tract.

Dissection

Cut across gluteus maximus and reflect it. This is made difficult because the vessels (superior and inferior gluteal) and the inferior gluteal nerve enter its deep surface and are easily destroyed before they are seen. Avoid this by passing two fingers deep to the lower edge of the muscle 2–3 cm medial to its femoral insertion, and cutting upwards between the fingers to the upper border superior to the greater trochanter.

Reflect the lateral part of the muscle to its insertion. Identify the bursae which separate it from the greater trochanter and the upper part of vastus lateralis close to the gluteal tuberosity.

Reflect the medial part of the muscle. Keep close to the deep surface of the muscle to avoid injury to the posterior cutaneous nerve of the thigh [Fig. 140]. Find the inferior gluteal vessels and nerve entering the lower part of the muscle, and the superficial parts of the superior gluteal vessels entering its upper part. As the ischial tuberosity is uncovered, look for the bursa superficial to the origin of the hamstring muscles from the tuberosity. Carefully detach the muscle from the surface of the rigid sacrotuberous ligament. While doing this, you may find the perforating cutaneous nerve [Fig. 140].

Trace the branch of the superior gluteal artery towards its source. It emerges between the muscles gluteus medius (superiorly) and piriformis (inferiorly). Remove the fascia from the conical piriformis muscle to its attachment to the greater trochanter. Find and follow the posterior cutaneous nerve of the thigh upwards to the point where it emerges at the lower border of piriformis. A perineal branch of this nerve curves medially, below the ischial tuberosity, towards the perineum.

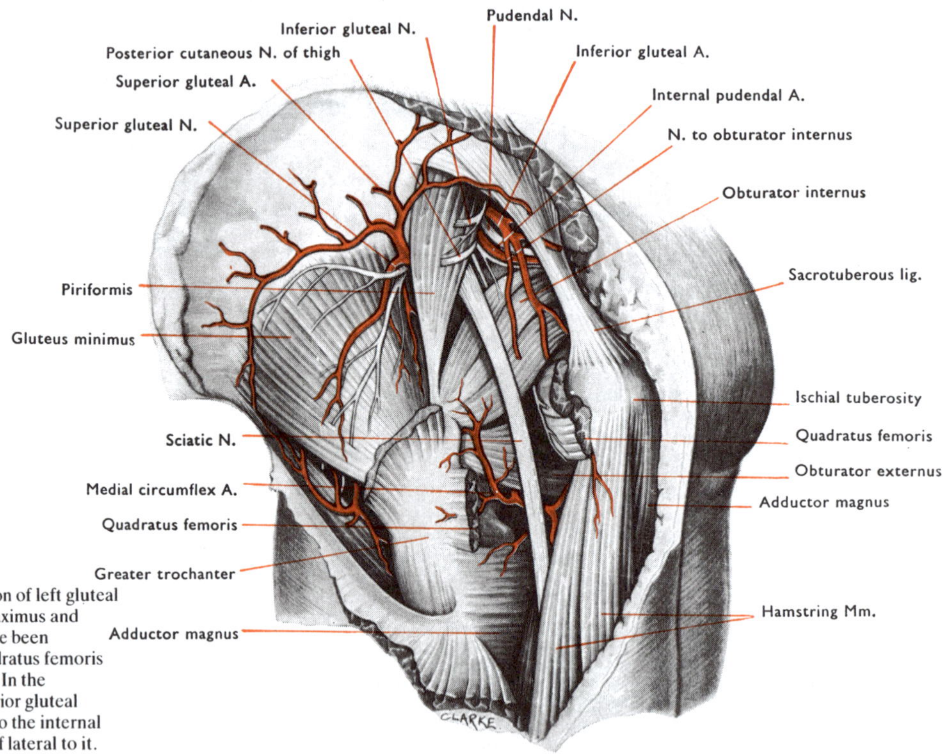

Fig. 142. Dissection of left gluteal region. Gluteus maximus and gluteus medius have been removed, and quadratus femoris has been reflected. In the specimen, the inferior gluteal artery was medial to the internal pudendal instead of lateral to it.

Structures deep to gluteus maximus

Begin by studying an articulated pelvis, preferably with the sacrotuberous and sacrospinous ligaments attached [Fig. 144]. The **sacrotuberous ligament** passes from the medial side of the ischial tuberosity to the posterior iliac spines thus turning the sciatic notches into a B-shaped foramen. This foramen is subdivided by the **sacrospinous ligament** into an upper, **greater sciatic foramen** and a lower, **lesser sciatic foramen**. The sacrospinous ligament passes from the ischial spine to the side of the lower part of the sacrum and coccyx, deep to the sacrotuberous ligament, and lies edge to edge with the levator ani muscle which also arises from the ischial spine. Together with the corresponding muscle of the opposite side, levator ani forms the sloping muscular floor of the pelvis which separates its contents from the perineum. Hence, the greater sciatic foramen, which lies superior to the ischial spine and the muscular floor of the pelvis, leads from the pelvis into the gluteal region; the lesser sciatic foramen, which lies inferior to the ischial spine, leads from the gluteal region into the perineum. It follows that nerves, arteries, and a muscle (piriformis) can enter the gluteal region from the pelvis through the greater sciatic foramen and corresponding veins can enter the pelvis in the opposite direction.

Vessels and nerves which enter the gluteal region from the pelvis may either (1) remain in the gluteal region, or (2) descend from the gluteal region into the back of the thigh, or (3) turn forwards through the lesser sciatic foramen into the perineum. The first group includes the gluteal vessels and nerves. The second group includes the sciatic nerve, the posterior cutaneous nerve of the thigh, and branches of the inferior gluteal vessels. The third group (the internal pudendal vessels, the pudendal nerve, and the nerve to obturator internus) curve over the posterior surface of the ischial spine and sacrospinous ligament into the lesser sciatic foramen. This foramen also transmits the **oburator internus** into the gluteal region from the lateral wall of the perineum.

Sacrotuberous ligament
[Figs. 144, 146, 158]

This strong band passes upwards from the medial side of the ischial tuberosity to the margins of the sacrum and coccyx, and to both posterior iliac spines. The lateral edge of the ligament forms the posteromedial border of the greater and lesser sciatic foramina. The medial edge, between coccyx and ischial tuberosity, forms the posterior boundary of the perineum. The ligament holds down the posterior part of the sacrum and thus prevents the weight of the body depressing its anterior part. When the loading on the anterior part of the sacrum is severe, e.g. in landing on the feet when jumping from a height, the ligament gives resilience to the slight movement at the sacro-iliac joint.

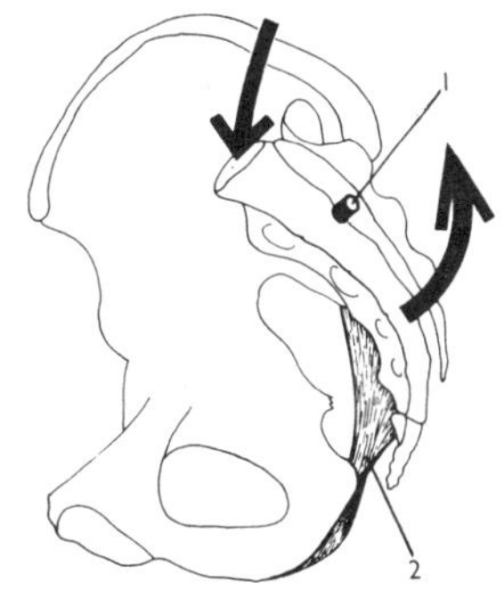

Fig. 143. Diagram to show the forces applied to the sacrum due to the weight of the body acting through the vertebral column. Note how the sacrotuberous ligament (2) will act as a shock absorber permitting only slight movement of the sacrum at the sacro-iliac joint around its axis of movement (1).

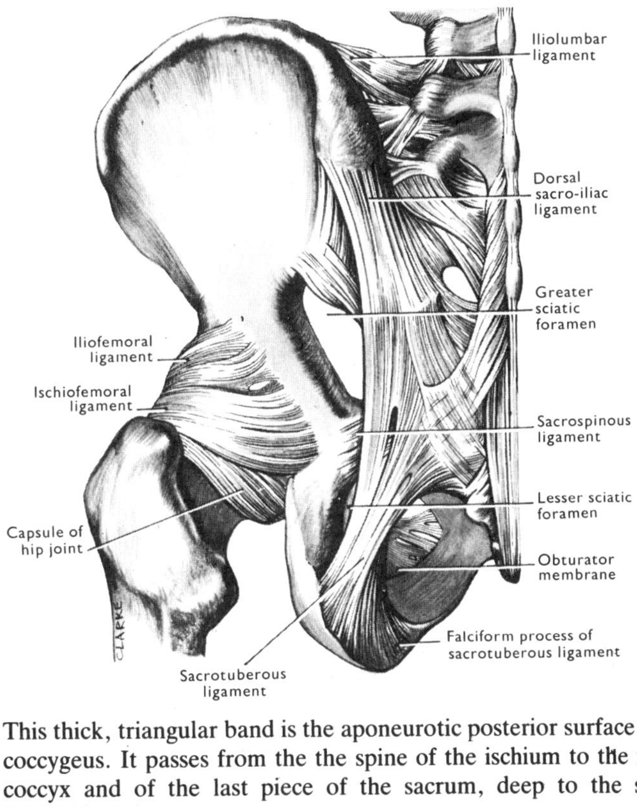

Fig. 144. Dorsal view of the pelvic ligaments and the hip joint.

Sacrospinous ligament

This thick, triangular band is the aponeurotic posterior surface of the muscle coccygeus. It passes from the the spine of the ischium to the margin of the coccyx and of the last piece of the sacrum, deep to the sacrotuberous ligament.

Sciatic foramina

The **greater** sciatic foramen is bounded by the greater sciatic notch of the hip bone, the sacrotuberous ligament, and the sacrospinous ligament. It transmits structures between the pelvis and the gluteal region (see above).

The **lesser** sciatic foramen is bounded by the lesser sciatic notch of the ischium and the sacrospinous and sacrotuberous ligaments. It transmits structures between the gluteal region and the perineum (see above).

Dissection

Find the large sciatic nerve anterior to the posterior cutaneous nerve of the thigh. Carefully split the fascia surrounding the nerve. Trace the nerve upwards to the lower border of piriformis and downwards to the point where its branches to the hamstring muscles arise, near the level of the ischial tuberosity. The vessels running with these branches arise from the medial circumflex femoral artery.

Lift the upper part of the sciatic nerve laterally. The bone which is exposed is the posterior surface of the acetabulum. The slender nerve to quadratus femoris lies here. Trace this nerve distally. It disappears anterior to the obturator internus tendon overlapped by the superior and inferior gemelli.

Medial to the upper part of the sciatic nerve, identify the ischial spine and the sacrospinous ligament. The ligament can be felt as a tough resistance medial to the spine. On the surface of these, find the nerve to obturator internus with the internal pudendal vessels and the pudendal nerve medial to it. A slender branch of the nerve to obturator internus may be found passing to the superior gemellus.

Remove the fascia from the muscles anterior to the sciatic nerve. From above downwards these are [Fig. 142]: (1) the tendon of obturator internus overlapped by the gemelli. Split the gemelli apart and expose the tendon. Follow it to the greater trochanter. (2) The quadratus femoris passing from the ischial tuberosity to the back of the femur [Fig. 136]. (3) Inferior to quadratus femoris is the posterior surface of adductor magnus. Branches of the medial circumflex femoral artery appear both above and below quadratus femoris [Figs. 137, 142]. Inferior to this, the first perforating artery (a branch of the profunda femoris) may be found piercing adductor magnus close to the gluteal tuberosity of the femur [Fig. 152].

Separate gemellus inferior from quadratus femoris. Lift the gemelli and obturator internus and cut across them lateral to the nerve to quadratus femoris. Follow the nerve to quadratus femoris and its branch to the inferior gemellus. Lift the medial part of obturator internus to expose the bursa between it and the lesser sciatic notch. Separate quadratus femoris from adductor magnus and remove quadratus femoris to expose the lesser trochanter of the femur, the medial circumflex artery, the lower, posterior part of the capsule of the hip joint, and the tendon of obturator externus.

Inferior gluteal nerve
(L. 5; S. 1, 2)

This branch of the sacral plexus enters the gluteal region with the posterior cutaneous nerve of the thigh, inferior to piriformis. It breaks into a number of twigs which enter the deep surface of gluteus maximus—the only structure it supplies.

Inferior gluteal artery

This branch of the internal iliac artery emerges from the pelvis below piriformis. It sends large branches into the deep surface of gluteus maximus and cutaneous branches to the buttock and to the back of the thigh with the posterior cutaneous nerve of the thigh [p. 166]. The artery also gives rise to the slender **companion artery of the sciatic nerve**, and anastomoses with the circumflex femoral arteries [p. 158].

Sciatic nerve
[L. 4, 5; S. 1, 2, 3]

This is the thickest nerve in the body. It arises from the sacral plexus and passes through the lower part of the greater sciatic foramen into the gluteal region, deep to gluteus maximus. From above downwards, it lies on: (1) the ischial wall of the acetabulum [Fig. 128] and the nerve to quadratus femoris; (2) the obturator internus muscle [Fig. 158] with the two gemelli; (3) the quadratus femoris, between the ischial tuberosity and the greater trochanter of the femur. Here, one or more nerves leave its medial side to pass to the hamstring muscles. The sciatic nerve then enters the thigh on the posterior surface of adductor magnus [Fig. 161] and descends between it and the hamstring muscles. The sciatic nerve usually ends half-way down the back of the thigh by dividing into the **common peroneal** and **tibial nerves**. These are mainly concerned with the supply of structures from the knee distally. The

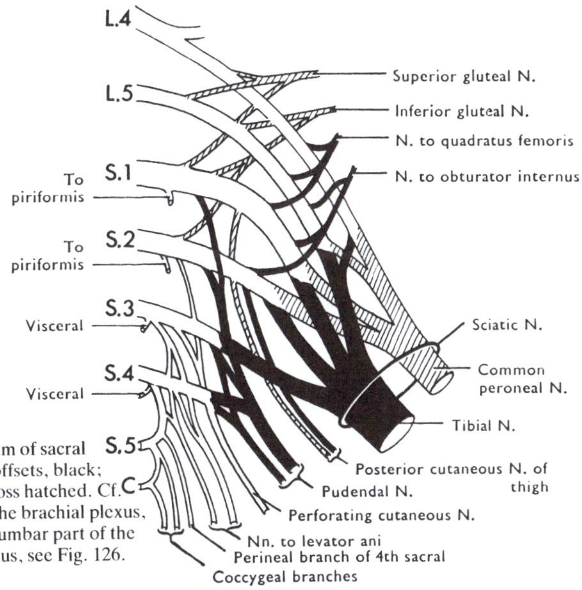

Fig. 145. Diagram of sacral plexus. Ventral offsets, black; dorsal offsets, cross hatched. Cf. arrangement of the brachial plexus, Fig. 24. For the lumbar part of the lumbosacral plexus, see Fig. 126.

position of this division of the sciatic nerve is variable. If it occurs before the nerve leaves the pelvis, the tibial nerve emerges below piriformis while the common peroneal nerve pierces that muscle.

Pudendal nerve, internal pudendal artery, and nerve to obturator internus [Fig. 142]

These structures enter the gluteal region through the lowest part of the greater sciatic foramen. They lie on the posterior surface of the junction of the ischial spine and the sacrospinous ligament with the artery between the nerve to obturator internus laterally and the pudendal nerve medially. They then curve forwards to enter the perineum through the lesser sciatic foramen and run on to the medial surface of obturator internus.

Small muscles on the back of the hip joint

Most of these muscles are only partly exposed in the gluteal region.

Piriformis arises in the pelvis from the pelvic surface of the middle three pieces of the sacrum. This conical muscle passes through the greater sciatic foramen to the upper border of the greater trochanter of the femur [Fig. 134] immediately lateral to the tendon of obturator internus. **Nerve supply:** branches of the first and second sacral nerves in the pelvis.

Obturator internus is a large, fan-shaped muscle which arises from the

Fig. 146. The medial aspect of the right hip bone. Muscle attachments, red; ligamentous attachments and cartilage, blue.

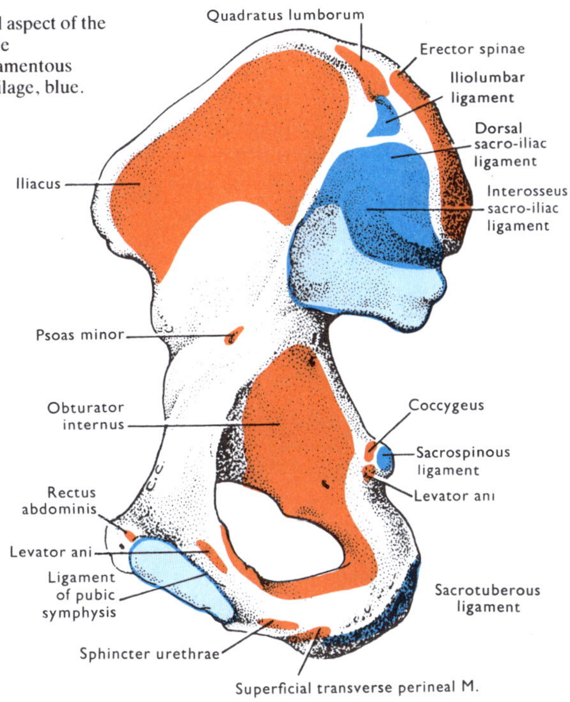

pelvic surface of the dense obturator membrane, which is stretched across the obturator foramen, and most of the bone surrounding the foramen [Figs. 146, 157–159]. The **levator ani muscle** arises from the fascia covering the pelvic surface of the obturator internus in front of the ischial spine. Thus obturator internus is in the lateral wall both of the pelvis and of the perineum. The muscle fibres converge posteriorly to the lesser sciatic foramen. The deeper fibres become tendinous and hook over the lesser sciatic notch to run laterally behind the hip joint to the upper medial part of the greater trochanter [Figs. 134, 158]. The tendon is separated from the notch by a bursa. **Nerve supply:** the nerve to obturator internus (L. 5; S. 1, 2).

The **gemelli** are essentially continuations of the muscular part of obturator internus on either side of its tendon. They arise from the superior and inferior margins of the lesser sciatic notch and are inserted into the posterior surface of the tendon. **Nerve supply:** the superior gemellus from the nerve to obturator internus; the inferior gemellus from the nerve to quadratus femoris.

Quadratus femoris passes from the lateral margin of the ischial tuberosity to the back of the greater trochanter of the femur in the region of the quadrate tubercle [Fig. 136]. The muscle lies between the inferior gemellus and the superior margin of adductor magnus. **Nerve supply:** nerve to quadratus femoris (L. 4, 5; S. 1).

Obturator externus arises from the external surface of the obturator membrane and the lower bony margin of the obturator foramen [Fig. 135]. It passes backwards inferior to the hip joint and then turns upwards and laterally on the lateral half of the posterior surface of the neck of the femur. Here its tendon is lateral to the capsule of the hip joint and deep to the quadratus femoris and the obturator internus. Obturator externus is inserted into the trochanteric fossa. **Nerve supply:** obturator nerve.

Actions. Various actions may be attributed to these muscles depending on the degree of flexion or extension of the hip joint. However, their main function is to act as ligaments of variable length and tension which can help to maintain the head of the femur in the acetabulum. Many of them act as lateral rotators of the thigh, more especially quadratus femoris.

Medial circumflex femoral artery

This artery arises from the profunda femoris (or femoral) artery in the femoral triangle. It passes backwards between pectineus and iliopsoas and then inferior to obturator externus and the hip joint, above the adductor muscles [Fig. 137]. It sends branches downwards between the adductor muscles, a branch to the acetabulum, and anastomoses with the obturator artery. Posteriorly the artery divides into an **ascending branch** to the trochanteric fossa with the tendon of obturator externus and a **transverse branch** to the hamstring muscles between quadratus femoris and adductor magnus. The latter branch *anastomoses* with: (1) the terminal part of the transverse branch of the lateral femoral circumflex artery; (2) the inferior gluteal artery; (3) the first perforating artery. This complex is the **cruciate anastomosis** [p. 168]. The ascending branch anastomoses with branches of both gluteal arteries and sends branches to the back and posterosuperior surface of the neck of the femur. It is the latter branches which supply a large part of the **femoral head**.

Dissection

Remove the fascia from the superficial surface of gluteus medius and define its attachments. Lift the posterior border of the muscle away from piriformis and define the plane of separation between it and the gluteus minimus beneath. Separate the muscles from behind forwards by pushing your fingers between them. Pull the tensor fasciae latae forwards so that the separation can be seen anteriorly.

Cut across the gluteus medius 5 cm above the greater trochanter and reflect its parts. Find the bursa between the tendon of insertion and the greater trochanter and confirm the insertion. Find the branches of the superior gluteal vessels and nerve deep to the upper part of the muscle. Trace these between gluteus medius and minimus to the deep surface of tensor fasciae latae. Here the artery anastomoses with the ascending branch of the lateral femoral circumflex artery and the nerve enters and supplies the tensor.

Gluteus medius

This powerful muscle arises from the ilium between the anterior and posterior gluteal lines [Figs. 114, 141]. It is overlapped posteriorly by gluteus maximus and anteriorly by tensor fasciae latae. Between these it is easily felt in the living body through the skin and iliotibial tract. Check this on yourself by feeling it contracting when the opposite foot is raised from the ground. The flattened tendon is inserted into the posterosuperior angle of the greater trochanter and the oblique ridge on its lateral surface [Fig. 136]. A small bursa lies between the tendon and the trochanter in front of the insertion. **Nerve supply:** the superior gluteal nerve.

Gluteus minimus

This thick muscle arises from the ilium between the anterior and inferior gluteal lines [Fig. 141]. It is inserted into the front of the greater trochanter [Fig. 134] and fuses with the adjacent part of the fibrous capsule of the hip joint. A bursa separates the tendon from the upper anterior part of the trochanter. **Nerve supply:** the superior gluteal nerve.

Actions of the gluteus medius and minimus

These muscles abduct the thigh when the limb is free to move. When the limb is supporting the weight of the body, their action is reversed. They can then tilt the pelvis on the hip joint sufficiently to raise the opposite foot from the ground. Their continued contraction prevents the pelvis from sagging to the unsupported side so long as the foot on that side is raised from the ground. They are, therefore, very important muscles in walking for, without them, the opposite foot cannot be raised from the ground unless the centre of gravity is moved so as to lie lateral to the hip joint of the supporting limb by flexing the trunk to that side. Thus bilateral paralysis of these muscles, or bilateral congenital dislocation of the hip joints which prevents the muscles from acting, produces a waddling gait in which the trunk is flexed from side to side with each step. The anterior fibres of both these muscles are also medial rotators of the thigh.

Superior gluteal nerve
(L. 4, 5; S. 1)

This branch of the sacral plexus enters the gluteal region through the uppermost part of the greater sciatic foramen. It turns forwards between gluteus medius and minimus and divides into a number of branches. The upper branches enter gluteus medius. The lowest branch crosses the middle of minimus, gives twigs to both muscles, and emerges between their anterior borders to supply tensor fasciae latae.

Superior gluteal vessels
[Fig. 142]

The artery arises from the posterior division of the internal iliac artery and enters the gluteal region with the corresponding nerve. Here it divides. A **superficial branch** passes between gluteus medius and piriformis to gluteus maximus. A **deep branch** divides and follows the branches of the superior gluteal nerve. This supplies gluteus medius and minimus and sends branches to the hip joint. Anteriorly it reaches the deep surface of tensor fasciae latae and anastomoses with the ascending branch of the lateral circumflex femoral artery. Together they give branches to the anterior surfaces of the neck and greater trochanter of the femur.

Arterial anastomosis in the proximal part of the thigh

There are many anastomoses between the arteries arising from the internal and external iliac arteries in this region. (1) Between the medial femoral circumflex artery and (a) the obturator artery, (b) both gluteal arteries, (c) the lateral circumflex femoral artery, and (d) the perforating branches of the profunda femoris. (2) Between the superior gluteal artery and (a) the lateral femoral circumflex artery and (b) the superficial circumflex iliac artery. (3) Between the internal pudendal artery and the deep and superficial external pudendal branches of the femoral artery in the perineum. Also, in the abdomen, the external iliac artery anastomoses with, or may form, the obturator artery and it communicates with the subclavian artery through the superior and inferior epigastric arteries in the abdominal wall.

Dissection

Detach gluteus minimus from its origin and turn it downwards. Separate it inferiorly from the fibrous capsule of the hip joint and examine this part of the capsule. Find the tendon of rectus femoris attached to the anterior inferior iliac spine. Follow the tendon to its reflected head. This is attached to a groove immediately above the margin of the acetabulum hidden by superficial fibres of the hip joint capsule.

The popliteal fossa

Surface anatomy

The popliteal fossa lies behind the knee. It is posterior to the lower third of the femur, the knee joint, and the upper part of the tibia. It forms a hollow when the knee is flexed, because the tendons which form its superior boundaries stand out from the femur on their way to the leg bones. The fossa bulges slightly when the knee is straight, because the tendons then lie close to the femur.

Review again the major structures which can be felt in the vicinity of the knee joint [p. 128] by examining your own knee. In addition, find the **tendon of biceps** behind the lateral condyle of the femur. With the knee extended, press your finger against the posterior surface of the lateral condyle immediately medial to the biceps tendon. When the finger is moved from side to side, a rounded cord, the **common peroneal nerve**, can be felt. Follow the tendon of biceps to the head of the fibula and repeat the process on the back of that head. The same nerve can be felt again. Slide the finger down to the posterolateral side of the neck of the fibula. Move the finger up and down, maintaining some pressure. Again the nerve can be felt turning forwards on the fibular neck. With the knee flexed and the lateral side of the foot pressed against the floor, the **fibular collateral ligament** of the knee joint can be felt as a firm resistance between the head of the fibula and the lateral femoral condyle.

Place a finger in the middle of the popliteal fossa with the knee bent. Press firmly and feel the pulsations of the popliteal artery. In the lower part of the fossa, the two heads of gastrocnemius form rounded swellings which merge inferiorly in the calf.

Immediately above the popliteal fossa, the back of the thigh is smooth and rounded, but the distal part of the belly of semimembranosus may be seen to bulge near the midline as it contracts in walking [Fig. 147].

Dissection

Make skin incision 7 [Fig. 139] and reflect the skin flaps leaving the superficial fascia intact. Now strip the superficial fascia from the deep fascia starting proximally. Look for any branches of the posterior cutaneous nerve of the thigh piercing the deep fascia in the proximal part of the fossa and for the small saphenous vein with the terminal part of that nerve in the distal part of the fossa. Rarely the sural nerve may pierce the deep fascia at this level also.

Follow the medial anterior cutaneous nerve of the thigh downwards in the posteromedial part of the calf [Fig. 140]. The peroneal communicating nerve (a branch of the common peroneal nerve) may be found in the lower lateral part of the popliteal area. It may pierce the deep fascia at a much lower level and will be found later.

Fascia of the popliteal region

There is relatively little fat in the superficial fascia. The deep fascia, though thin, is strong and firmly bound to the tendons which form the boundaries of the popliteal fossa.

Boundaries of the popliteal fossa

Though diamond-shaped when dissected, the popliteal fossa is a narrow interval between the diverging hamstring muscles superiorly and the converging heads of gastrocnemius inferiorly. Biceps femoris forms the

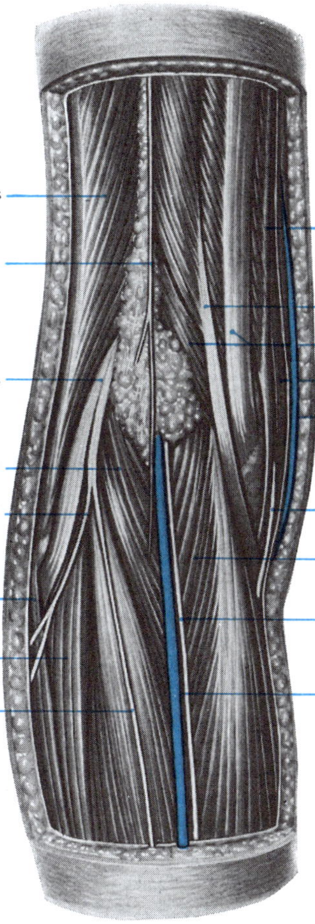

Fig. 147. Left popliteal region after removal of the deep fascia—the muscles and fat being left undisturbed.

upper lateral boundary, semimembranosus and semitendinosus the upper medial boundary. The last two have the gracilis, the sartorius, and the tendon of adductor magnus close to them as they approach the knee. The two lower boundaries are the heads of gastrocnemius. Because the space between the boundaries is slight, only a small part of the popliteal vessels (just above the knee joint level) is not covered by muscles. The posterior wall of the fossa is the deep fascia; its anterior wall is the popliteal surface of the femur, the posterior capsule of the knee joint, and the fascia covering popliteus.

Dissection

Cut through the deep fascia along the biceps femoris. Expose the muscle and its tendon to the insertion. Make a similar incision over semitendinosus and semimembranosus. Follow the tendon of semitendinosus to the medial surface of the tibia, then lift the semimembranosus and follow it distally. Find the bursa between semimembranosus and the medial head of gastrocnemius. Find and follow the gracilis and its tendon. As you free gracilis from the posterior surface of sartorius, look for the saphenous nerve and its accompanying artery which emerge between them. Follow the nerve and artery downwards with the great saphenous vein.

Follow the posterior cutaneous nerve of the thigh upwards to the upper angle of the popliteal fossa. Strip the deep fascia from the posterior surface of the popliteal fossa and remove the fat from its upper angle to expose the tibial nerve. Follow this large nerve downwards and find its branches. The cutaneous branch—the sural nerve—lies between the two heads of gastrocnemius. Of the three articular branches (superior medial, inferior medial, and middle genicular) the superior arises near the upper angle of the fossa, the others below this. Trace them as far as possible. The muscular branches to gastrocnemius, plantaris, soleus, and popliteus arise near the middle of the fossa. Separate the heads of gastrocnemius and follow these branches as far as possible.

Find the common peroneal nerve medial to the tendon of biceps femoris. Trace the nerve to the upper angle of the fossa and to the back of the head of the fibula. Find the genicular branches which arise near the upper limit of the fossa. The superior lateral genicular leaves the fossa above the lateral femoral condyle, the inferior lateral genicular accompanies the trunk of the nerve. The peroneal communicating nerve and the lateral cutaneous nerve of the calf arise near the lateral angle of the fossa. Follow these branches downwards.

Remove the fascia from the heads of gastrocnemius. Identify and separate the plantaris from the posteromedial surface of the lateral head but avoid injury to the nerve to the lateral head which passes between them.

Lift the upper part of the tibial nerve from the popliteal vessels. The vein is posterolateral to the artery with the genicular twig of the obturator nerve in the groove between them. If this nerve is found, trace it proximally and distally.

Remove the fascia from the popliteal vein. It also encloses the artery and parallel venous channels which run on it. Remove these separate channels to expose the artery, but retain the small saphenous vein.

Find the large muscular branches of the popliteal artery and divide these. They pass with the nerves to the muscles. Gently scrape the fat from the popliteal surface of the femur and find the genicular branches [Fig. 151]. Follow the lateral and medial pairs and find the middle genicular branch passing forwards into the posterior capsule of the knee joint.

Contents of the popliteal fossa
[Figs. 148–150]

The popliteal fossa transmits the branches of the sciatic nerve and the popliteal vessels. These vessels lie close to the posterior surface of the knee joint and so are minimally affected by its movements. They are the continuation of the femoral vessels which enter the fossa through the tendinous opening in adductor magnus. Hence they lie anterior to the nerves which descend behind that muscle. The tibial nerve runs with the vessels; the common peroneal nerve deviates laterally following the medial side of the biceps femoris. The fossa also contains some lymph nodes close to the

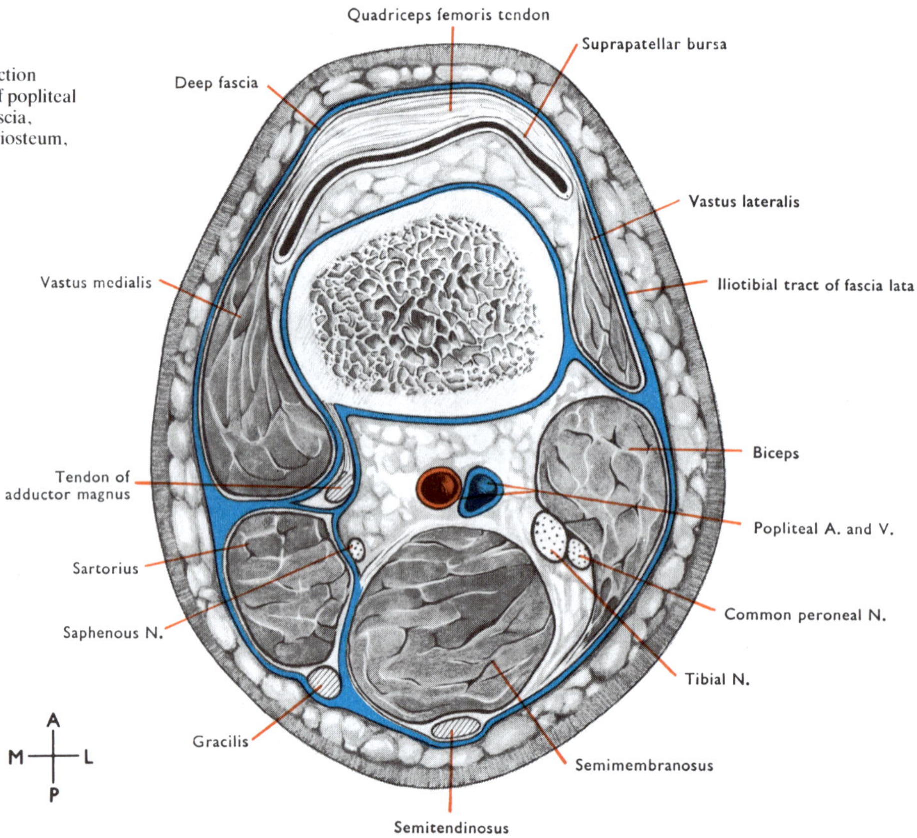

Fig. 148. Transverse section through proximal part of popliteal region of thigh. Deep fascia, intermuscular septa, periosteum, and popliteal vein, blue.
A. Anterior.
P. Posterior.
M. Medial.
L. Lateral.

vessels. They drain the deep tissues of the leg and foot and the knee joint. They also receive superficial lymph vessels from the lateral side of the foot, the heel, and the back of the calf [Fig. 180]. These drain along the line of the small saphenous vein and pierce the deep fascia over the lower part of the popliteal fossa where there may be one or two nodes just under the deep fascia.

The **posterior cutaneous nerve of the thigh** passes through the fossa immediately deep to the deep fascia. It gives branches to the overlying skin and finally enters the superficial fascia with the small saphenous vein.

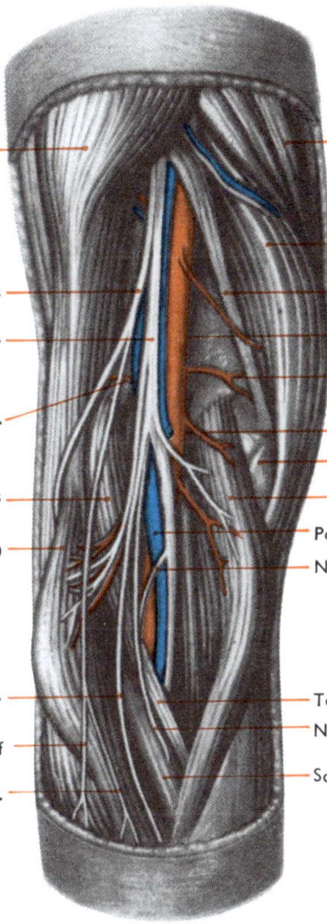

Fig. 149. Dissection of left popliteal fossa. The upper boundaries have been pulled apart and the aponeurosis to which the two heads of the gastrocnemius are attached has been split and the heads separated. For deeper dissection see Fig. 150.

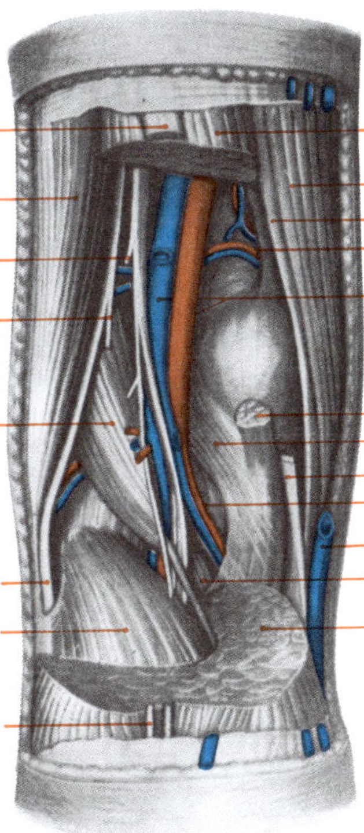

Fig. 150. Dissection of left popliteal fossa. The two heads of the gastrocnemius and portions of the semimembranosus and semitendinosus have been removed. For more superficial dissections, see Figs. 147, 149.

Tibial nerve
(L. 4, 5; S. 1, 2, 3)

This is the larger of the two terminal branches of the sciatic nerve which separate about the middle of the back of the thigh. It runs vertically through the popliteal fossa, posterior to the popliteal vessels [Fig. 149]. The tibial nerve supplies the muscles of the back of the leg and the sole of the foot, and the skin of the lower half of the back of the leg and the lateral side and sole of the foot [Fig. 218].

Branches in the popliteal fossa

The **sural nerve** is the cutaneous branch. It arises in the middle of the fossa and descends in the groove between the heads of gastrocnemius. It pierces the deep fascia about the middle of the back of the leg. From this point it supplies a strip of skin on the back of the leg to the lateral malleolus, and then along the lateral side of the dorsum of the foot to the little toe.

Muscular branches arise in the distal part of the fossa and pass to gastrocnemius, plantaris, soleus, and popliteus. That to soleus passes between the lateral head of gastrocnemius and plantaris to enter the superficial surface of soleus. The nerve to popliteus descends over the muscle and its inferior border to reach its anterior surface. This nerve also supplies the **superior tibiofibular joint** and sends twigs to the **interosseous membrane** [Fig. 183].

The *articular branches* arise in the upper part of the fossa, or even above it. They descend to join the corresponding arteries [Fig. 151]. The **superior medial genicular nerve** runs above the medial condyle of the femur, deep to the muscles. The **middle genicular nerve** pierces the posterior capsule of the knee joint and supplies the structures lodged in the intercondylar notch of the femur. The **inferior medial genicular nerve** runs inferomedially on the upper border of popliteus and then forwards inferior to the medial tibial condyle, deep to the superficial part of the tibial collateral ligament of the knee.

Common peroneal nerve
(L. 4, 5; S. 1, 2)

This nerve, smaller than the tibial nerve, supplies the muscles on the lateral and anterior surfaces of the leg and the dorsum of the foot and skin on the lateral side of the leg and the greater part of the dorsum of the foot. It runs along the medial border of the biceps femoris to the back of the head of the fibula. It then curves forwards between the neck of the fibula and the upper fibres of the peroneus longus muscle which arise from it. Here the nerve divides into **superficial** and **deep peroneal nerves**. The common peroneal nerve is easily rolled under the finger on the back of the lateral condyle of the femur and of the head of the fibula, and on the posterolateral side of the neck of the fibula. In all these positions it may be damaged by a blow on the bone.

Branches in the popliteal fossa

Cutaneous branches. The **peroneal communicating nerve** arises in the upper part of the popliteal fossa. It descends on the posterolateral side of the calf [Fig. 140] and joins the sural nerve at a variable level. The **lateral cutaneous nerve of the calf** arises on the lateral head of gastrocnemius. It descends to the skin on the lateral surface of the upper half of the leg.

Articular branches. The **superior** and **inferior lateral genicular nerves** are small. They accompany the corresponding arteries [Fig. 151]. The **recurrent genicular nerve** arises where the common peroneal nerve divides. It ascends anterior to the knee joint.

Genicular branch of the obturator nerve

This slender continuation of the posterior branch of the obturator nerve pierces the distal part of the adductor magnus, descends on the popliteal artery, and pierces the posterior surface of the fibrous capsule of the knee joint.

Popliteal artery
[Fig. 151]

This artery begins at the tendinous opening in adductor magnus. Here it is continuous with the femoral artery. It ends at the lower border of the popliteus muscle where it divides into **anterior** and posterior tibial arteries. The artery lies on the anterior wall of the popliteal fossa. From above downwards, it is anterior to semimembranosus, the popliteal vein and tibial nerve, and gastrocnemius with plantaris [Fig. 150].

Branches

Muscular branches pass to the lower parts of the hamstring muscles and to the upper parts of the muscles of the calf. These are large and give rise to

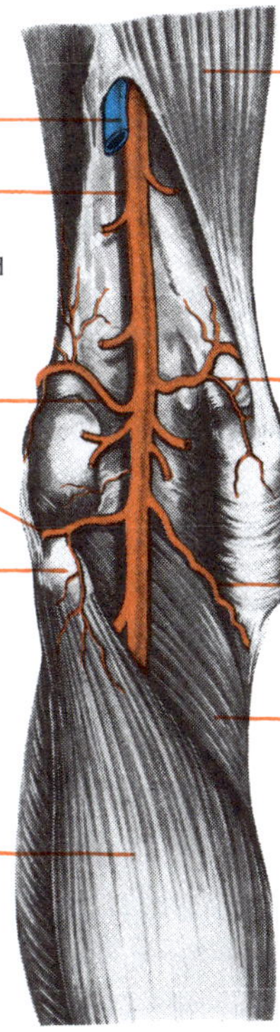

Fig. 151. Left popliteal artery and its branches.

cutaneous twigs, one of which accompanies the sural nerve. The hamstring branches anastomose superiorly with the perforating branches of the profunda femoris artery.

Superior, inferior, and **middle genicular arteries** lie on the anterior wall of the popliteal fossa. Their course and the anastomoses they form are shown in Figs. 151 and 187 and are described on p. 201. *The popliteal artery is the only significant route through which blood can reach the leg and foot from the thigh*. It is subject to compression when sitting on a hard edged seat and when the legs are crossed. Obliterative arterial disease affecting the popliteal artery seriously prejudices the blood supply to the large muscles of the leg and leads to ischaemic pain in them on exercise which is relieved by standing still—a condition known as intermittent claudication.

Popliteal vein

This is formed by the junction of the anterior and posterior tibial veins near the lower border of the popliteus muscle. The vein ascends on the posterior surface of the popliteal artery, moving gradually towards its lateral side. The tributaries of the popliteal vein correspond to the branches of the artery with the addition of the small saphenous vein. Open the popliteal vein and note its numerous **valves**.

The back of the thigh

Dissection

Make a vertical incision through the skin remaining on the back of the thigh. Strip the skin and superficial fascia from the deep fascia by blunt dissection. Look for the branches of the posterior cutaneous nerve of the thigh as you do so. Find and follow the branches of the medial anterior and lateral cutaneous nerves of the thigh into this region [Fig. 140].

Divide the deep fascia vertically. Find the posterior cutaneous nerve of the thigh and trace it to the gluteal region. Remove the fascia from the posterior surfaces of the hamstring muscles. Follow the sciatic nerve downwards from the gluteal region. Trace its branches into the hamstring muscles, including the short head of biceps, and adductor magnus. Find the branches of the perforating arteries which run with the nerves.

Separate the hamstring muscles from each other and trace them to their attachments.

Posterior cutaneous nerve of the thigh
(S. 1, 2,3)

This nerve leaves the pelvis through the lower part of the greater sciatic foramen close to the inferior gluteal vessels and nerve. In the gluteal region, it is deep to gluteus maximus and lies on the sciatic nerve or along its medial border. It then runs down the middle of the back of the thigh immediately deep to the deep fascia, and is separated from the sciatic nerve by the long head of biceps. It pierces the deep fascia at the back of the knee and descends as far as the middle of the back of the calf.

Branches

All are cutaneous. (a) In the gluteal region: (1) **Gluteal** branches wind around the lower border of gluteus maximus and supply a small area of skin in the lower part of the buttock. (2) A **perineal** branch turns medially across the back of the hamstring muscles to the perineum. It supplies skin on the upper, medial side of the thigh and the external genital organs. (b) A series of small branches pierce the deep fascia to the medial side and *back of the thigh* and the upper half of the posterior surface of the *calf of the leg* [Fig. 218].

Flexor muscles

These muscles form the mass on the back of the thigh. Their tendons in the ham, or back of the thigh, give them the name of **hamstrings**. All arise from the ischial tuberosity, except the short head of biceps, and all are inserted into the bones of the leg. They are, therefore, extensors of the hip joint and flexors of the knee joint. It is their inability to stretch sufficiently when the hip joints are flexed and the knees extended which prevents the untrained from touching their toes in this position. The structural changes which result from training and which permit a greater range of movement are not clear in these or other muscles.

Biceps femoris

The **long head** arises with semitendinosus from the medial part of the ischial tuberosity [Fig. 141] and is partly continuous with the sacrotuberous ligament. The **short head** arises from the linea aspera and the upper half of the lateral supracondylar line. The two heads unite and cross the posterolateral surface of the knee joint to the head of the fibula [Fig. 251]. Near its insertion, the tendon of biceps overlies the **fibular collateral ligament** of the knee joint. This ligament passes obliqely through the tendon dividing it into two unequal parts. **Nerve supply:** the long head is supplied by the tibial part of the sciatic nerve, the short head by the common peroneal part. Thus each head may be separately paralysed as a result of a wound. **Action:** it extends the hip joint, flexes the knee joint, and rotates the leg laterally when the knee is flexed. The short head acts only on the knee joint.

Semitendinosus

This muscle arises with the long head of biceps [Figs. 141, 251]. In the distal third of the thigh, the muscle forms a cylindrical tendon. This descends on the semimembranosus to the medial side of the knee. Here the tendon turns forwards and spreads out to be inserted into the upper part of the medial surface of the tibia, posterior to the tendons of gracilis and sartorius. A complex **bursa** separates these tendons from one another and is continuous with a bursa between semitendinosus and the tibial collateral ligament of the knee. **Nerve supply:** it receives two branches from the tibial part of the sciatic nerve, one above and one below an incomplete tendinous intersection. **Action:** it extends the hip joint, flexes the knee, and medially rotates the leg when the knee is flexed.

Semimembranosus

This muscle arises from the lateral part of the ischial tuberosity [Fig. 141]. The broad tendon of origin passes downwards and medially deep to the biceps and semitendinosus and forms a groove in which the semitendinosus lies. At the back of the knee, it forms a thick, flattened tendon which is inserted chiefly into the groove on the posteromedial surface of the medial condyle of the tibia [fig. 253]. The tendon also has extensions which form: (1)

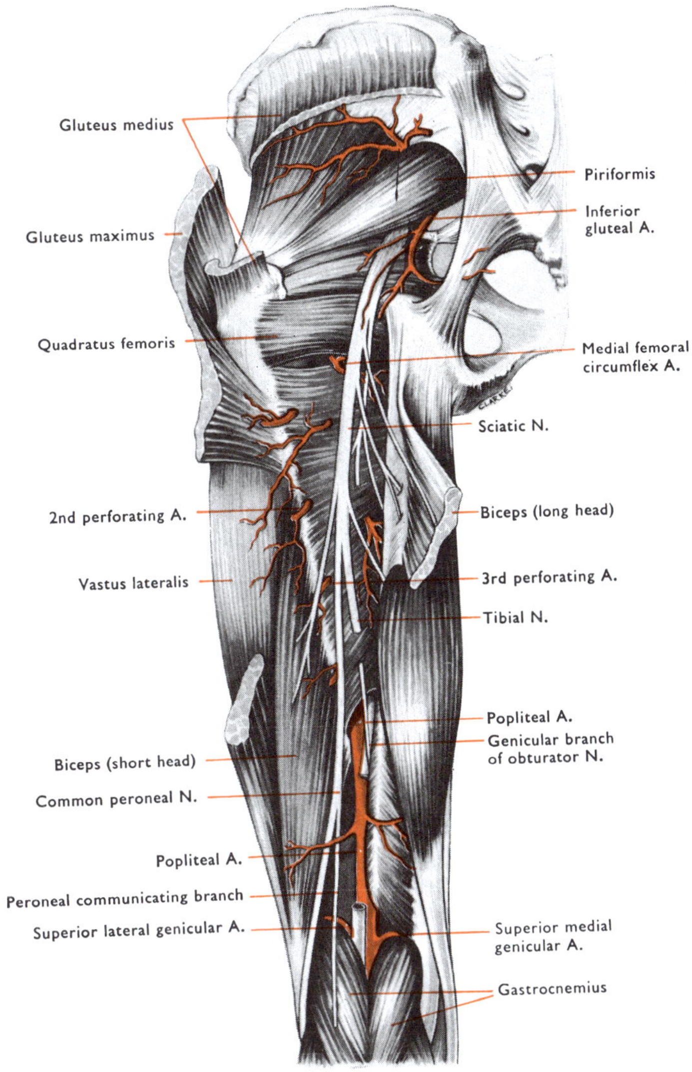

Fig. 152. Dissection of gluteal region and back of thigh. Most of the tibial N has been removed. Veins uncoloured.

the **oblique popliteal ligament** of the knee joint [p. 217] and (2) the **fascia covering popliteus** through which it is inserted into the soleal line of the tibia [Fig. 163]. The semimembranosus bursa lies between the tendon and the medial head of gastrocnemius. It is often continuous with the bursa between that head and the back of the knee joint. **Nerve supply:** the tibial part of the sciatic nerve. **Action:** as semitendinosus.

Sciatic nerve

The sciatic nerve leaves the pelvis through the greater sciatic foramen. It descends through the inferomedial part of the gluteal region between gluteus maximus, posteriorly, and the ischium, obturator internus and the gemelli, and quadratus femoris, anteriorly. In the back of the thigh, the nerve lies deep to the long head of biceps on the posterior surface of adductor magnus. It ends by dividing into the tibial and common peroneal nerves at a variable point above the popliteal fossa.

Branches

The branches that spring from the trunk of the nerve (tibial part) supply the **ischial** (hamstring) **part of adductor magnus** and the **hamstrings** except the short head of biceps femoris which is supplied by the common peroneal nerve. The semitendinosus receives two branches and those to the semimembranosus and adductor magnus often arise by a common stem.

Dissection

Detach the hamstring muscles from the ischial tuberosity and turn them aside. This exposes the posterior surface of adductor magnus. Remove the fascia from this muscle but preserve the branch from the sciatic nerve which enters the muscle near its medial border. Expose the insertion of the adductor magnus and the perforating arteries which pass between the muscle and the femur. Trace the perforating arteries laterally into vastus lateralis.

From the front, identify adductor longus and follow it to its insertion into the linea aspera. Turn the muscle forwards and follow the profunda vessels which pass downwards behind it. They are close to the femur. Remove the fascia from the profunda vein, which is anterior to the artery, then cut its tributaries to expose the artery and its branches. Divide the muscular branches of the profunda artery, but preserve the perforating arteries which lie close to the femur. Demonstrate their continuity with the vessels found on the posterior surface of adductor magnus.

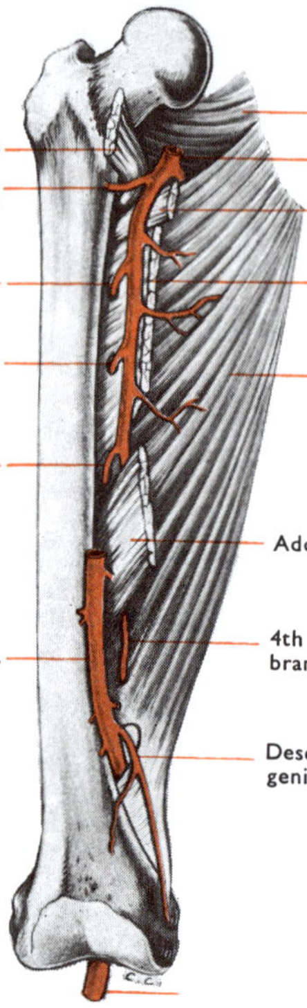

Fig. 153. Profunda femoris artery and its branches. The upper part of adductor longus has been removed to expose the artery.

Profunda femoris artery

This is the chief artery of supply to the muscles of the thigh. It arises from the femoral artery in the femoral triangle and curves medially behind the femoral vessels giving off the lateral and medial circumflex arteries. It then passes posteriorly between pectineus and adductor longus, and descends close to the femur, posterior to adductor longus. Here the first three perforating arteries arise and the vessel continues as the fourth perforating artery from a point a little below the middle of the thigh.

Branches

The circumflex arteries have been seen already [pp. 144, 158]. Muscular branches supply the adductor muscles. The four perforating arteries arise in series from the profunda [Fig. 153]. They wind round the back of the femur to vastus lateralis, grooving the linea aspera under tendinous arches formed by the muscles attached to it [Fig. 249]. They give branches to the adductor and hamstring muscles and the second or third supplies the **nutrient artery to the femur**. A further nutrient artery may arise from the fourth.

Arterial anastomoses

There is a longitudinal anastomosis between branches of the internal iliac, the femoral, and the popliteal arteries in the back of the thigh. The inferior gluteal artery anastomoses with the terminal branches of the circumflex arteries which link up with the perforating arteries (cruciate anastomosis, p. 158), anastomosing on the hamstring muscles and joining branches of the popliteal artery to these muscles. Thus an alternative supply to the limb exists by this route, but it can only communicate effectively with the leg through the popliteal artery.

The hip joint

This is the most perfect example in the body of a ball-and-socket joint. The range of movement which it permits is less than that at the shoulder joint, but the strength and stability are much greater. These features arise from: (1) the depth of the **acetabulum** which is increased by the **labrum acetabulare;** (2) the strength of the ligaments and the surrounding muscles. The long, narrow **neck of the femur** increases the range of movement but produces a weak zone which is liable to fracture, especially in the aged.

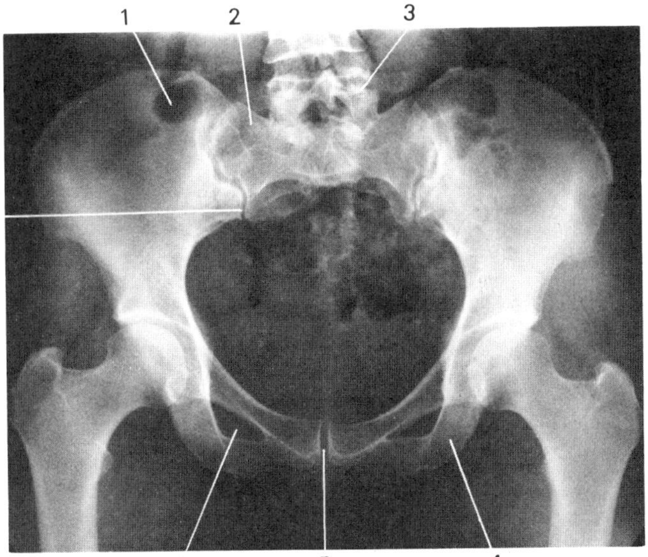

Fig. 154. Anteroposterior radiograph of adult pelvis, female.
1. Gas in caecum overlying ilium.
2. Lateral part of sacrum.
3. 5th lumbar vertebra.
4. Ischial tuberosity.
5. Public symphysis.
6. Obturator foramen.
7. Sacro-iliac joint.

Ligaments of the hip joint

Articular capsule

The fibrous capsule is exceedingly strong anteriorly, and surrounds the joint on all sides. Proximally, it is attached to the margin of the acetabulum and its transverse ligament. Distally, it is attached anteriorly to the whole length of the intertrochanteric line and to the root of the greater trochanter. Posteriorly, it falls short of the intertrochanteric crest by about a finger-breadth, and its attachment to the neck of the femur is weak.

The fibre bundles which comprise the fibrous capsule run in two different directions. The majority run obliquely from the acetabulum to the femur. Other bundles encircle the capsule more or less parallel to the margin of the acetabulum. These form the **zona orbicularis** and are best seen on the posterior and inferior parts of the fibrous capsule. The oblique fibres are best seen on the anterior surface.

The fibrous membrane has three main thickenings.

Iliofemoral ligament [Figs. 155, 158].

This ligament lies on the front of the joint. It is the thickest and most powerful part of the articular capsule. Proximally, it is attached to the inferior part of the anterior inferior iliac spine and to the surface of the ilium immediately lateral to the spine. Distally, it widens to be attached to the intertrochanteric line of the femur. It is thicker at the sides than in the middle. This gives the ligament the appearance of an inverted Y [Fig. 155].

The iliofemoral ligament is more than 0.5 cm thick. It is one of the strongest ligaments in the body—its only rival being the interosseous sacro-iliac ligament. A stress varying from 250 to 750 lb is required to rupture it. Thus it is rarely torn asunder in dislocation of the hip joint, and the surgeon may use it as a stay in levering the head of the femur back into the acetabulum.

In the erect posture, a vertical line through the centre of gravity of the body falls slightly behind a line joining the centres of the two hip joints. The tendency of the body to fall backwards on the hip joints is resisted by the iliofemoral ligaments which maintain the erect posture without muscular activity at these joints.

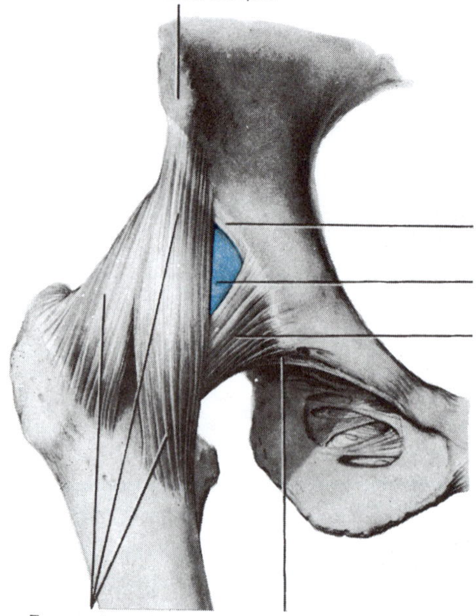

Fig. 155. Dissection of hip joint from the front.

Pubofemoral ligament

This ligament arises from the pubic bone and the obturator membrane [Fig. 155]. It lies in the lower and anterior part of the fibrous capsule. When the bursa deep to iliopsoas is continuous with the cavity of the hip joint, the communication lies between this band and the iliofemoral ligament.

Ischiofemoral ligament

This is a weak band which arises from the ischium below the acetabulum. It passes upwards and laterally into the fibrous capsule.

Movements at the hip joint

Test the range of movement of your own joint. **Flexion** is very free. It is only prevented by the thigh coming into contact with the anterior abdominal wall. **Extension** is extremely restricted by the iliofemoral ligament. The ability to carry the limb posteriorly to the horizontal plane is only achieved by tilting the pelvis fowards on the opposite femur. **Abduction** is restricted by the pubofemoral ligament. **Adduction** (as in crossing one thigh over the other) is limited by the lateral portion of the iliofemoral ligament and the upper part of the fibrous capsule. **Medial rotation** tightens the ischiofemoral ligament, while **lateral rotation** is limited by the pubofemoral ligament and the lateral parts of the iliofemoral ligament.

Dissection

If the hip joint is to be dissected in your specimen, cut through the femoral vessels and nerve immediately inferior to the inguinal ligament. Divide the sartorius and the rectus femoris about 5 cm from their origins and turn them downwards. Cut through iliopsoas near its insertion and turn the two parts upwards and downwards thus exposing the psoas bursa [Fig. 155] and the capsule of the hip joint through which the bursa and hip joint are usually continuous. Remove the bursa and identify the margins of the thick iliofemoral ligament. Make incisions through the articular capsule (fibrous capsule and synovial membrane) along the borders of the iliofemoral ligament, then remove all other parts of the capsule. This demonstrates the thickness and strength of the iliofemoral ligament.

Transverse ligament of the acetabulum

This strong band of fibres bridges the acetabular notch. It completes the rim of the acetabulum, and converts the notch into a foramen through which vessels and nerves enter the acetabular fossa and the ligament of the head of the femur.

Labrum acetabulare

This fibrocartilaginous ring, attached to the rim of the acetabulum and the transverse ligament, deepens the cavity of the acetabulum and, slightly narrows its mouth by sloping inwards. The labrum is a tight fit on the head of the femur and, sealing it in the acetabulum, exercises an important function

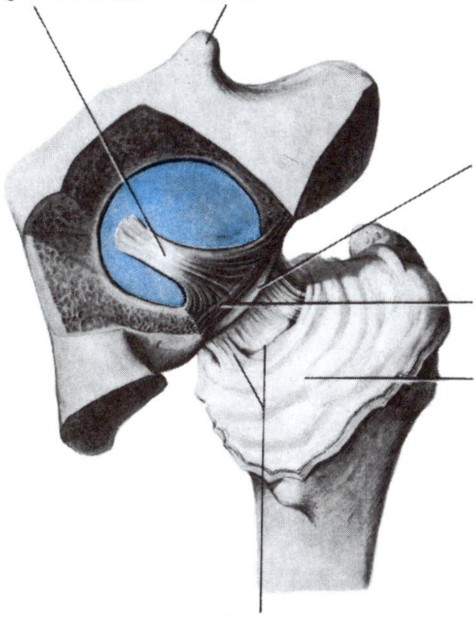

Fig. 156. Dissection of right hip joint from pelvic side. The floor of the acetabulum has been removed, and the articular capsule of the joint thrown laterally towards the trochanters.

in retaining the head within the acetabulum. Both surfaces of the labrum are covered by synovial membrane; the free margin is relatively thin, the attached margin much thicker.

Ligament of the head of the femur

This is a relatively weak band of connective tissue surrounded by snovial membrane. Its narrow, cylindrical end is implanted into the **pit on the head of the femur;** its broad, flattened end is attached to the transverse ligament and the adjacent margins of the acetabular fossa. This attachment may be defined by removing the synovial membrane which covers the ligament.

The ligament is too weak to play any mechanical part in the hip joint. It may help to spread synovial fluid on the head of the femur and act as part of the soft pad which can adjust the acetabular volume during movement by extrusion beneath the transverse ligament. Sometimes it transmits a small blood vessel to the head of the femur.

Synovial membrane and retinacula

A mass of fat occupies the non-articular fossa of the acetabulum. It is covered by synovial membrane which extends to the inner margin of the lunate surface and is reflected on to the ligament of the head of the femur at the acetabular notch. Acetabular branches from the obturator and medial circumflex arteries and the obturator nerve enter the fat and the ligament by passing through the acetabular notch.

The synovial membrane lines the inner surface of the fibrous capsule and covers the neck of the femur as far as the margin of the articular cartilage of the head. On the neck of the femur are a number of bundles of fibres which turn back along the neck from the attachment of the fibrous membrane. These **retinacula** may help to hold the fragments of the neck together when it is fractured within the articular capsule. Small arteries and veins pass along the retinacula to supply the neck and head of the femur (note the multiple foramina in the bone, especially on the posterosuperior surface of the neck). If the retinacula are torn when the neck is fractured, the *blood supply of the head of the femur* may be destroyed and normal repair of the fracture made impossible.

At the acetabular attachment of the articular capsule, the synovial membrane is reflected on to the labrum acetabulare and the transverse ligament and passes from the latter on to the ligament of the head of the femur.

Blood vessels and nerves

The hip joint is supplied from an anastomosis which is formed around the neck of the femur by: (1) ascending branches of the medial and lateral circumflex arteries; (2) acetabular branches of the obturator and medial circumflex arteries; (3) branches of the superior and inferior gluteal arteries.

Twigs which enter the ligament of the head of the femur from the acetabular branches sometimes enter the head of the femur but are not a significant supply to it.

Nerves enter the joint from : (1) the nerve to quadratus femoris; (2) the femoral, through the nerve to rectus femoris; (3) the anterior division of the obturator nerve and, occasionally, the accessory obturator nerve.

Dissection

If it is necessary to remove the lower limb to permit dissection of the perineum, this may be done by dividing the iliofemoral ligament and the ligament of the head of the femur. Otherwise the limb should be left attached to the hip bone.

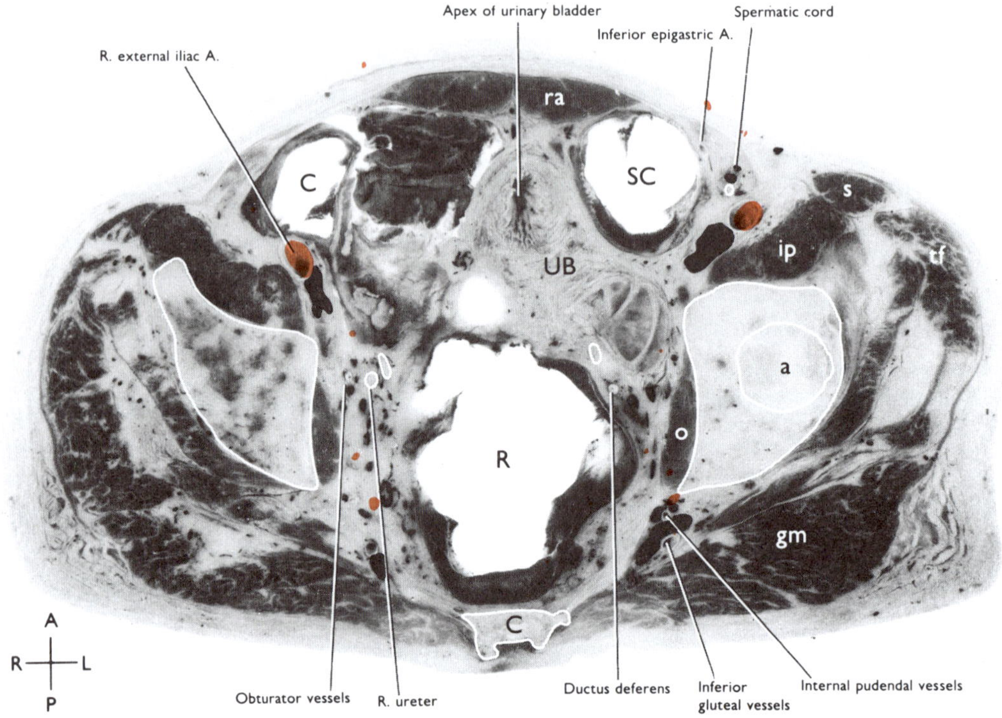

Fig. 157. Section through the coccyx, and upper part of the left hip joint, and urinary bladder (left side and apex). Outlined in white is each ureter and ductus deferens. The right ductus deferens (left side of illustration) lies immediately anteromedial to the right ureter, the left is in the spermatic cord. The left inferior gluteal and internal pudendal vessels lie immediately posterior to the sacrospinous ligament, the spine of the ischium lying below the level of the section.

a. Head of femur in acetabulum.
C. Caecum.
C. Coccyx.
gm. Gluteus maximus.
ip. Iliopsoas.
o. Obturator internus.
R. Rectum (distended).
ra. Rectus abdominis.
s. Sartorius.
tf. Tensor fasciae latae.
UB. Urinary bladder.
SC. Sigmoid colon.
A. Anterior.
P. Posterior.
L. Left.
R. Right.

It is the conventional arrangement to view CT and ultrasound scans from below. Hence the illustrations are of the lower surfaces of trunk sections so as to fit in with the attached CT scan (A).

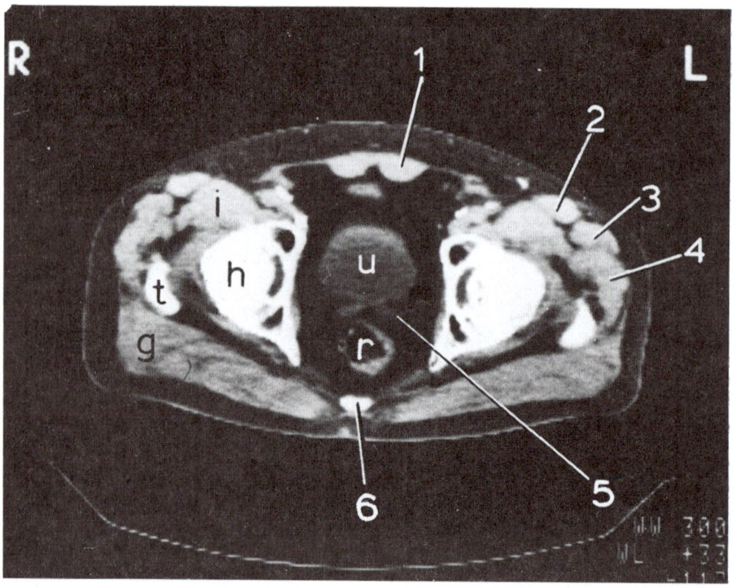

Fig. 157 (A). A computerized axial tomograph (CAT) taken through the hip joints during life. It is not exactly in the same plane as the cadaver section (above) but shows the anatomical detail which can be obtained by this radiological technique.

g. Gluteus maximus.
h. Head of femur in acetabulum.
i. Iliopsoas muscle. r. Rectum.
u. Urinary bladder.
t. Tip of greater tochanter of femur.
1. Rectus abdominis muscle.
2. Sartorius.
3. Tensor fasciae latae.
4. Gluteus medius and minimus.
5. Seminal vesicle. 6. Coccyx.

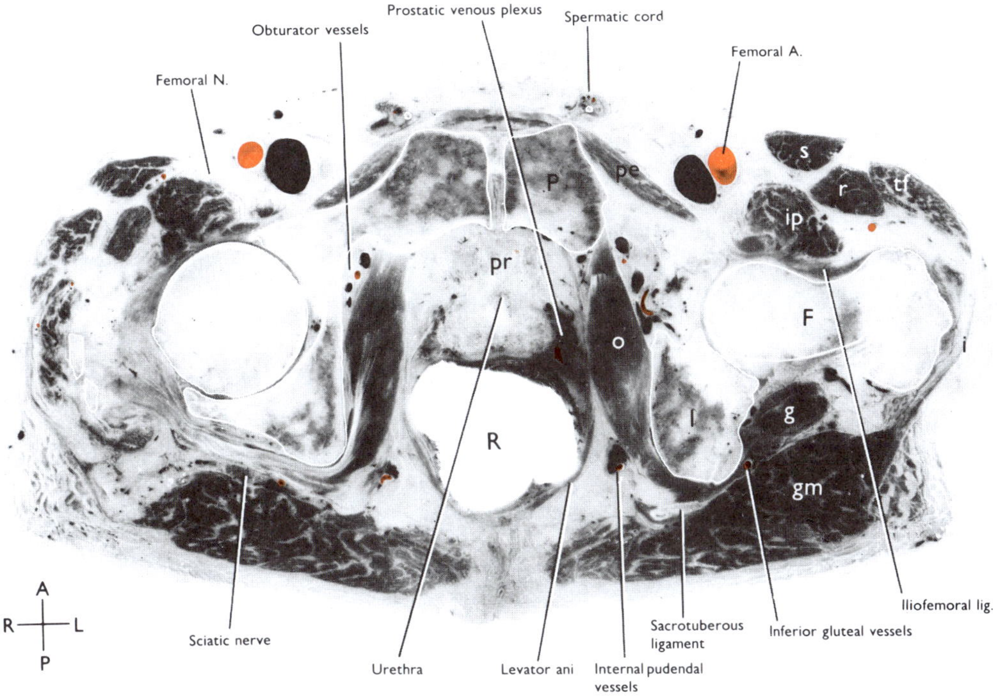

Fig. 158. Section through the pubic symphysis and the two hip joints. The left hip joint appears incomplete because the section passes through the acetabular notch. The entire length of the obturator internus is shown on the right side of the body, its tendon lying posterior to that of obturator externus as it approaches its insertion. The ductus deferens is outlined in white in each spermatic cord.

g. Gemellus inferior.
gm. Gluteus maximus.
i. Iliotibial tract.
ip. Iliopsoas.
o. Obturator internus.
P. Body of pubic bone.
pe. Pectineus.
pr. Prostate gland.
r. Rectus femoris.
R. Rectum (distended).
s. Sartorius.
tf. Tensor fasciae latae.
A. Anterior.
P. Posterior.
R. Right. L. Left.

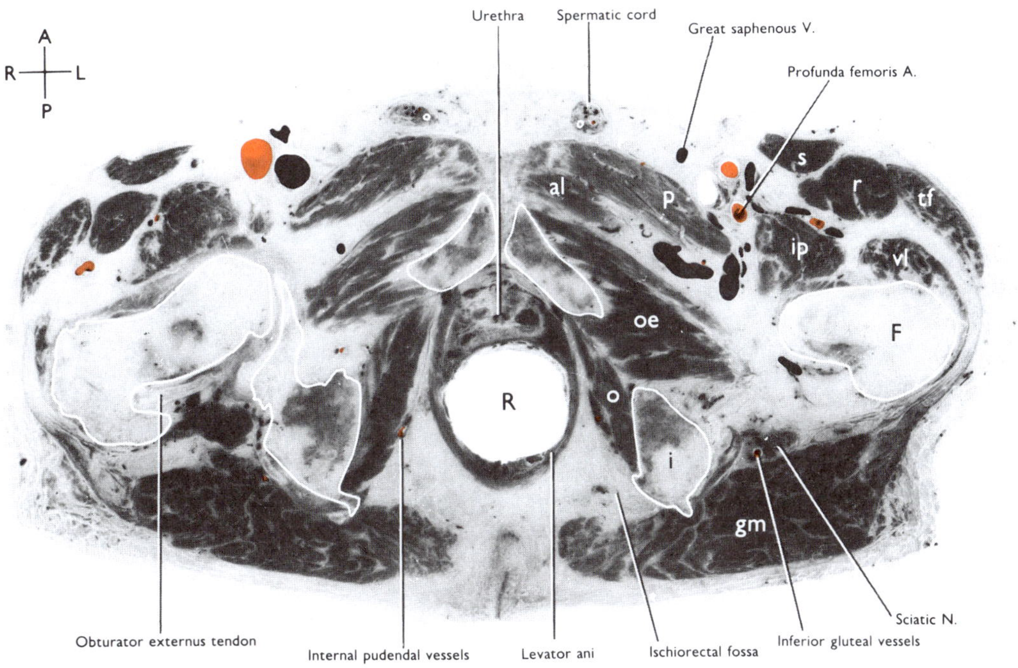

Fig. 159. Section through the trochanters of the femora, the greater on the right side of the body (left of illustration), the lesser on the left. Each ductus deferens is outlined in white.

al. Adductor longus.
F. Femur.
gm. Gluteus maximus.
ip. Iliopsoas.
o. Obturator internus.
oe. Obturator externus.
p. Pectineus.
r. Rectus femoris.
R. Rectum.
s. Sartorius.
tf. Tensor fasciae latae.
vl. Vastus lateralis.
A. Anterior.
P. Posterior.
R. Right.
L. Left.

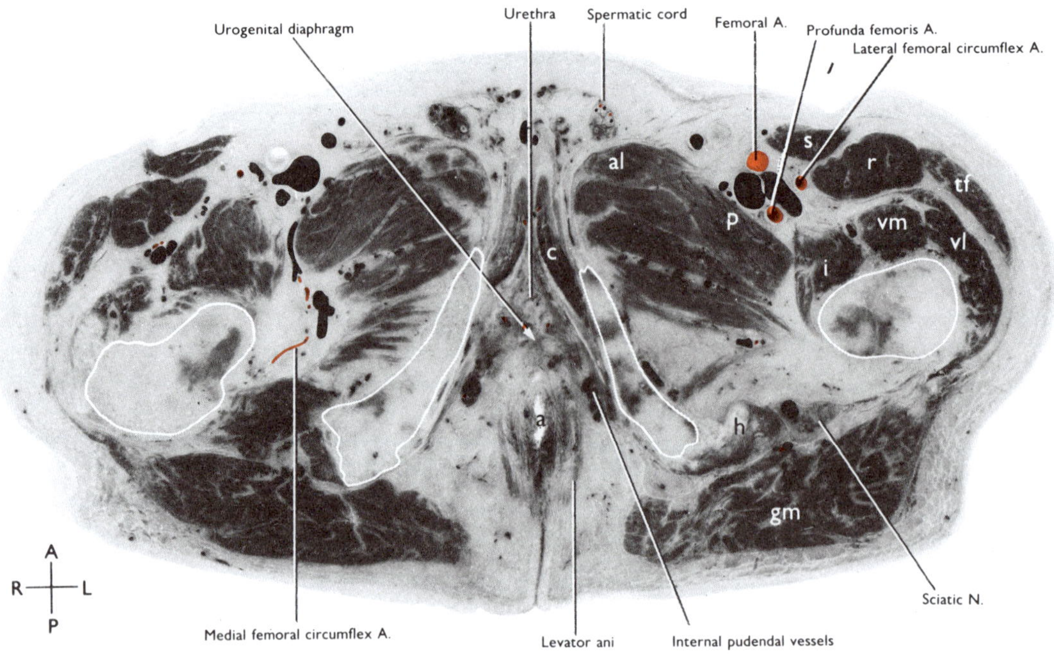

Fig. 160. Section through the inferior pubic and ischial rami, mainly in the plane of the urogenital diaphragm. Each ductus deferens is outlined in white.
a. Anal canal.
al. Adductor longus.
c. Crus of penis.
gm. Gluteus maximus.
h. Hamstring muscles.
i. Iliacus.
p. Pectineus.
r. Rectus femoris.
s. Sartorius.
tf. Tensor fasciae latae.
vl. Vastus lateralis.
vm. Vastus medialis.
A. Anterior.
P. Posterior.
R. Right.
L. Left.

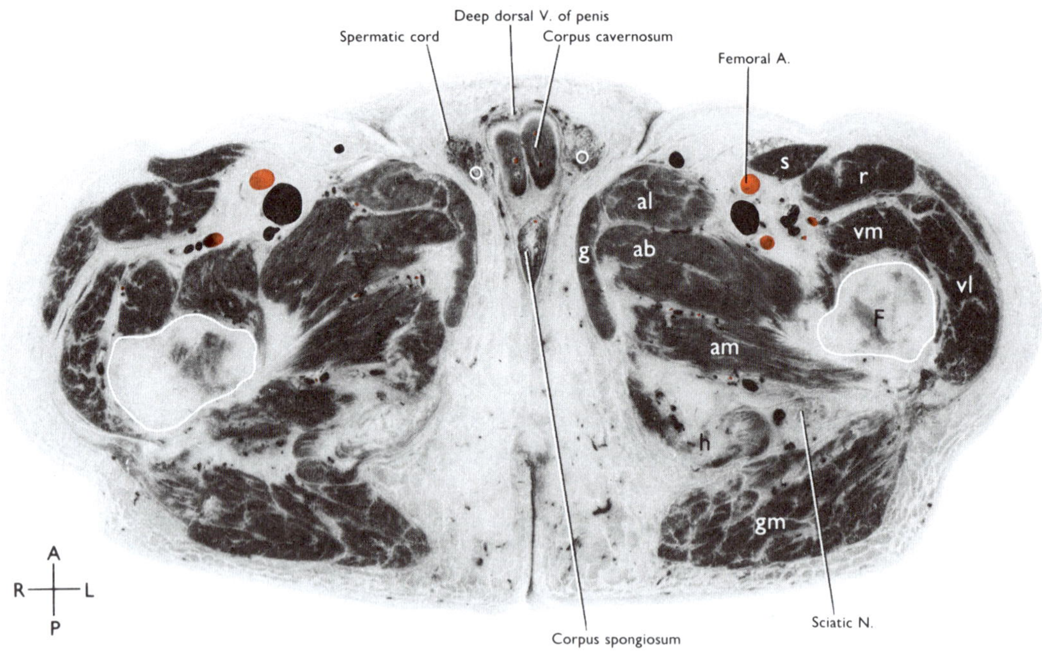

Fig. 161. Section through the proximal parts of the thighs and the root of the penis.
ab. Adductor brevis.
al. Adductor longus.
am. Adductor magnus.
F. Femur.
g. Gracilis.
gm. Gluteus maximus.
h. Hamstring muscles.
r. Rectus femoris.
s. Sartorius.
vl. Vastus lateralis.
vm. Vastus medialis.
A. Anterior.
P. Posterior.
R. Right.
L. Left.

The leg and the foot

Bones and surface anatomy

In the leg, the bones are the tibia medially and the fibula laterally [p. 124]. The body of the **tibia** is roughly triangular in transverse section with medial, posterior, and lateral surfaces. The medial surface is subcutaneous [Fig. 169] except in its upper quarter where the tendons of sartorius, gracilis, and semitendinosus are inserted into it towards the tibial tuberosity [Fig. 251]. Here the superficial part of the tibial collateral ligament of the knee is attached to a long, rough area immediately in front of the medial border. Inferiorly the medial surface is directly continuous with the medial surface of the medial malleolus —a thick downwards projection of the distal end of the tibia.

The plateau-like medial and lateral **condyles of the tibia** lie on the expanded upper end of the body. They are limited inferiorly by an almost horizontal line which, traced anteriorly, sweeps downwards to the junction of the smooth and rough parts of the **tibial tuberosity**. Here they mark the meeting of the fibrous capsule of the knee joint with the edge of the patellar ligament which is attached to the smooth part of the tuberosity. Inferiorly the tibial tuberosity is continuous with the sharp **anterior border of the tibia** [Fig. 162]. This is palpable throughout its length, though it becomes less sharp in the lower third of the bone, and deviates medially to the anterior surface of the medial malleolus. The posteromedial surface of the medial condyle has a

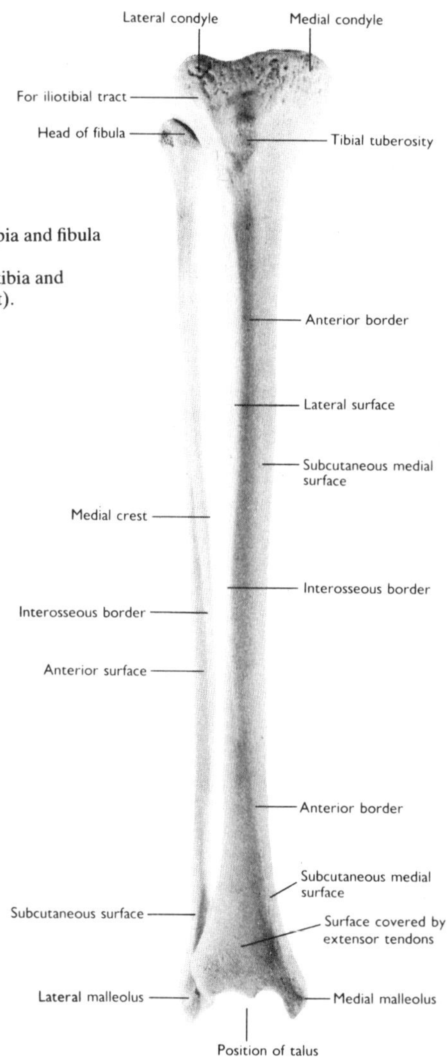

Fig. 162 (*left*) Right tibia and fibula (anterior aspect).
Fig. 163 (*right*) Right tibia and fibula (posterior aspect).

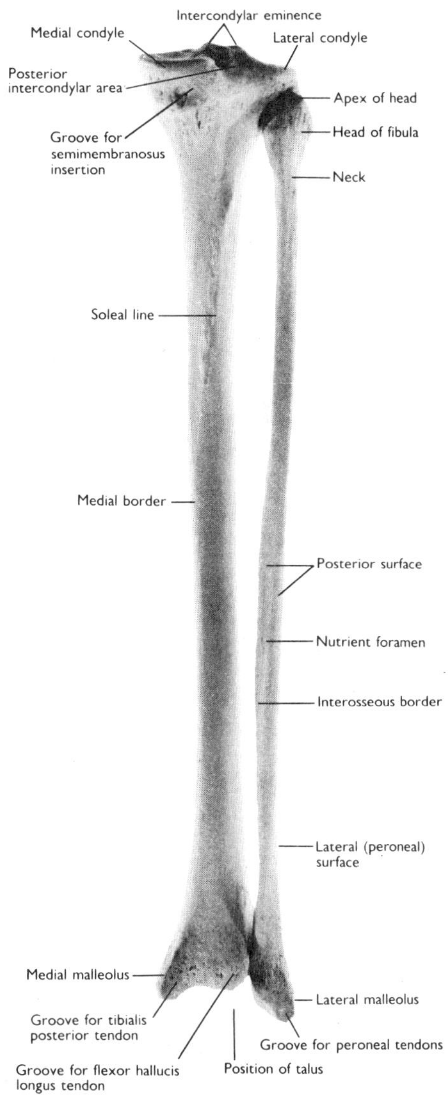

long, horizontal groove with a roughened area below it for the attachment of semimembranosus [Fig. 253]. In a similar but slightly lower position, the inferior surface of the lateral condyle has a smooth area for articulation with the **head of the fibula**. The upper surface of each condyle has a smooth, oval, concave area for articulation with the corresponding condyle of the femur. Between these is the **intercondylar area** which is divided into anterior and posterior parts by an **intercondylar eminence** on which there are medial and lateral **intercondylar tubercles**.

Immediately inferior to the articular area for the fibula, two ridges descend on the body of the tibia. (1) The vertical ridge is the **interosseous border** [Fig. 162] to which the interosseous membrane between the tibia and fibula is attached. At the distal end of the tibia, the interosseous border becomes continuous with a rough, triangular, concave area for the thickened part of the interosseous membrane (interosseous tibiofibular ligament) which binds the tibia firmly to the body of the fibula immediately above the ankle joint. The **interosseous membrane** separates the lateral from the posterior surface of the body of the tibia and hence the areas from which the anterior (extensor [Fig. 169B]) and posterior (flexor [Fig. 169E, G, H]) muscles of the leg arise. (2) The oblique ridge (soleal line [Fig. 163]) passes across the posterior surface of the tibia to meet the medial border at the junction of the upper and middle thirds of the body. The line gives attachment to the tibial head of the muscle soleus and to the popliteal fascia on the posterior surface of the **popliteus muscle** which is attached to the triangular area proximal to the soleal line. The nutrient artery to the body of the tibia enters the bone midway between the distal part of the soleal line and the interosseous border. Medial to the foramen is a vertical ridge which joins the middle of the soleal line to the interosseous border further distally. The area between these three ridges gives attachment to **tibialis posterior** [Fig. 253].

The **medial border** of the tibia is sharp distal to the point at which the soleal line meets it. Distally the border is continuous with the medial edge of a groove for the tendon of tibialis posterior on the posterior surface of the medial malleolus [Fig. 163]. Immediately lateral to this there may be a shallower, shorter groove for the tendon of flexor hallucis longus.

The **inferior articular surface** on the distal end of the tibia is concave anteroposteriorly, with a slight, central anteroposterior ridge. It is continuous medially with the articular surface on the lateral aspect of the medial malleolus. Both surfaces articulate with the body of the talus at the ankle joint.

The **medial malleolous** projects anteriorly (apex) and has a smooth notch posterior to this. The notch and the lateral surface of the apex give attachment to the powerful **medial** (deltoid) **ligament of the ankle joint**.

The **fibula** has an expanded head at its proximal end, with a narrower **neck** immediately below the head. The area for articulation with the tibia is on the superomedial surface of the head, with the **apex of the head** lateral to it. The distal end is the expanded **lateral malleolus** which projects beyond the medial malleolus and has a larger, triangular surface on its medial aspect for articulation with the body of the talus. The tibial and fibular malleoli grip the body of the talus between them. Posterior to the articular area on the malleolus is the **fossa of the lateral malleolus**.

The **body** of the fibula is buried in muscles and is moulded by them so that its shape varies considerably with the degree of muscularity. However, there are certain common characters.

The anterolateral surface of the lateral malleolus is continuous above with a rough, triangular, **subcutaneous area** which is easily palpated. This is continuous superiorly with the **anterior border** of the bone which marks the attachment of an intermuscular fascial plane separating the muscles of the anterior compartment of the leg (extensors) from those of the lateral compartment (peroneal muscles). Superior to the articular surface of the lateral malleolus is a rough triangular area for attachment of the **interosseous tibiofibular ligament** continuous above with the **interosseous border** of the fibula. This border inclines forwards as it ascends so that it comes close to the anterior border and leaves only a very narrow **medial surface** between them to which the extensor muscles are attached. Posterior to the interosseous border is the **posterior surface** of the fibula. Between the medial and posterior parts of this surface is a curved vertical ridge (**medial crest**) which meets the interosseous border inferiorly and is produced by the strong intermuscular septum immediately posterior to the tibialis posterior muscle [Fig. 169 E]. Behind the medial crest, the posterior surface gives rise to soleus above and flexor hallucis longus below [Fig. 253].

The **peroneal muscles** arise from the lateral surface. Inferiorly they follow the surface backwards, behind the subcutaneous triangular area, to run over the posterior surface of the lateral malleolus.

On your own leg, identify again the head of the fibula and the condyles and tuberosity of the tibia. Feel the anterior and medial borders of the tibia and the subcutaneous medial surface between them. Follow this surface to the **medial malleolus** and note that it is difficult to feel the apex and notch because of the medial ligament of the ankle joint attached to them. The **great saphenous vein** and the **saphenous nerve** run along the upper two-thirds of the medial border of the tibia.

Find the **neck of the fibula** and roll the peroneal nerve on its posterolateral surface [p. 160]. Trace the fibula downwards, feeling it through the muscles. Press on the middle of the bone and note that it can be pushed inwards to a slight extent, like a firm spring. Find the **lateral malleolus** and confirm that it projects further distally than the medial malleolus.

On the back of your leg, feel the fleshy mass of the **gastrocnemius** and **soleus**. These two muscles are thrown into contraction by standing on the toes. When this is done, the two heads of the superficial gastrocnemius stand out on the flat soleus which bulges laterally and medially beyond it and extends further inferiorly than gastrocnemius. Trace these muscles to the **tendo calcaneus**—the thick tendon through which they are inserted into the tip of the heel. Note that the tendo calcaneus lies more than 2 cm posterior to the bones of the leg. Place your fingers in the hollows anterior to the tendo calcaneus and press forwards. The malleoli are felt indistinctly through the tendons which cover their posterior surfaces. These tendons are passing from the leg into the foot. On the back of the medial malleolus, feel the pulsations of the **posterior tibial artery**.

Bones of the foot

The general arrangement has been given already [p. 124]. Make use of a set of foot bones to confirm the following points, and identify the palpable parts in your own foot.

The **talus** consists of a cuboidal **body** with a **neck** and **head** projecting forwards and slightly medially from it. The body articulates, superiorly, by its convex **trochlea** with the distal end of the tibia, medially, with the medial malleolus through a flat, comma-shaped surface, laterally, with the lateral malleolus through a large, triangular area. The last area is concave from above downwards, its lower end projecting as the **lateral process of the talus.** Posterior to the trochlea, the lower part of the talus projects backwards (**posterior process**). This is grooved by the tendon of flexor hallucis longus producing the lateral and medial **tubercles of the posterior process**. On the inferior surface, the body of the talus articulates with the calcaneus at the cylindrical **subtalar joint**. Anterior to this, and separated from it by the **sulcus tali**, is a long, oblique articular surface on the body, neck, and lateral part of the inferior surface of the head. The posterior part of this surface articulates with a medial projection of the calcaneus, the **sustentaculum tali**, the anterior part with a separate area on the distal, superior surface of the calcaneus. These two surfaces on the talus are angled to each other but are continuous. Medial to and between them is another articular area on the inferomedial part of the head. This articulates, with the powerful **plantar calcaneonavicular** (spring) **ligament** which binds the sustentaculum tali to the navicular and supports the head of the talus. The distal surface of the head forms a shallow ball-and-socket joint with the navicular. This complex is the **talocalcaneonavicular** joint.

Thus the talus is firmly gripped between tibia and fibula at the ankle joint. Only movements in the sagittal plane (**dorsiflexion** and **plantar flexion**) are possible here. Note that the **malleolar surfaces on the talus** are wider apart anteriorly than posteriorly. Thus in dorsiflexion, the talus is more firmly

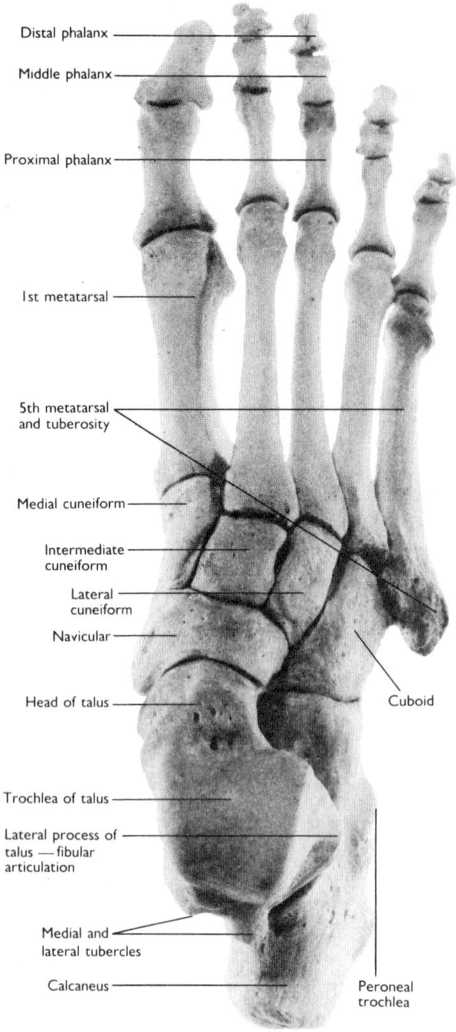

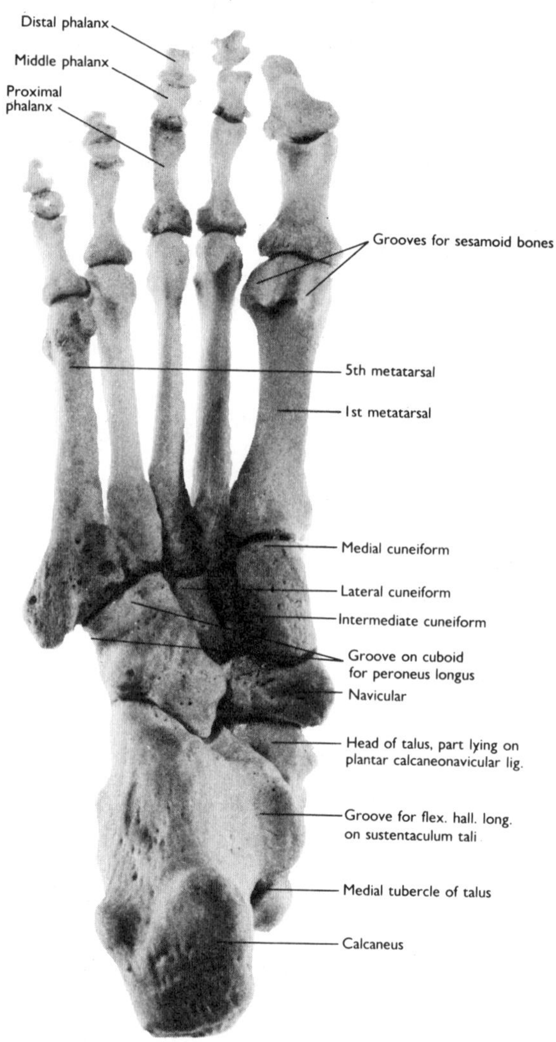

Fig. 164 (*above left*). Superior or dorsal surface of bones of right foot.
Fig. 165 (*above right*). Inferior or plantar surface of bones of right foot.

gripped than in plantar flexion. The slight spring which is present in the body of the fibula allows the lateral malleolus to move outwards to a slight degree in dorsiflexion. If the talus is twisted in the ankle joint in this position, the lateral malleolus may be forced so far laterally that the springiness of the body of the fibula is overcome and it is fractured in the leg. The fulcrum for this movement is the thick interosseous tibiofibular ligament.

The joints between talus, calcaneus, and navicular permit the calcaneus and navicular to move round the talus on an almost horizontal axis (carrying

Fig. 166. Right talus (inferior surface). The groove of talus is the salcus tali.

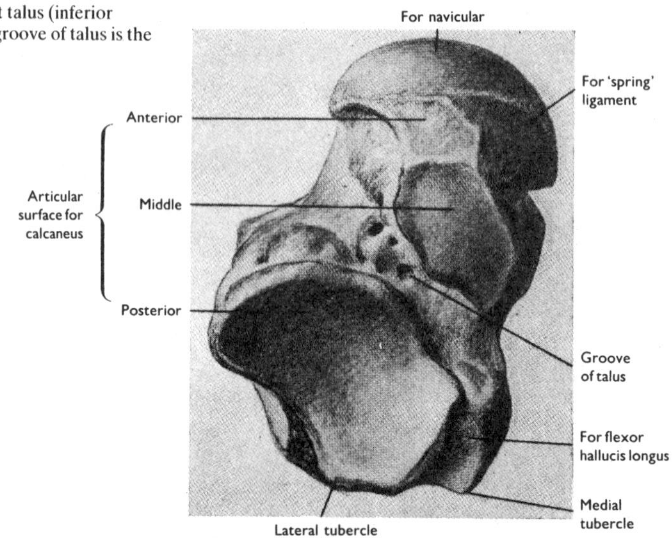

the remaining bones of the foot and toes with them). Movement of the calcaneus and navicular medially around this axis, turns the foot so that the sole faces medially (**inversion**). The opposite movement is **eversion** and is more limited.

The **cuboid** articulates with the distal end of the calcaneus by a curved, saddle-shaped joint which permits a moderate amount of movement. It also articulates medially with the navicular and the lateral cuneiform bone by flat surfaces. The remaining joints, between the navicular and the three cuneiform bones, and between these cuneiform bones and the medial three metatarsals, as well as those between the cuboid bone and the lateral two metatarsals, are all flat surfaces. These permit relatively little movement. This, combined with the close fitting of the first metatarsal to the medial cuneiform bone by two surfaces angled to one another and the manner in which the second metatarsal is keyed between the medial and lateral cuneiform bones, makes the foot a relatively rigid structure which has some resilience because of the presence of the joints. *The principal movements in the foot occur at the subtalar and talocalcaneonavicular joint complex.*

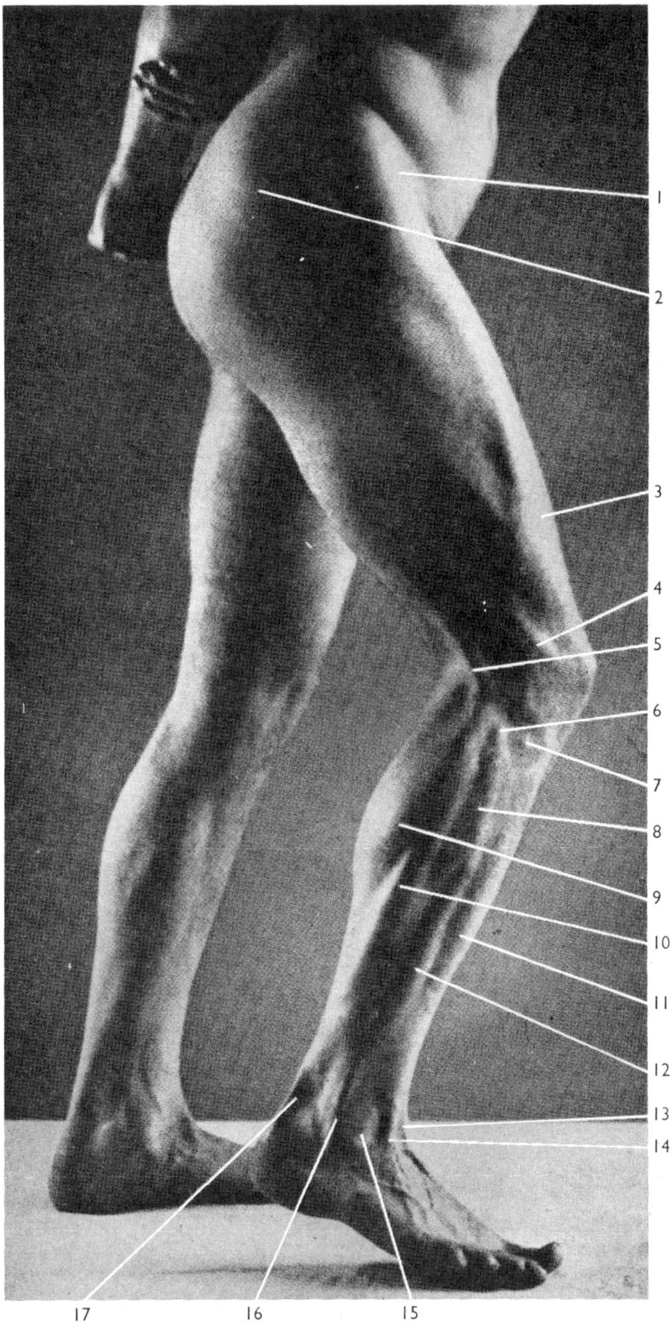

Fig. 167. The subject is 'setting' the muscles of the leg. Note the concavity of the popliteal fossa behind the flexed knee and the fullness of that region behind the straight knee. (From *Living anatomy* by R. D. Lockhart, 6th edn. Faber and Faber, London (1963).)

1. Tensor fasciae latae.
2. Gluteus medius.
3. Vastus lateralis.
4. Iliotibial tract.
5. Tendon of biceps femoris.
6. Head of fibula.
7. Prominence of side of condyle of tibia.
8. Peroneus longus.
9. Gastrocnemius.
10. Soleus.
11. Extensor digitorum longus.
12. Peroneus brevis.
13. Extensor hallucis longus.
14. Extensor digitorum longus.
15. Lateral malleolus.
16. Peroneus longus superficial to peroneus brevis.
17. Tendo calcaneus.

Note too that the foot may be split into lateral and medial parts. The *lateral part* consists of the calcaneus, the cuboid, and the lateral two metatarsals. This forms a relatively flat **lateral longitudinal arch** with the cuboid at the high point. The inferior surface of the cuboid is grooved by the **tendon of peroneus longus** which passes transversely across the foot beneath it. The *medial part* of the foot consists of the calcaneus, the talus, the navicular, the cuneiform bones, and the medial three metatarsals. This forms a high arch, especially medially. The head of the talus is at the summit resting on the plantar calcaneonavicular ligament. The anterior pillar of this **medial longitudinal arch** is the powerful **first metatarsal** bone. Its head rests on the ground through two **sesamoid bones** which transmit the pull of the short muscles of the great toe and form a tunnel between them through which the

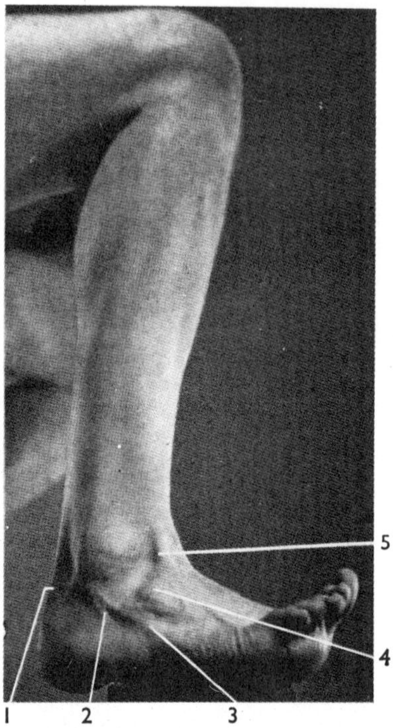

Fig. 168. Eversion with dorsiflexion of foot. The tendons of the peronei and extensor digitorum longus stand out actively. (From *Living anatomy* by R. D. Lockhart, 6th edn. Faber and Faber, London (1963).)
1. Tendo calcaneus.
2. Peroneus longus.
3. Peroneus brevis.
4. Extensor digitorum brevis.
5. Extensor digitorum longus.

long tendon may pass. This prevents compression of these structures when the full weight of the body is thrust forwards by pushing off on the head of the first metatarsal in walking or running. The other **metatarsals** are relatively thin and weak, except the fifth which forms the lateral end of a **transverse arch** in which the metatarsals and the distal row of the tarsal bones take part. This arched arrangement of the foot, which has approximately the shape of a half dome, permits the structures in the sole of the foot to avoid compression—a situation which no longer holds when the arches sag in *flat foot*.

On your own foot, identify the following palpable structures.

Grip the posterior part (**tuber**) of the **calcaneus**. Feel its lateral and medial **processes**. These are blunt prominences on each side of its plantar surface. Feel the subcutaneous lateral surface of the calcaneus and the resistance of the peroneal tendons immediately postero-inferior to the lateral malleolus. Follow the tendons inferiorly to the **peroneal trochlea**—a projection of the calcaneus a finger-breadth below the malleolus.

Find the **tuberosity on the base of the fifth metatarsal**. It lies midway between the point of the heel and the little toe. The **head of the fifth metatarsal** is felt as a rounded bulge at the root of the little toe. When the foot is shod, the head of the fifth metatarsal is so far from the point of the shoe that it may be mistaken for the tuberosity of the base. The **cuboid bone** can only be felt indistinctly proximal to the base of the fifth metatarsal.

Extend the toes firmly. A bulge appears on the lateral side of the dorsum of the foot a thumb-breadth anterior to the lateral malleolus. This is the muscle **extensor digitorum brevis** which arises from the dorsal surface of the distal part of the calcaneus.

Repeatedly plantar and dorsiflex the foot at the ankle joint. The anterior part of the **trochlea tali** can be felt appearing from under cover of the anterior part of the distal end of the tibia in plantar flexion. It is covered anteriorly by the tendons of the extensor muscles of the toes and tibialis anterior. Invert the foot firmly. The **tendon of tibialis anterior** becomes very prominent as it passes to the junction of the medial cuneiform and the base of the first metatarsal. A lump appears on the dorsum of the foot distal to the lateral malleolus. This is the lateral part of the **head of the talus**. Confirm that it disappears on eversion when the tendons of extensor digitorum become prominent.

On the medial side of the ankle, feel the resistance of the sustentaculum tali a thumb-breadth below the medial malleolus. Note that this moves with the posterior part of the calcaneus as the foot is inverted and everted. Evert the foot as far as possible and feel a bony lump antero-inferior to the medial malleolus. This is the medial surface of the head of the talus. Keep your finger on it and invert the foot. Note that it disappears and that the proximal edge of the **navicular** becomes prominent distal to it. Follow the navicular edge to its **tuberosity** on the plantar aspect. The tendon which passes forwards to this tuberosity, and stands out where the head of the talus lay in eversion, is the **tendon of tibialis posterior**.

Note the parts of the foot which are normally in contact with the ground and that it is the head of the first metatarsal which takes the pressure contact when you push off to take a step.

Toes

The arrangement of the phalanges and their joints with each other and with the metatarsals is similar to that in the fingers. The main difference lies in the massive phalanges in the big toe and the relatively small phalanges in the others. In the little toe, the middle and distal phalanges are commonly fused. The appearance of these bones indicates that the major stresses are carried by the big toe.

Front of the leg and dorsum of the foot

Dissection

Place the limb in a convenient position, e.g. with a block under the knee and the foot bent down (plantar flexed). Make incision 11 [Fig. 118]. Reflect the skin only from the front of the leg and the dorsum of the foot, but retain the superficial fascia so as not to destroy the veins.

Find the lateral cutaneous nerve of the calf and the great saphenous vein with the saphenous nerve beside it. Follow all three towards the foot [Fig. 123]. Note the branches of the nerves and the tributaries of the vein.

The great saphenous vein is continuous with the medial extremity of the dorsal venous arch of the foot. This lies transversely on the anterior parts of the metatarsals. Follow the arch to the lateral side of the foot, finding its dorsal metatarsal tributaries. Laterally the arch is continuous with the small saphenous vein. Trace this vein to a point below the lateral malleolus and find the sural nerve beside it. Follow the sural nerve along the lateral side of the foot to the little toe. It gives a communicating branch to the superficial peroneal nerve.

Find the superficial peroneal nerve as it pierces the deep fascia at the junction of the middle and distal thirds of the leg 2–3 cm medial to the fibula. Trace the nerve and its branches into the dorsum of the foot and the toes. Note that the most medial branch is to the medial side of the big toe, and that a branch does not pass to the first interdigital cleft. Find the dorsal digital nerves of the adjacent sides of the big and second toes. Follow them proximally. They arise from a branch of the deep peroneal nerve proximal to the cleft.

Superficial veins

There are two **dorsal digital veins** in each toe. Each joins the corresponding vein of the adjacent toe to form a **dorsal metatarsal vein** which enters the dorsal venous arch. The dorsal digital veins on the medial side of the big toe and the lateral side of the little toe join the ends of the arch to form the great and small saphenous veins respectively.

The **dorsal venous arch** lies on the distal parts of the bodies of the metatarsals. It drains the dorsum of the foot and toes.

The **small saphenous vein** runs posteriorly, passing first inferior and then posterior to the lateral malleolus. It ascends to the popliteal fossa in the back of the leg [Fig. 176].

The **great saphenous vein** passes posteriorly on the medial side of the foot. It ascends anterior to the medial malleolus, then obliquely across the distal third of the medial surface of the tibia. It receives most of the superficial veins of the medial side of the foot and leg, and communicates through the deep fascia with the deep veins: (a) on the medial side of the foot (medial plantar veins); (b) anterior to the ankle (anterior tibial veins); (c) behind the medial border of the tibia along which it ascends (posterior tibial veins). Slit open these **communicating veins** when they are found and note any valves within them. These **valves** are said only to permit the flow of blood from the superficial to the deep veins if they are functioning. Thus blood from the superficial veins can flow into the deep veins when these are emptied by the pressure of muscle contraction, but not vice versa. In fact, many of the communicating veins, especially in the foot, have no valves.

Cutaneous nerves

The upper two-thirds of the *front of the leg* is supplied by the **saphenous nerve** (L. 3, 4) medially, and the **lateral cutaneous nerve of the calf**, laterally. The lower third is supplied by the **superficial peroneal** and **saphenous nerves**.

The *dorsum of the foot* is mainly supplied by the medial and intermediate cutaneous branches of the **superficial peroneal nerve**. However, the lateral margin is supplied by the **sural nerve** and the medial margin by the **saphenous nerve** proximally and the **superficial peroneal** distally. The first interdigital cleft and the skin immediately proximal to it are supplied by the **deep peroneal nerve** [Fig. 218].

The *dorsum of the toes* is supplied by the digital branches of these nerves, except the saphenous. On the terminal phalanges, the supply is from the plantar nerves.

Superficial peroneal nerve (L. 4, 5; S. 1)

This arises from the common peroneal nerve on the lateral side of the neck of the fibula. It descends through the peroneal muscles supplying them. It enters the superficial fascia at the junction of the middle and distal thirds of the leg, and then branches into the **medial** and **intermediate dorsal cutaneous nerves**. Each of these supplies skin in the lower part of the front of the leg and the dorsum of the foot and divides into two **dorsal digital nerves of the foot**. Those from the medial nerve pass respectively to the medial side of the big toe and the adjacent sides of the second and third toes. Those from the intermediate nerve pass to the adjacent surfaces of the third, fourth, and fifth toes. All lie deep to the dorsal venous arch.

Sural nerve (S. 1, 2)

It descends in the back of the leg from the tibial nerve in the popliteal fossa to the posterior surface of the lateral malleolus. It lies first on gastrocnemius and then with the small saphenous vein (lower half of leg) in the superficial fascia supplying the overlying skin. Here it is joined by the **peroneal communicating** branch of the common peroneal nerve [Fig. 140]. It then turns forwards along the lateral border of the foot and little toe supplying the skin of both [Fig. 218].

Dissection

Remove the remainder of the superficial fascia and expose the deep fascia of the front of the leg and the dorsum of the foot and define its thickenings, the superior and inferior extensor retinacula [Fig. 173].

Deep fascia

The deep fascia of the leg is very strong. It is fused with the periosteum where the bones are subcutaneous. Thus it is attached to the borders of these areas on the tibia, fibula, and their malleoli. At the ankle it forms thickened bands (retinacula) which hold the tendons close to the joint and prevent them from springing forwards in dorsiflexion of the ankle [p. 177].

Retinacula

The **superior extensor retinaculum** is a broad band which extends between the triangular subcutaneous area of the fibula and the anterior border of the tibia.

The **inferior extensor retinaculum** is Y-shaped. The stem of the Y is attached to the upper surface of the anterior part of the calcaneus, medial to the extensor digitorum brevis. A superficial part of it continues over that muscle to the inferior peroneal retinaculum [Figs. 170, 174]. Medially, the limbs of the Y separate. The upper is attached to the medial malleolus, the lower passes to the medial side of the foot and fuses with the fascia of the sole. The deep fibres of the retinaculum turn back on themselves forming loops around the tendons. There are two loops: (a) around the extensor digitorum longus and peroneus tertius; (b) around the extensor hallucis longus. Thus the retinaculum also prevents the tendons from springing medially when the foot is inverted. In this position, there is a marked, medial angulation of the tendon of extensor hallucis at the retinaculum. The superior and inferior **peroneal retinacula** hold the tendons of peroneus longus and brevis in position as they pass, respectively, postero-inferior to the lateral malleolus, and on the lateral surface of the calcaneus [Fig. 174]. A similar **flexor retinaculum**, postero-inferior to the medial malleolus, holds the tendons of the deep muscles of the back of the leg in position as they pass into the foot [Fig. 186].

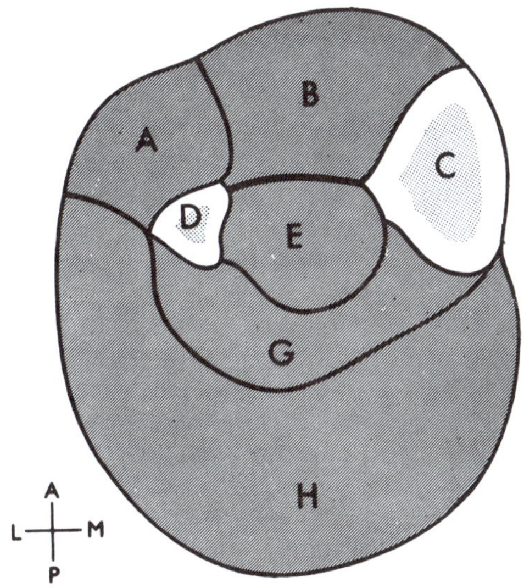

Fig. 169. Diagram of osteofascial compartments of leg. The interosseus membrane lies between B and E.

A. Peroneal muscles — Superficial Peroneal N.
B. Extensors — Deep peroneal N.
C. Tibia
D. Fibula
E. Tibialis posterior
G. Long flexors of toes
H. Superficial muscles of calf
(E, G, H) — Tibial N.
A. Anterior.
P. Posterior.
M. Medial.
L. Lateral.

Intermuscular septa
[Fig. 169]

These have already been mentioned in connection with the bones [p. 176]. They separate the various groups of muscles, give attachments to their fibres proximally, and place each group within a tight fascial box. Thus, when the muscles contract they are compressed by the fascia so that blood is pumped upwards from them in the veins—an essential part of the mechanism of venous return from the lower limb. Extensive division of the fascia or wasting of the muscles within the fascia impairs this venous return and leads to swelling of the limb because of the accumulation of fluid (oedema) [Fig. 124].

There are three named intermuscular partitions in the leg. (1) The interosseous membrane between B and E in Fig. 169. (2) The anterior septum between A and B. (3) The posterior septum between A and H. In addition the muscles of the back of the leg are divided into three layers by two coronal sheets of fascia.

Dissection

Divide the deep fascia of the front of the leg longitudinally between the tibia and fibula. Leave the extensor retinacula intact. As the division approaches the superior retinaculum, pass a blunt seeker deep to these retinacula. This will allow you to define their margins more easily. Try to avoid injury to the synovial sheaths of the tendons which lie deep to the retinacula and extend inferiorly beyond them [Fig. 170].

Turn the deep fascia medially and laterally and confirm its attachments to the bones. Open the synovial sheaths of the tendons and pass a blunt probe along them to define their extent. Note that a seeker in the compartment containing the extensor digitorum longus tendons under the inferior extensor retinaculum cannot be passed medially into that of extensor hallucis because of the loop passing from the deep surface of the retinaculum back towards the attachment to the calcaneus and to the tarsal bones. A similar restriction exists in the compartment of the extensor hallucis longus tendon.

Follow the tendons upwards and downwards. Define the individual muscles and their attachments to the bones. Separate tibialis anterior from the other three muscles down to the interosseous membrane. Find the anterior tibial vessels and the deep peroneal nerve on the membrane. Trace these upwards and downwards.

Draw the peroneus tertius muscle aside, and find the perforating branch of the peroneal artery as it pierces the lower part of the interosseous membrane. Follow it into the foot [Fig. 172].

Find the extensor digitorum brevis muscle on the dorsum of the foot. Trace its tendons to the medial four toes [Fig. 173]. Follow the anterior tibial artery and the deep peroneal nerve into the foot. Here the artery is known as the dorsalis pedis artery.

On the second or third toe, clean the extensor expansion formed by the extensor tendons. Trace the expansion, which is similar to that in fingers, to the distal phalanx.

Fig. 170. Synovial sheaths of dorsum of foot.

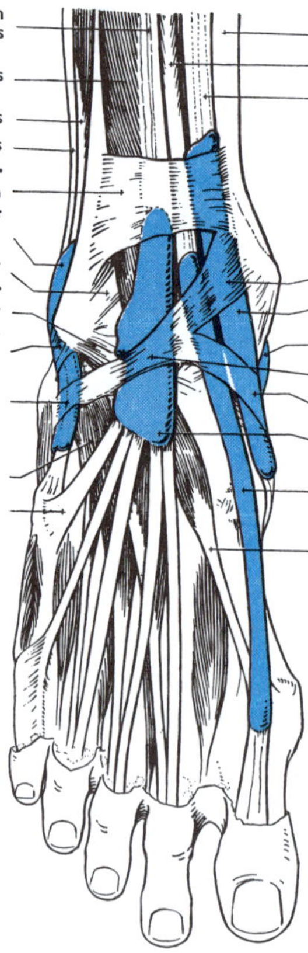

Synovial sheaths of the extensor tendons

There are three separate synovial sheaths [Fig. 170]. (1) That surrounding the tendon of **tibialis anterior** extends from the upper border of the superior extensor retinaculum almost to the insertion of the tendon. (2) That on the **extensor hallucis longus** tendon begins between the retinacula and reaches to the proximal phalanx of the big toe. (3) The third surrounds the tendons of **extensor digitorum longus** and **peroneus tertius**. It extends from the lower part of the superior extensor retinaculum to the middle of the dorsum of the foot.

Contents of the anterior compartment of the leg

The muscles arise from the tibia (tibialis anterior), the fibula (extensor digitorum longus, extensor hallucis longus, peroneus tertius), and from the adjacent parts of the interosseous membrane, the deep fascia, and the intermuscular septa. The compartment also contains the anterior tibial vessels and the deep peroneal nerve. These supply the muscles and continue into the dorsum of the foot and toes.

Tibialis anterior

It arises from the upper half of the lateral surface of the tibia and from the interosseous membrane. The tendon passes deep to the retinacula and inclines medially to the medial surface of the medial cuneiform and adjacent part of the first metatarsal close to their plantar aspects. This insertion is almost continuous with that of **peroneus longus** (q.v.). **Nerve supply:** the deep peroneal and recurrent genicular nerves. **Action:** it is a dorsiflexor and powerful invertor [p. 179] of the foot when the foot is raised from the ground. When the foot is on the ground, the muscle helps to balance the leg and talus on the other tarsal bones so that the leg is kept vertical even when walking on uneven ground.

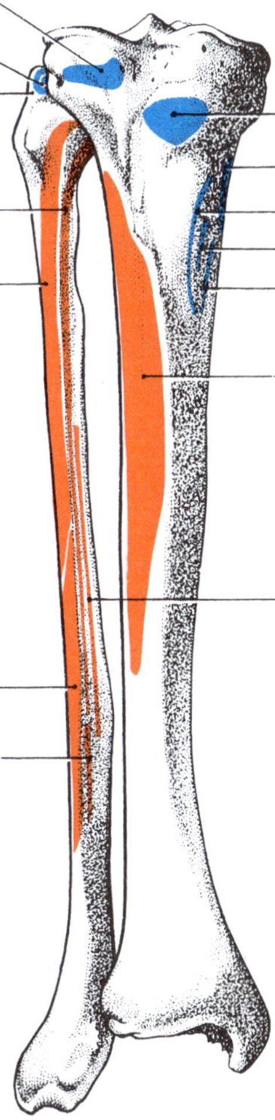

Fig. 171. Anterior aspect of bones of leg to show attachments of muscles.

Extensor digitorum longus

This long, thin muscle arises mainly from the upper three-fourths of the medial surface of the fibula. The tendon passes deep to the retinacula. Anterior to the ankle joint, it divides into four parts which pass to the lateral four toes. As each tendon approaches the metatarsophalangeal joint, it forms an **extensor expansion** similar to that in the fingers [p. 100]. This expansion forms the fibrous capsule on the dorsal surface of the metatarsophalangeal joint and extends on each side of the joint to the deep transverse metatarsal ligament. The thick, central part of the expansion continues on the dorsal surface of the proximal phalanx. Here it is joined by the greater part of the tendon of **extensor digitorum brevis** to the toe (second to fourth toes only) and is inserted into the base of the middle phalanx. The lateral and medial parts of the expansion continue distally, fused to the median portion. They cross the dorsolateral surfaces of the proximal interphalangeal joint and, approaching each other, are inserted into the base of the distal phalanx. The tendons of the **lumbricals** may join the medial side of the expansion in each toe; the interossei may send delicate expansions into it also, though, in the foot, they are principally inserted into the proximal phalanx.

The little toe has only the long extensor tendon, but the expansion is otherwise the same as in the second to fourth toes.

Nerve supply: the deep peroneal nerve. **Action:** it extends the interphalangeal and metatarsophalangeal joints of the lateral four toes. The failure of the interossei (q.v.) to be inserted to a significant degree into the extensor expansion means that extension of the interphalangeal joints when the metatarsophalangeal joints are extended depends on the **lumbricals**. If these muscles weaken or fail to join the extensor expansion the toes tend to be pulled into extension at the metatarsophalangeal joints (extensor digitorum longus and brevis) with flexion at the interphalangeal joints—a condition known as *hammer toe*. See also p. 209. The extensor digitorum longus also dorsiflexes the ankle joint, and acts with the peroneal muscles to evert the foot, i.e. it turns the foot on the talus so that the sole faces inferolaterally.

Peroneus tertius

This small muscle is continuous at its origin with the extensor digitorum longus and appears to be a part of it. It arises from the distal fourth of the medial surface of the fibula and the adjacent interosseous membrane. It is inserted into the base of the fifth metatarsal bone. Not infrequently it is partly fused with the tendon of extensor digitorum longus to the fifth toe. **Nerve supply:** deep peroneal nerve. **Action:** it everts the foot and dorsiflexes the ankle.

Extensor hallucis longus

It arises from the middle two-fourths of the medial surface of the fibula, medial to extensor digitorum longus. The tendon passes deep to the retinacula, and crosses in front of the distal part of the anterior tibial artery between them. The inferior retinaculum holds the tendon laterally so that it inclines forwards and medially to the big toe. On the distal part of the metatarsal the tendon forms an **extensor expansion**. The central part of the expansion passes to the distal phalanx, and a slip of the tendon may pass to the proximal phalanx. The lateral part of the expansion passes to the deep transverse metatarsal ligament, the medial part joins the tendon of **abductor hallucis** (q.v.). It is this part of the expansion which is stretched over the head of the first metatarsal when the big toe deviates laterally in the condition known as *hallux valgus*. The exposed medial part of the head of the metatarsal then forms the basis of a 'bunion'. The obliquity of the tendon of extensor hallucis longus, and more particularly that of brevis, plays a part in this lateral deviation of the phalanges of the big toe. **Nerve supply:** the deep peroneal nerve. **Action:** it extends the phalanges of the big toe and dorsiflexes the ankle joint. It may be used in inversion if the big toe is extended.

Deep peroneal nerve

This nerve arises from the common peroneal nerve between the neck of the fibula and the peroneus longus muscle. It pierces the anterior intermuscular septum and extensor digitorum longus, and descends in the anterior compartment of the leg with the anterior tibial vessels. It lies on the interosseous membrane between tibialis anterior and the long extensors of the toe. Near the ankle joint it is crossed superficially by the extensor hallucis longus [Fig. 173] and enters the dorsum of the foot midway between the malleoli. Here it is between the tendons of extensor digitorum longus and extensor hallucis longus with the dorsalis pedis artery. It almost immediately divides into two. (1) A medial branch continues towards the first interdigital space. It gives twigs to the adjacent joints and the first dorsal interosseous muscle. It ends by forming the **dorsal digital nerves** for the adjacent sides of the big and second toes. (2) The lateral branch passes between extensor digitorum brevis and the tarsal bones. Here a swelling on it gives branches to the **extensor digitorum brevis** and the surrounding joints. The deep peroneal

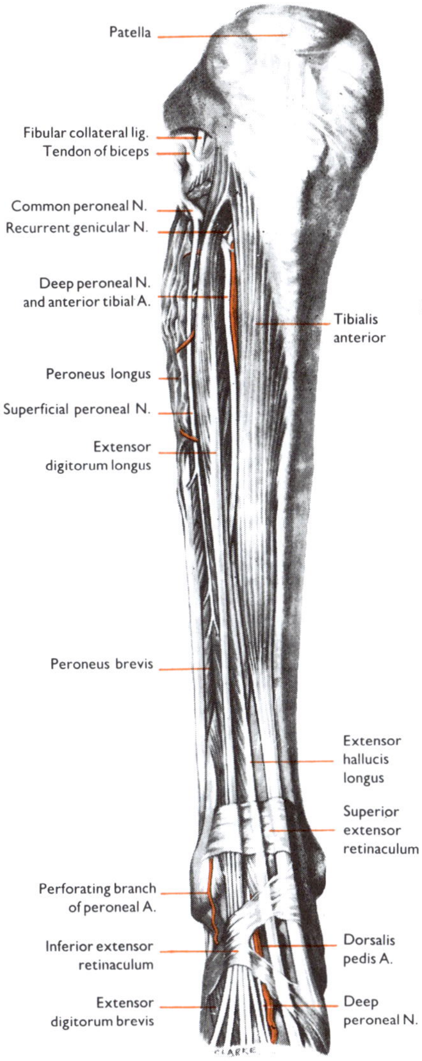

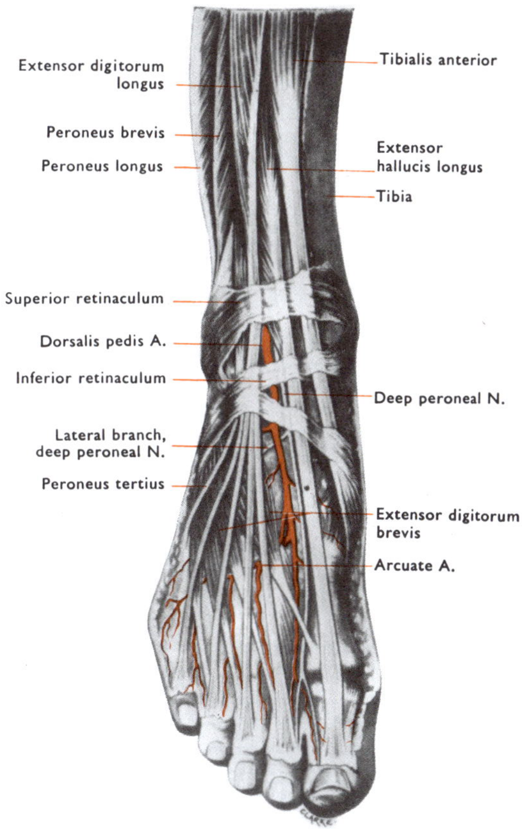

Fig. 172 (*left*). Dissection of front and lateral side of leg.

Fig. 173 (*above*). Dissection of dorsum of foot. Unusually the deep peroneal nerve is medial to the dorsalis pedis artery.

nerve supplies all the muscles of the anterior compartment of the leg and extensor digitorum brevis. If the nerve is destroyed, dorsiflexion of the ankle and extension of the metatarsophalangeal joints is lost, and inversion is weakened—the condition known as 'drop foot' [Table 12, p. 240].

Anterior tibial artery

This arises from the popliteal artery at the lower border of popliteus. It passes forwards above the interosseous membrane, close to the neck of the fibula, and turns downwards on the anterior surface of that membrane with the deep peroneal nerve. It becomes progressively more superficial as it descends and forms the dorsalis pedis artery, midway between the malleoli. The anterior tibial veins are closely applied to the artery.

Branches

It supplies twigs to the muscles of the anterior compartment of the leg and sends an anterior tibial recurrent artery upwards to the knee joint [Fig. 187]. Medial and lateral anterior malleolar arteries help to form a rete on each malleolus. The lateral one anastomoses with the perforating branch of the peroneal artery [p. 197].

Dorsalis pedis artery

It is the continuation of the anterior tibial artery. It begins on the anterior surface of the ankle joint, and runs with the deep peroneal nerve, deep to the inferior extensor retinaculum and the extensor hallucis brevis, to the proximal end of the first intermetatarsal space. Here it divides into the **arcuate artery** and the **first dorsal metatarsal artery**. On the dorsum of the foot it lies on the tarsal bones and is readily palpated against them between the tendons of extensor hallucis longus and extensor digitorum longus.

Branches

It gives medial and lateral **tarsal branches** to the tarsal bones and extensor digitorum brevis. The **arcuate artery** runs laterally across the bases of the metatarsals deep to the extensor tendons. It gives a dorsal metatarsal artery to each of the other intermetatarsal spaces. Each of these communicates through the proximal end of the intermetatarsal space with the plantar arch in the sole of the foot through the perforating branches of that arch. The perforating artery in the first space (**deep plantar branch** of the arcuate artery) is larger than the others and carries blood to the medial end of the plantar arch [Figs. 194, 195]. Each dorsal metatarsal artery then runs forwards over the corresponding dorsal interosseous muscle and forms the dorsal digital artery in each of two adjacent toes. The first and last of these dorsal metatarsal arteries sends a branch to the medial side of the big toe and the lateral side of the little toe respectively.

Extensor digitorum brevis

This muscle arises from the anterior part of the dorsal surface of the calcaneus and from the stem of the inferior extensor retinaculum and forms four tendons. The most medial is the **extensor hallucis brevis**. Its tendon runs obliquely across the dorsum of the foot to the base of the proximal phalanx of the big toe. **Action:** it extends the metatarsophalangeal joint of the big toe [p. 238].

The remaining three tendons join the long extensor tendons of the second to fourth toes. They are inserted into the middle and terminal phalanges of these toes through the extensor expansions [p. 186]. **Nerve supply:** the deep peroneal nerve. **Action:** extension of the interphalangeal and metatarsophalangeal joints of the second, third, and fourth toes.

Dissection

Cut through and reflect the extensor retinacula so that their attachments and the mechanism by which the tendons are held in position can be seen.

The lateral side of the leg

The muscles which cover the lateral surface of the fibula are the peroneus longus and brevis. They lie between the anterior and posterior intermuscular septa and partly take origin from them.

Peroneal muscles

The **peroneus longus** arises from the upper two-thirds of the lateral surface of the fibula. It overlaps the **peroneus brevis** which arises from the lower two-thirds of the same surface. They descend, closely applied to the lateral surface of the fibula, with longus superficial, and follow that surface as it spirals behind the triangular subcutaneous area of the fibula to reach the posterior surface of the lateral malleolus which is slightly grooved near its tip by them. Here they are in a **common synovial sheath**, and are held in position

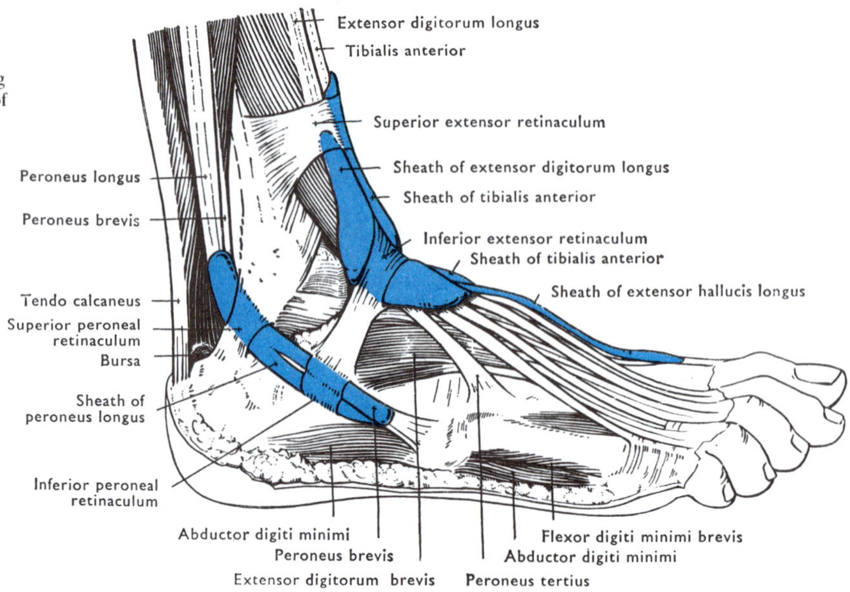

Fig. 174. Dissection showing synovial sheaths of tendons of lateral aspect of foot.

by the **superior peroneal retinaculum**. This is a thickened part of the deep fascia which passes from a ridge on the fibula, lateral to the peroneal tendons, to the calcaneus [Fig. 174]. The tendons emerge from the retinaculum and run antero-inferiorly below the lateral malleolus, on the lateral surfaces of the calcaneus and cuboid, with peroneus brevis superior to peroneus longus. They reach the lateral border of the foot near the base of the fifth metatarsal to which peroneus brevis is attached. Just proximal to this, peroneus longus turns over the lateral margin of the cuboid to enter the groove on its plantar surface. It then runs obliquely across the sole of the foot and is inserted into the medial cuneiform and the base of the first metatarsal. On the lateral surface of the calcaneus, the tendons are separated by the **peroneal trochlea** to which the inferior peroneal retinaculum is attached [Fig. 174]. **Nerve supply:** the superficial peroneal nerve. **Action:** peroneus longus and brevis are both evertors of the foot and plantar flexors of the ankle joint. Peroneus longus also draws the lateral and medial borders of the foot together by its transverse course across the sole. Like a tie-beam, it helps to maintain the transverse arch of the foot. The tendon of peroneus brevis is readily visible on the lateral side of the everted foot.

Peroneus tertius, p. 186.

Dissection

Divide the deep fascia over the peroneal muscles by a longitudinal incision in the leg. Turn the flaps aside and demonstrate their continuity with the anterior and posterior intermuscular septa. Retain the peroneal retinacula.

Separate the muscles from each other. Determine their attachments and find the nerves supplying them. Trace the common peroneal nerve to peroneus longus, and divide the muscle to follow the nerve between the muscle and the fibula. Trace the recurrent genicular branch of the nerve upwards and the superficial peroneal nerve downwards. Follow the deep peroneal nerve into continuity with the part already found in the anterior compartment of the leg.

Find and open the common **synovial sheath of the peroneal muscles.** It begins 3–5 cm above the superior peroneal retinaculum. Pass a blunt seeker into it and try to define its extent. Distally it divides to surround each tendon separately, and continues into the sole of the foot around the tendon of peroneus longus. Do not follow the latter tendon into the sole, but follow the tendon of peroneus brevis to its insertion and define the inferior peroneal retinaculum.

Terminal branches of the common peroneal nerve

This nerve turns round the lateral surface of the neck of the fibula between the deeper fibres of peroneus longus. Here it gives off a small recurrent genicular branch which pierces extensor digitorum longus and passes through tibialis anterior with the anterior tibial recurrent artery to the knee joint. It gives a branch to tibialis anterior and to the superior tibiofibular joint. The common peroneal nerve then divides into the superficial and deep peroneal nerves. The deep peroneal nerve pierces extensor digitorum to enter the anterior compartment of the leg [p. 186].

Superficial peroneal nerve

This nerve descends in peroneus longus till it reaches peroneus brevis. It then passes over the anterior border of brevis and descends between it and extensor digitorum longus, immediately deep to the deep fascia. It pierces the deep fascia in the distal third of the leg and divides into **medial** and **intermediate dorsal cutaneous nerves**. It supplies the peroneus longus and brevis, and the skin of the lower part of the front of the leg, the greater part of the dorsum of the foot, and most of the dorsal surfaces of the toes [p. 241].

The medial side of the leg

This consists of the medial surface of the tibia. It is subcutaneous except for a small part at the upper end which is covered by the tibial collateral ligament of the knee joint and the tendons of sartorius, gracilis, and semitendinosus [Fig. 171].

Dissection

Trace the tendons of sartorius, gracilis, and semitendinosus to their attachments. Turn them forwards and note the complex bursa which lies between them and separates them from the tibial collateral ligament of the knee joint as the tendons approach their insertion. Turn the tendons forwards and clean the surface of the ligament. Note that the tendon of semimembranosus and the inferior medial genicular vessels and nerves pass deep to the superficial part of the ligament. The deep part is attached to the margin of the tibial condyle, superior to the insertion of semimembranosus.

The back of the leg

The muscles in this region are divided into three layers by two layers of fascia [Fig. 169]. The *superficial layer* of muscles is inserted into the point of the heel by the large **tendo calcaneus** which can be felt and seen in the lower quarter of the back of the leg. This layer consists of the powerful plantar flexors of the ankle joint (gastrocnemius and soleus, with plantaris) which raise the weight of the body on to the toes, using the heads of the metatarsals as a fulcrum, e.g. in the push-off of walking. These muscles move independently of the middle layer of muscles; hence they are separated from it by a well-defined fascial layer which stretches from the medial border of the tibia to the posterior border of the fibula. This fascia encloses the deeper muscles, together with their vessels and nerve, and is attached above to the soleal line on the tibia. At the ankle it is thickened to form part of the **flexor retinaculum** [Fig. 186].

The *middle layer* consists of the long flexors of the toes, flexor hallucis longus and flexor digitorum longus. The *deepest layer* is formed by tibialis posterior. It lies on the interosseous membrane between the tibia and fibula. The fascia covering the posterior surface of tibialis posterior is attached above to the soleal line, laterally to the medial crest of the fibula, and medially to the vertical ridge on the tibia [p. 176].

Dissection

Make a transverse incision through the skin on the distal part of the heel. Carry the incision along the borders of the foot to join the previous incisions. Find the sural nerve and the small saphenous vein again below the lateral malleolus. Strip the skin and superficial fascia upwards from the back of the leg retaining the nerve and vein, together with their tributaries and branches. Small, medial calcanean nerves may be found as the skin is removed from the medial side of the heel [Fig. 175]. Find the junction between the sural and peroneal communicating nerves. Follow both upwards through the deep fascia to the tibial and common peroneal nerves respectively. Trace the small saphenous vein to its entry into the popliteal vein. Note at least one considerable communication between the small and great saphenous veins.

Great saphenous vein
[Figs. 123, 131, 175, 176]

This important vein begins at the medial border of the foot by the junction of the **dorsal venous arch** and the **medial dorsal digital vein** of the big toe. It ascends in front of the medial malleolus, passes obliquely across the distal third of the medial surface of the tibia, and runs along the medial border of the tibia to the posteromedial side of the knee. In this part of its course, it lies in a membranous sleeve of fascia which separates it from the more superficial venous channels, and it has an unusually thick wall. From the knee, it ascends obliquely through the superficial fascia of the thigh to the **saphenous opening**. Here it pierces the cribriform fascia and enters the femoral vein.

The great saphenous vein receives many tributaries throughout its length, and **anastomoses** through them with the small saphenous vein so that it may occasionally receive most of the blood from the small saphenous vein. The great saphenous vein contains many **valves** which diminish the pressure on the distal parts of its walls by dividing up the column of blood within it, while the communications with the deep veins [p. 182] permit individual segments to drain into these veins when they have been emptied by muscle contraction. If these valves become incompetent, the pressure on the walls of the great

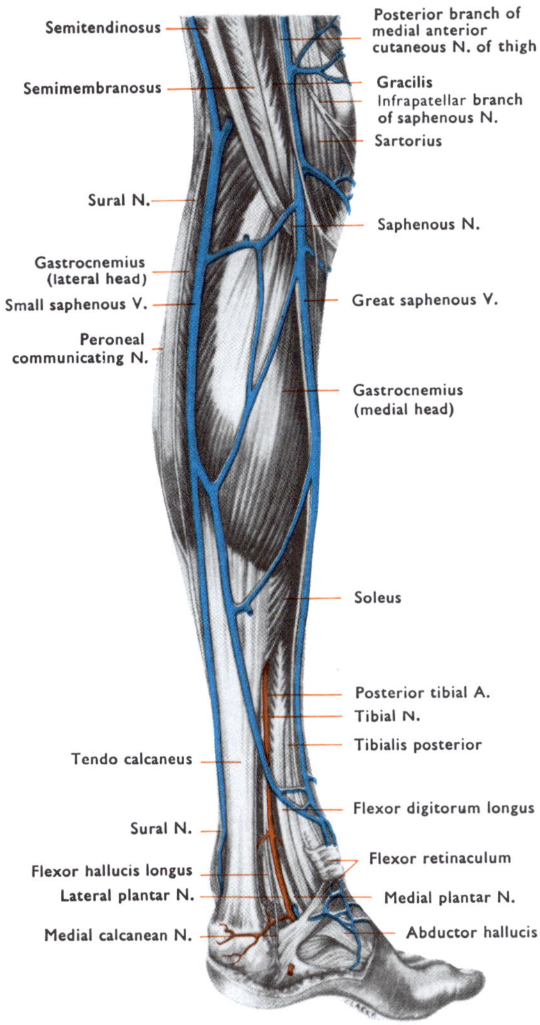

Fig. 175. Superficial dissection of leg viewed from posteromedial side, showing veins and nerves. Note the numerous anastomoses between the great and the small saphenous veins.

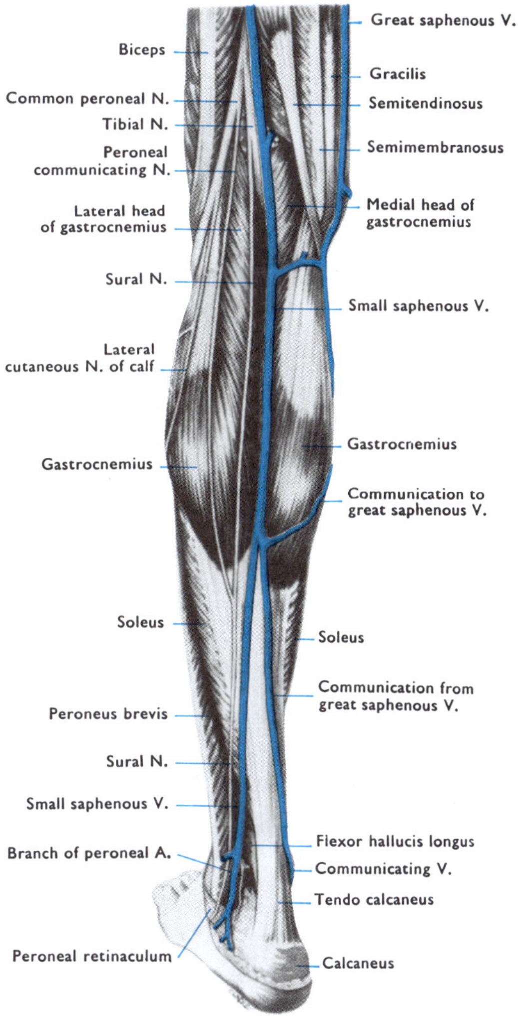

Fig. 176. Superficial dissection of leg viewed from posterolateral side, showing veins and nerves. In the specimen there were numerous large anastomosing channels between the small and the great saphenous veins.

saphenous vein increases, with the result that it becomes distended and tortuous (varicose veins). This condition is greatly aggravated if the pumping action of the muscles is transmitted to the superficial veins as a result of incompetent valves in the communicating veins.

Small saphenous vein

This is formed by the junction of the dorsal venous arch of the foot with the lateral dorsal digital vein of the little toe. It passes backwards, inferior to the lateral malleolus, and then ascends in the back of the leg, at first lateral to the tendo calcaneus and then in the midline on gastrocnemius. It pierces the deep fascia at the lower border of the popliteal fossa and enters the popliteal vein. It drains the lateral side of the foot and ankle and the back of the leg.

Saphenous nerve (L. 3, 4)

This is the longest branch of the femoral nerve. It arises in the femoral triangle and accompanies the femoral artery into the adductor canal. It leaves the canal through its roof in the distal quarter of the thigh, and lies deep to sartorius. Here it gives off the **infrapatellar branch**, which pierces sartorius to reach the patellar plexus, and then emerges between sartorius and the tendon of gracilis a little above the knee. The saphenous nerve lies posteromedial to the knee and pierces the deep fascia inferior to it, beside the great saphenous vein. In the leg and foot it accompanies the great saphenous vein, and ends in the skin of the medial side of the foot. It supplies skin on the medial side of the knee, leg, and proximal part of the dorsum of the foot [Fig. 218].

Sural nerve (S. 1, 2)

It arises from the tibial nerve in the popliteal fossa, and descends on the posterior surface of gastrocnemius to enter the superficial fascia about the

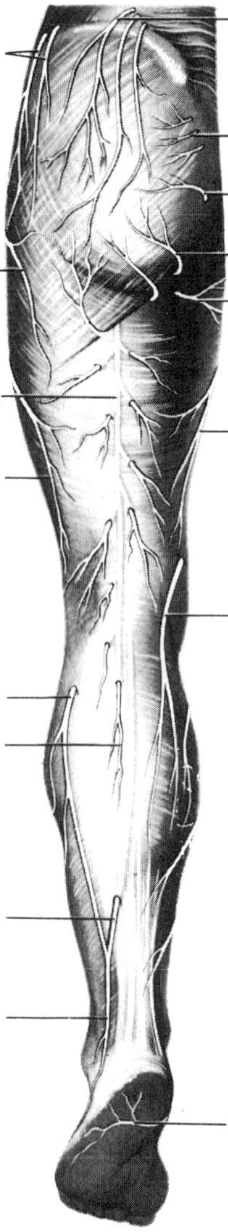

Fig. 177. Cutaneous nerves on back of lower limb.
See also Fig. 123.

middle of the back of the leg. It is then joined by the **peroneal communicating nerve** [Fig. 177] and accompanies the small saphenous vein to the lateral side of the foot. The sural nerve supplies skin on the lower lateral part of the back of the leg, the lateral border and adjoining part of the dorsum of the foot, and the lateral side of the little toe [Fig. 218].

Peroneal communicating nerve (L. 5; S. 1, 2)

This nerve arises from the common peroneal nerve in the popliteal fossa, often with the lateral cutaneous nerve of the calf. It pierces the deep fascia over the lateral head of gastrocnemius, and descends to join the sural nerve [Fig. 177]. *Area of supply:* the skin on the proximal two-thirds of the posterolateral surface of the leg and the territory of the sural nerve.

The posterior branch of the **medial anterior cutaneous nerve of the thigh** (L. 2, 3) descends into the calf and supplies skin in the upper posteromedial part.

Lymph vessels and lymph nodes of the lower limb

Very little of this extensive system can be demonstrated by dissection. Even the lymph nodes are poorly seen, especially in the elderly, unless enlarged by disease. However, a knowledge of the routes taken by the lymph vessels and of the nodes to which they drain is essential if the site of an infection or tumor is to be traced after the finding of an enlarged lymph node. It follows that this important vascular system has to be understood principally from diagrams and from the text. The source of the information is twofold: (1) the experimental injection of lymph vessels and nodes in the living or dead; (2) the spread of disease in patients.

The student should study Figs. 179 and 180 and note the following points.

1. The **superficial lymph vessels and nodes** drain the skin and subcutaneous tissues. They are separated from the **deep lymph vessels and nodes** by the deep fascia. The superficial and deep systems communicate with each other only at restricted regions, usually where a major superficial vein pierces the deep fascia. In the lower limb, this is through the cribriform fascia and the popliteal fascia, c.f. axilla and the point where the basilic vein pierces the deep fascia in the upper limb.

2. The superficial vessels are much more numerous than the deep vessels. There are few lymph vessels in muscle, but very many in skin, synovial membranes, synovial sheaths, and bursae.

3. Superficial lymph vessels take a direct course to the superficial (occasionally deep) lymph nodes. Deep lymph vessels run with the deep blood vessels and enter deep nodes.

4. **Superficial nodes** in the lower limb are virtually restricted to the inguinal region. These drain the superficial tissues of the lower limb, perineum, and trunk below the level of the umbilicus. The only exception is the group of lymph vessels which accompany the small saphenous vein through the popliteal fascia to the deep lymph nodes in the popliteal fossa. The area drained by these lymph vessels corresponds approximately to the drainage area of the small saphenous vein.

5. The **superficial inguinal lymph nodes** are arranged in the shape of a T. The nodes forming the stem of the T are concerned with the lower limb. The lateral nodes of the cross-member of the T drain the upper lateral gluteal region and the posterior and lateral parts of the trunk; the medial ones receive lymph from the upper medial part of the thigh, the perineum (including the external genitalia), the medial gluteal region, and the anteromedial part of the abdominal wall below the umbilicus.

6. There is a '*lymphshed*' along the back of the lower limb. Vessels from the medial half of the limb pass round the medial surface of the limb, those from the lateral half pass round the lateral surface of the limb to converge on the inguinal lymph nodes [Fig. 180]. This 'lymphshed' is split distally by the vessels flowing to the popliteal nodes.

7. **Deep lymph vessels** of the leg and foot also enter the **popliteal nodes**, though those passing with the anterior tibial vessels may have traversed a node on these vessels in the anterior compartment of the leg. The drainage of

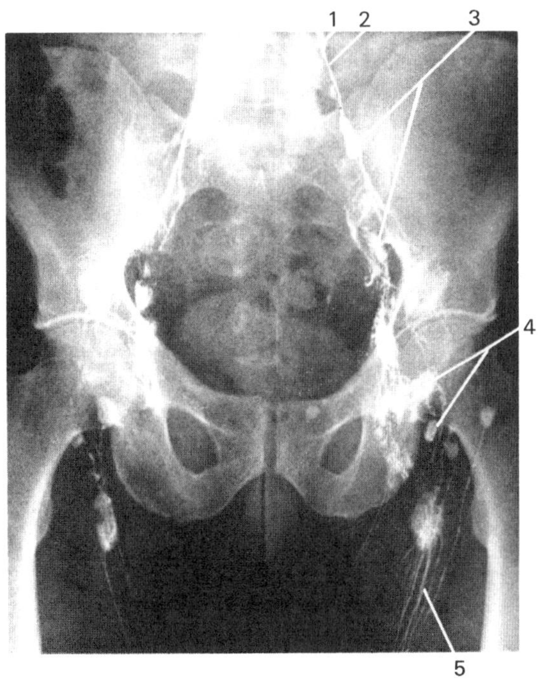

Fig. 178. Lymphangiogram of some of the lymph vessels and nodes draining the thigh. This is produced by the injection of some lymph vessels with X-ray-opaque dye followed by a radiograph after an interval to permit the dye to ascend in the vessels and through the nodes. Only the lymph vessels and nodes which drain lymph from the injected region are shown; the remainder are invisible.
1. Lumbar lymph node.
2. Lumbar lymph trunk.
3. Common and external iliac nodes.
4. Inguinal nodes.
5. Lymph vessels of thigh.

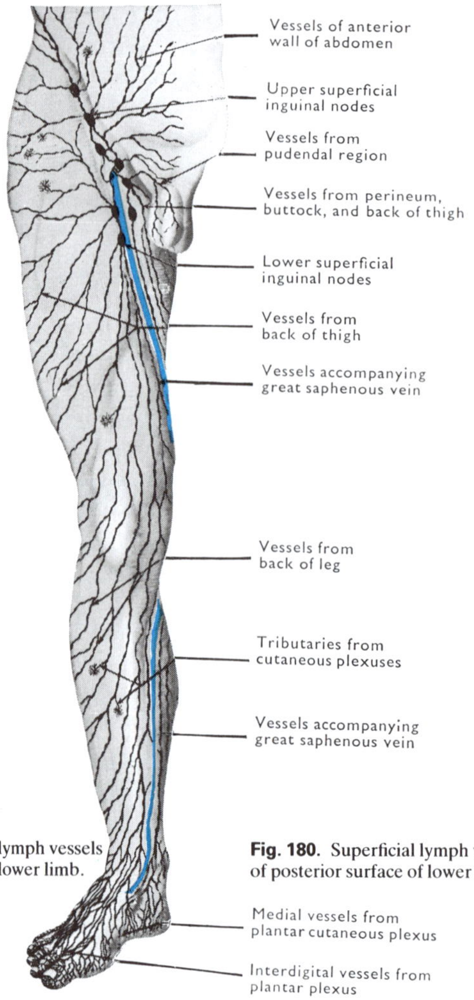

Fig. 179. Superficial lymph vessels of anterior surface of lower limb.

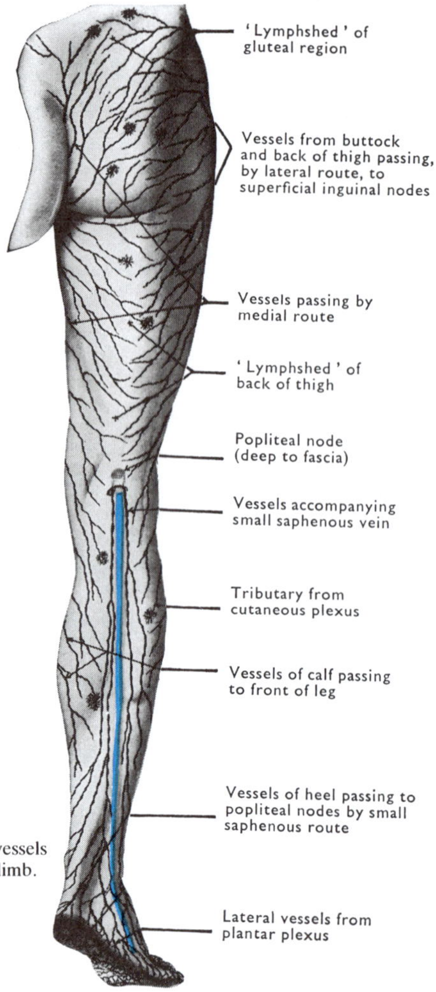

Fig. 180. Superficial lymph vessels of posterior surface of lower limb.

the popliteal nodes is mainly along the femoral vessels. Here they are joined by most of the deep vessels of the thigh and pass together to the **deep inguinal lymph nodes** in the femoral triangle. These also receive the efferent vessels from the superficial inguinal lymph nodes, and drain to the **external iliac nodes** by passing behind the inguinal ligament into the abdomen. The exception to this route is that taken by the deep lymph vessels of the perineum and gluteal region. These drain with the corresponding blood vessels (gluteal and internal pudendal) through the greater sciatic foramen into the pelvis (**internal iliac nodes**).

Deep fascia

The importance of the dense deep fascia of the leg has already been mentioned [p. 182]. *At the ankle*, the deep fascia is thickened to form the peroneal and flexor retinacula [Fig. 185] on the lateral and medial sides respectively. The **flexor retinaculum** stretches from the calcaneus to the medial malleolus. It covers the tendons of the deep flexor muscles of the back of the leg as they pass into the foot over the posterior and inferior surfaces of the medial malleolus with the tibial nerve and posterior tibial vessels. Distally, the flexor retinaculum gives partial attachment to the abductor hallucis muscle of the foot.

Dissection

Define the flexor retinaculum postero-inferior to the medial malleolus. The medial calcanean nerves and vessels may be found passing through it to the skin.

Extend the division of the deep fascia, which was made when the sural nerve was followed, down to the calcaneus. Reflect the fascia. Identify and follow the bellies of gastrocnemius to their attachments. Lift the muscle from the underlying soleus and cut across the medial head close to its attachment to the femur. Turn the medial belly laterally to expose the lower part of the popliteal vessels and tibial nerve in the popliteal fossa. Find the large muscular branches to gastrocnemius.

Lift the tendon of semimembranosus from the proximal part of the medial head of gastrocnemius and find the bursa which separates them. Lift this part of the medial head of gastrocnemius and find the bursa which separates it from the fibrous capsule of the knee joint. This bursa may be continuous with the bursa under semimembranosus and with the joint cavity through the articular capsule.

Trace the nerve to soleus from the tibial nerve. Find the plantaris, a small muscle posteromedial to the lateral head of gastrocnemius. Follow its tendon between gastrocnemius and soleus to the medial side of the tendo calcaneus. Remove the fatty connective tissue anterior to the tendo calcaneus. This uncovers the lower part of the first intermuscular fascial septum which is close to the deep fascia here.

Cut across the lateral head of gastrocnemius at the level of the knee joint. Turn its proximal part upwards. There may be a bursa between it and the fibrous capsule of the knee joint, and a small sesamoid bone may be felt within the head. Turn both bellies of gastrocnemius downwards. Note the way in which they are inserted into the tendo calcaneus. Expose the posterior surface of soleus and define its attachments. Note the tibial nerve and popliteal vessels passing deep to a tendinous arch from which the intermediate fibres of soleus arise. The lowest fibres of soleus can be followed on the deep surface of the tendo calcaneus almost to the calcaneus.

Superficial muscles of the calf

Gastrocnemius

This muscle arises by two tendinous heads from the femur—the **lateral head** from the lateral surface of the lateral condyle, the **medial head** from a rough area on the popliteal surface above the medial condyle [Fig. 181]. The medial head is separated from the tendon of semimembranosus and from the articular capsule of the knee joint by bursae. These may be continuous with each other and with the cavity of the knee joint. The lateral head frequently contains a small sesamoid bone (the **fabella**).

The two fleshy bellies, the medial larger and longer than the lateral, remain separate. They end, near the middle of the leg, on the posterior surface of a thin, common tendon. This tendon fuses with the superficial surface of the tendon of soleus to form the **tendo calcaneus**.

Soleus

This powerful, flat muscle arises (a) from the posterior surface of the head and upper third of the body of the fibula, (b) from the soleal line and middle third of the medial border of the tibia, and (c) from the tendinous arch posterior to the popliteal vessels and the tibial nerve. The stout tendon fuses with that of gastrocnemius to form the tendo calcaneus [Fig. 183].

Plantaris

This small muscle (8–10 cm long) arises from the popliteal surface of the femur [Fig. 181] and is partly hidden by the lateral head of gastrocnemius. The long, slender tendon passes between gastrocnemius and soleus and along the medial side of the tendo calcaneus to the calcaneus. It may fuse with the tendo calcaneus or with the fascia of the leg. The plantaris is occasionally absent, cf. palmaris longus.

Nerve supply of these three muscles is the tibial nerve.

Actions. Gastrocnemius and soleus are powerful plantar flexors of the ankle. They act around the fulcrum of the heads of the metatarsals, mainly the first, to raise the weight of the body on to the toes—a position which soleus maintains in running. They are responsible for the powerful push-off in running, jumping, and walking. They also act with the dorsiflexors of the ankle joint to stabilize the ankle in an anteroposterior plane.

Gastrocnemius also flexes the knee joint but it becomes ineffective as a plantar flexor of the ankle when the knee is bent. Soleus is then the main muscle concerned. If the femur is fractured a short distance proximal to the

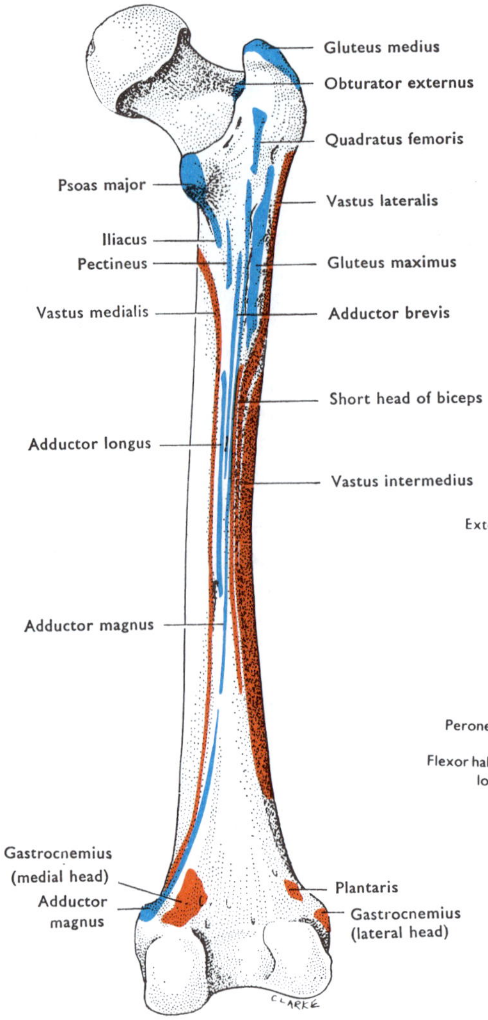

Fig. 181 (*left*). Right femur to show muscles attached to posterior aspect.
Fig. 182 (*below*). Transverse section through middle of leg.
A. Anterior.
P. Posterior.
M. Medial.
L. Lateral.

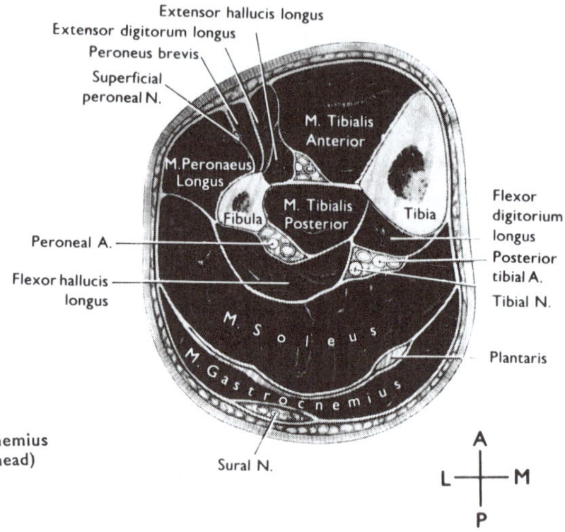

attachments of gastrocnemius (supracondylar fracture), that muscle pulls the distal fragment backwards. Such fractures, therefore, are treated with the knee flexed to relax gastrocnemius and prevent this displacement.

Gastrocnemius and soleus are an important element in the *muscle pump* returning venous blood from the lower limbs. Both muscles have a considerable blood supply and soleus contains a considerable venous plexus.

Plantaris can add very little to the strength of gastrocnemius and soleus. It is an important muscle in animals that walk on their toes for it then continues over the heel into the plantar aponeurosis, cf. palmaris longus. It may be that it is concerned with proprioception in man.

Tendo calcaneus

This powerful tendon is inserted into the smooth, intermediate part of the posterior surface of the calcaneus. The upper part of this surface is separated from the tendon by a small bursa. If the tendon is ruptured, the disability in walking is severe and running is impossible.

Dissection

Separate the soleus from the tibia and turn it laterally. Divide the blood vessels to the muscle, noting the large size of the veins which emerge from it, but retain its nerves. Look for any communicating veins from the great saphenous vein to the deep veins. Open these and check for any valves within them.

The first intermuscular septum is now exposed. Divide the septum longitudinally in its middle and reflect it to expose the second layer of muscles and the neurovascular bundles.

Trace the tibial nerve as far as the ankle. Find its muscular branches which arise mainly in the upper part of the leg. The small nerve to popliteus arises in the popliteal fossa and descends over popliteus to its lower border. It then turns round that border to enter the deep surface of the muscle [Fig. 183]. Define the lower border of popliteus and follow it to its tendon. Do not attempt to follow it into the knee joint at this stage.

Remove the fascia from the lowest part of the popliteal vessels. Find the anterior and posterior tibial branches of the artery and the corresponding veins. Check the continuity of the anterior tibial vessels with the vessels in the anterior compartment. Follow the posterior tibial artery as far as the ankle. Find the peroneal artery which arises from it. This artery descends posterior to the fibula, under cover of flexor hallucis longus.

Define and separate the long flexor muscles of the toes; flexor hallucis longus is lateral to and larger than flexor digitorum longus. Follow their tendons to the flexor retinaculum. Push the flexor hallucis longus laterally and separate its deep surface from the second intermuscular septum and the distal part of the interosseous membrane. Trace the peroneal artery deep to this muscle and find its perforating branch passing through the lower part of the interosseous membrane. The remainder of the artery is distributed to the lateral side of the calcaneus and the lateral malleolar rete.

Divide the second intermuscular septum covering tibialis posterior. Trace that muscle and its tendon as far as the flexor retinaculum. Note its close association with the medial malleolus. Palpate the tendon in your own foot between the medial malleolus and the navicular, first tightening it by plantar flexing and inverting the foot.

Tibial nerve

This nerve lies under of the first intermuscular septum with the posterior tibial vessels. In the upper part of the leg it lies on popliteus and then on the second intermuscular septum, posterior to tibialis posterior. In the lower third of the leg, it is close to the deep fascia midway between the tendo calcaneus and the medial border of the tibia and the tendons of flexor digitorum longus and flexor hallucis longus [Fig. 183]. The tibial nerve divides into medial and lateral plantar nerves, deep to the flexor retinaculum.

Branches inferior to popliteal fossa

Muscular branches pass to tibialis posterior, flexor hallucis longus, flexor digitorum longus, and the deeper part of soleus. They arise in the upper part of the leg.

Cutaneous, medial calcanean nerves (S. 1) arise at the ankle, pierce the flexor retinaculum, and supply the posterior and lower surfaces of the heel.

Small **articular** branches pass to the posterior aspect of the ankle joint.

Popliteal artery

The popliteal artery ends at the distal border of popliteus. Here it divides into the anterior and posterior tibial arteries. The anterior and posterior tibial veins unite to form the popliteal vein at the same point.

Anterior tibial artery

This vessel gives off a small posterior tibial recurrent artery to the back of the knee joint. It then passes forwards above the interosseous membrane to the anterior compartment of the leg.

Posterior tibial artery

This artery supplies the deep muscles of the back of the leg and is the main artery of the foot. It begins at the lower border of popliteus and descends with the tibial nerve. It ends by dividing into the medial and lateral plantar arteries deep to the flexor retinaculum.

Branches in the leg

1. **Peroneal artery**. This large branch arises close to the beginning of the parent artery and descends along the back of the fibula, deep to flexor hallucis longus. It supplies: (a) muscular branches; (b) the **nutrient artery to the fibula;** (c) the **perforating branch** which pierces the interosseous membrane just above the tibiofibular syndesmosis and anastomoses with the lateral tarsal branch of the dorsalis pedis artery. The peroneal artery ends by giving lateral malleolar and calcanean branches, and anastomoses with the posterior tibial on the back of the ankle joint.

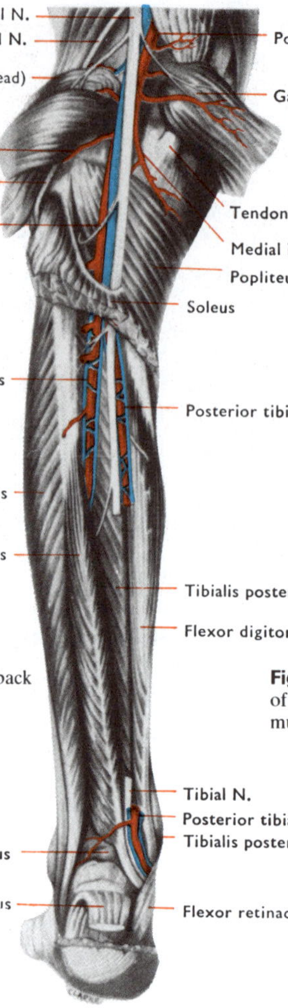

Fig. 183. Deep dissection of back of leg.

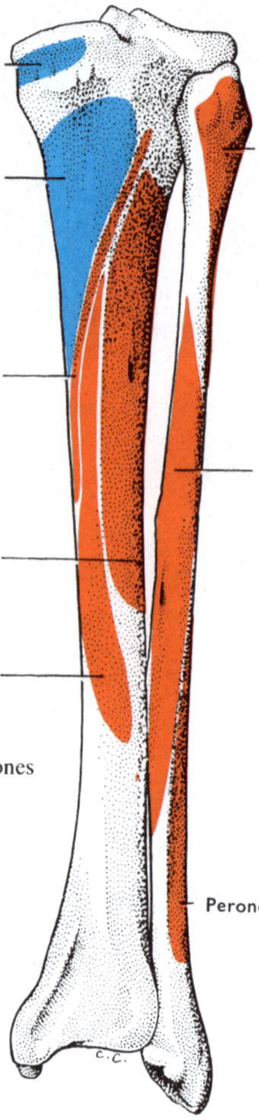

Fig. 184. Posterior aspect of bones of leg to show attachments of muscles.

The peroneal artery is sometimes enlarged. It may then become the major source of blood for the dorsalis pedis artery, through the lateral tarsal artery, or for the posterior tibial artery in the foot, through its communication with that artery at the ankle.

2. The circumflex fibular artery runs round the neck of the fibula to supply muscles and skin.

3. A large **nutrient artery to the tibia** arises from the upper end of the posterior tibial artery. It enters the tibia a short distance below the soleal line. Like other nutrient arteries it is the main supply to the bone, though it may be supplemented by arteries in the fleshy attachments of muscles when the bone is broken. Because there are no such attachments to the lower third of the tibia, fractures in this region, which destroy the marrow and the branches of the nutrient artery in it, grossly reduce the potential blood supply to the bone distal to the fracture and so reduce the rate of healing.

4. **Muscular branches** to the deep muscles of the back of the leg. **Cutaneous branches** to the medial side of the leg.

5. A **communicating branch** with the peroneal artery behind the ankle joint.

6. **Medial calcanean branches** with the corresponding nerves.

Deep muscles of the back of the leg

Popliteus

This muscle is attached to the lateral condyle of the femur at the anterior end of the popliteal groove [Fig. 247] and to the back of the lateral meniscus [Fig. 202] both within the capsule of the knee joint. It emerges from the capsule of the knee joint through the posterior part of the capsule, below the **arcuate popliteal ligament**. The tendon then expands into a triangular fleshy belly which is attached to the posterior surface of the tibia above the soleal line [Fig. 184].

Nerve supply: tibial nerve. **Action:** when the leg is free, it medially rotates the tibia on the femur at the beginning of knee flexion. When the foot is on the ground, it laterally rotates the femur on the tibia. Both movements 'unlock' the extended knee joint and allow flexion to occur. The attachment to the meniscus ensures that the meniscus moves with the femoral condyle in the rotation and is not caught between the femur and the tibia.

The remaining deep muscles have considerable attachments to the intermuscular septa and the interosseous membrane in addition to their bony origins. The use of the terms 'origin' and 'insertion' is inappropriate to these muscles since their distal attachments are often fixed because the foot is on the ground. This is true of all the muscles of the lower limb, especially of the muscles stabilizing the trunk on the hip joint and the femur on the tibia. The actions given for the following muscles are stated as though the distal attachment was free to move, but the reverse action occurs with equal frequency.

Flexor hallucis longus

This muscle is much larger than the flexor digitorum longus—a feature which indicates the relative forces applied to the hallux and the other toes. It arises chiefly from the posterior surface of the fibula, below the origin of soleus. Its tendon descends obliquely over the back of the ankle joint and curves forwards into the sole of the foot in an almost continuous bony groove (pulley) on the posterior surfaces of the tibia [Fig. 163] and talus, and the inferior surface of the **sustentaculum tali** of the calcaneus [Fig. 255]. It is inserted into the distal phalanx of the great toe.

Nerve supply: tibial nerve. **Action:** it flexes the metatarsophalangeal and interphalangeal joints of the great toe, and assists with plantar flexion of the ankle. These are important movements in the last phase of the 'push-off' especially in running.

Flexor digitorum longus
[Figs. 183, 186]

This muscle arises from the medial part of the posterior surface of the tibia, distal to the soleal line [Fig. 184]. It descends behind the tendon of tibialis posterior, and its tendon grooves the back of the tibia just medial to the medial malleolus. Passing deep to the flexor retinaculum, it enters the sole of the foot and divides into four tendons. One of these passes to the terminal phalanx of each of the lateral four toes.

Nerve supply: tibial nerve. **Action:** it flexes the metatarsophalangeal and interphalangeal joints of the lateral four toes, and assists with plantar flexion of the ankle joint. It may play a part in inversion of the foot.

Tibialis posterior

This muscle arises from the posterior surface of the interosseous membrane and the adjoining parts of the tibia and fibula [Figs. 182–184]. Proximally, the anterior tibial vessels pass between the upper ends of its two bony attachments. Distally, it passes inferomedially, between flexor digitorum longus and the tibia, and its tendon grooves the posterior surface of the medial malleolus. The tendon then passes deep to the flexor retinaculum, immediately inferior to the malleolus and, crossing the inferomedial surface of the head of the talus, is inserted mainly into the tuberosity of the navicular bone [Fig. 256]. It also sends strong slips to all the other tarsal bones (except the talus) and to the middle three metatarsals.

Nerve supply: tibial nerve. **Action:** it plantar flexes the foot and also inverts it because of its extensions to the lateral tarsal bones.

Flexor retinaculum

This thick band of fascia passes from the medial malleolus to the medial process of the tubercle of the calcaneus. It is continuous proximally with the deep fascia of the leg and with the first septum which covers the deep muscles and forms the major part of the retinaculum. Distally, it is continuous with the deep fascia of the sole and gives attachment to the abductor hallucis muscle.

Beneath the retinaculum lie the tendons of tibialis posterior, flexor digitorum longus, and flexor hallucis longus. The posterior tibial vessels and the tibial nerve, dividing into plantar vessels and nerves, lie between the tendons of the digital flexors.

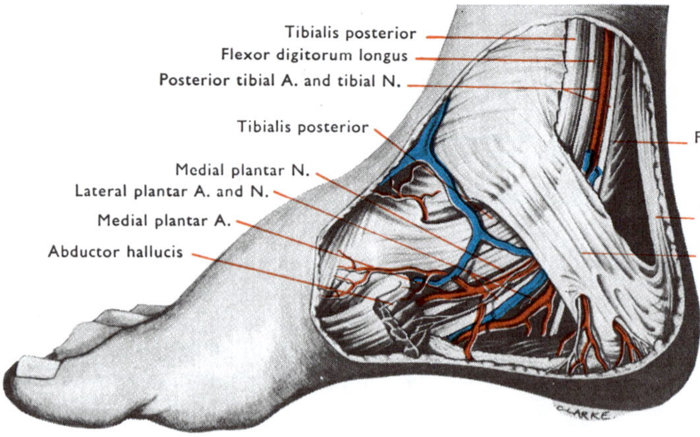

Fig. 185. Dissection of medial side of ankle, showing the structures adjacent to flexor retinaculum.

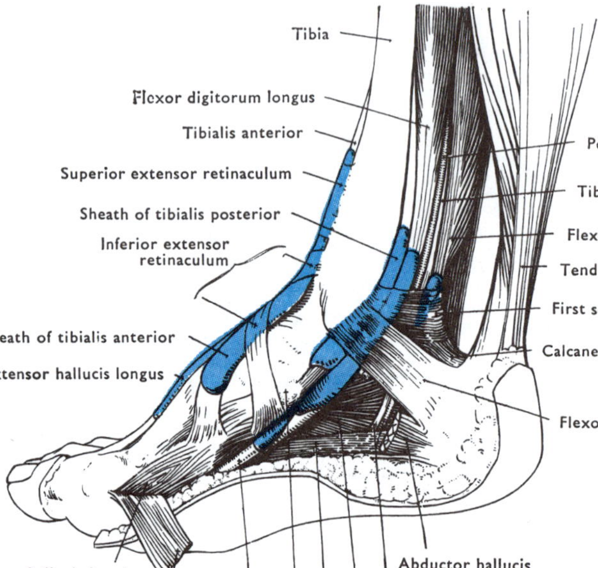

Fig. 186. Dissection of leg and foot showing synovial sheaths.

Synovial sheaths

Each of the tendons deep to the flexor retinaculum is separated from the others by a fibrous tissue sheath and each is surrounded by its own synovial sheath. The synovial sheaths begin approximately 2 cm above the tip of the medial malleolus. That on tibialis posterior extends to its insertion, on flexor digitorum longus to the middle of the foot, and on flexor hallucis longus either to the insertion or to the middle of the first metatarsal. The dissector should open and pass a probe along at least one of these sheaths.

Nerves and vessels of the knee joint

As a general rule, at any synovial joint (1) the nerves which supply the muscles that move the joint also supply the joint, and (2) all the arteries in the region of the joint send branches to it. The arteries form a circular anastomosis around the end of each bone that articulates at the joint [Fig. 187]. This supplies the articular capsule and the epiphysis of the bone while the epiphysis is separated from the diaphysis by the growth cartilage. These epiphysial arteries are represented in the adult by the multiple small foramina in the ends of long bones, more of which transmit the corresponding veins than the arteries.

Dissection

Now that most of the structures around the knee joint have been dissected, it is possible to follow the various nerves and arteries to the knee.

Find the nerves to the three vasti. Trace their articular filaments down through each muscle as far as the knee. Follow the descending branch of the lateral circumflex artery and the descending genicular artery from the femoral artery to the knee. Trace the branch of the posterior division of the obturator nerve to adductor magnus. Follow the longest filament to the back of the knee joint beside the popliteal artery.

Find again the genicular branches of the popliteal artery and of the tibial and common peroneal nerves. Follow the inferior lateral genicular artery to the fibular collateral ligament of the knee joint. Cut through the tendon of biceps above the knee and turn it downwards to expose the ligament. Follow the artery and nerve between the ligament and the articular capsule. Trace the inferior medial genicular artery and nerve along the upper border of popliteus till they disappear deep to the superficial part of the tibial collateral ligament of the knee joint. Turn the tendons of sartorius, gracilis, and semitendinosus forwards and find the artery and nerve emerging from beneath the ligament.

Find the posterior tibial recurrent branch of the anterior tibial artery. Follow it upwards, anterior to popliteus, by cutting through popliteus near its tendon and turning the belly of the muscle medially. This exposes the nerve to popliteus: its branch to the adjacent tibiofibular joint may also be found. Find the anterior tibial recurrent branch of the anterior tibial artery and the recurrent genicular branch of the common peroneal nerve on the front of the leg. It may be possible to trace them through the upper part of tibialis anterior to the knee joint.

Nerves of the knee joint

1. The **femoral nerve** supplies the anterosuperior part of the joint via the nerves to the three vastus muscles. That from the nerve to vastus medialis is the largest. It accompanies the descending genicular artery.

2. The **common peroneal nerve** supplies the lateral part of the joint via the superior and inferior lateral genicular nerves and the recurrent genicular nerve [p. 189].

3. The **tibial nerve** supplies the medial and posterior parts of the articular capsule and the central structures within the capsule via the superior and inferior medial and middle genicular nerves. The inferior medial is the largest of the genicular nerves. It runs with the corresponding artery as do the other genicular nerves [Figs. 151, 187].

4. The **obturator nerve** sends a twig to the posterior surface of the knee joint.

Anastomosis around the knee joint

This is formed by eight arteries [Figs. 151, 187]. Two lateral and two medial genicular arteries from the popliteal artery; a descending genicular artery from the femoral artery; a genicular artery from the lateral circumflex artery; and an anterior and a posterior tibial recurrent artery. They form anastomoses with each other mainly in front of the joint. The middle genicular artery plays little part since it supplies mainly the structures which lie within the articular capsule between the two femoral condyles. Though

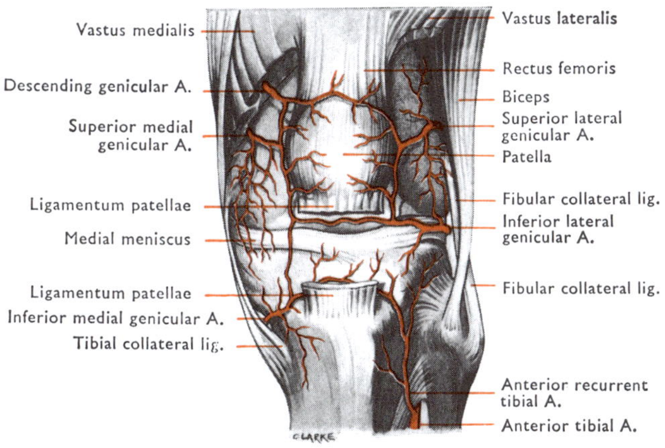

Fig. 187. Arterial anastomosis on front and sides of left knee joint.

this is a considerable anastomosis, the individual vessels are small and can scarcely make good for blockage of the popliteal artery. In any case, blockage of the popliteal artery almost invariably means blockage of one or more of its genicular branches.

Anastomosis around the ankle joint

On the lateral side, the lateral malleolar branch of the anterior tibial artery and the lateral tarsal branch of the dorsalis pedis artery anastomose with the perforating and terminal branches of the peroneal artery. On the medial side, the medial malleolar branch of the anterior tibial anastomoses with the medial calcanean branches of the posterior tibial. The posterior tibial also anastomoses with the peroneal artery posterior to the ankle joint.

Sole of the foot

Before beginning the dissection, revise the surface anatomy of your own foot [p. 180]. Make certain that you can identify the palpable parts of the bones and the major tendons entering the foot from the leg. Note also the parts of the foot which are in contact with the ground in standing, in the various phases of walking, and in running.

The foot has many features in common with the hand in its internal structure. The major differences arise from the function of the foot as a supporting structure which has to carry considerable static loads in standing and even greater loads at the point of application of severe thrust forces, e.g. in kicking, pushing off in running, and landing on the feet when jumping from a height. Strength and resilience have to be the main features of the foot rather than the type of mobility which is required in the hand for holding and grasping. Strength is obtained by having massive tarsal and big toe bones bound together by powerful ligaments, and by binding the metatarsal of the big toe to those of the other toes so that it has none of the mobility that the thumb has in its metacarpal. Thus there is no opposition either of the big toe or of the little toe and no muscles equivalent to the opponens muscles of the hand. Resilience is obtained by the presence of multiple joints each of which has very limited movement (except for those concerned with inversion and eversion) and by the arrangement of the bones in an arch held together by massive ligaments on the plantar surface and by a strong tie-beam (the **plantar aponeurosis**) which binds the ends of the arch together and has its tension altered in different positions of the foot. When standing, the weight is supported on the heel and on the heads of the metatarsals (mainly the first metatarsal) and to a lesser extent on the lateral border of the sole of the foot. When the foot is used in thrusting, the force is carried principally on the head

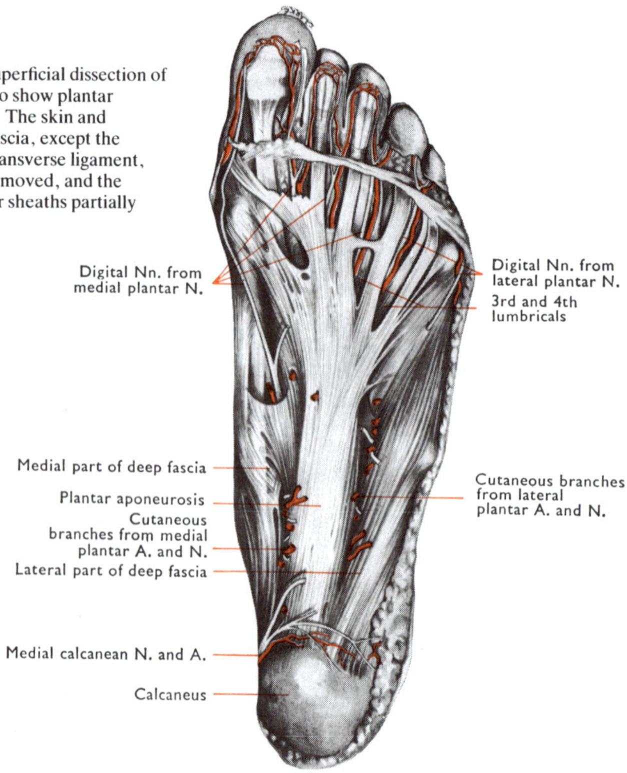

Fig. 188. Superficial dissection of sole of foot to show plantar aponeurosis. The skin and superficial fascia, except the superficial transverse ligament, have been removed, and the fibrous flexor sheaths partially opened.

of the first metatarsal and the big toe. The remaining metatarsals and toes are relatively weak and can be looked upon as a stabilizing flap. Without them the foot would have an unstable, two-point contact with the ground on the calcaneus and the ball of the great toe. The arched shape of the foot has the added advantage of giving protection to the structures in the sole which would otherwise be subjected to pressure. One special development to resist the pressures on the head of the first metatarsal, e.g. in running, is the presence on its plantar surface of two **sesamoid bones**. These transmit the pull of the small muscles of the big toe without subjecting them to pressure, and also make a tunnel between them through which the long flexor tendon can reach the toe.

Many of the other differences between the foot and the hand arise from the presence of the heel. This gives attachment to several of the muscles of the foot and to the plantar aponeurosis, which has no muscle of the leg inserted into it. It also forces the long tendons from the leg muscles to enter the foot around the heel. Thus flexor digitorum longus is out of line with the toes on which it acts—a situation no doubt responsible for the presence of an extra muscle, the **flexor accessorius**, which passes from the calcaneus into the tendon of flexor digitorum longus and helps to straighten the direction of its pull. Also the flexor digitorum brevis, which corresponds to the flexor digitorum superficialis in the upper limb, is confined to the foot and arises from the heel. This is possible because of the relatively small range of movement of the short toes in comparison with the long fingers.

Dissection

Cut longitudinally through the skin and superficial fascia of the sole from the heel to the root of the middle toe. Avoid cutting into the deep fascia (plantar aponeurosis). Strip the skin and superficial fascia from the deep fascia with a knife. The superficial fascia, like that of the palm, is dense and firmly bound to the deep fascia. The superficial fascia has fat packed tightly in its interstices so that it forms a firm pad, especially over the weight bearing areas. Stripping the skin and superficial fascia in one piece removes the cutaneous vessels and nerves [Fig. 188] but they are difficult to follow through the dense fascia. On the lateral and medial sides, remove the fascia with care so as to retain the digital nerves to the medial side of the big toe and the lateral side of the little toe. These become superficial further proximally than the other plantar digital nerves [Fig. 188].

Make a longitudinal incision through the skin on the plantar surface of each toe. Reflect the skin and find the plantar digital vessels and nerves. Follow them to the ends of the toes. Between these, expose the deep fascia of the toes. This is thickened to form the fibrous flexor sheath—a dense tunnel enclosing the flexor tendons in the toes.

Define the plantar aponeurosis and note the furrows at its edges. The branches of the medial and lateral plantar vessels and nerves pass through these furrows to the skin of the sole. As you approach the toes, take care not to damage the plantar metatarsal arteries and common plantar digital nerves which become superficial between the slips of the plantar aponeurosis passing to the toes. As far as possible, trace these slips into the toes.

Superficial fascia

This is a dense fascia, especially over the heel and the ball of the foot. It contains loculi of fat in the dense fascial pockets. These make it firm and resilient but also make isolated pockets within which infections of the sole may become trapped.

The skin and superficial fascia of the sole is supplied by the **medial calcanean nerves** and vessels in the region of the heel, by branches of the **medial** and **lateral plantar nerves** and **vessels** in the greater part of the sole, and by the **plantar digital nerves** and vessels in the toes [Fig. 188].

Deep fascia

Fibrous flexor sheaths

In each toe this is a thick, fibrous tunnel. It is attached to the margins of the proximal and middle phalanges (proximal only in the big toe), to the base of the distal phalanx, and to the palmar ligaments of the digital joints. It is relatively thin at the level of the interphalangeal joints and so does not restrict flexion at them. It contains the long and short flexor tendons enclosed in a synovial sheath in the lateral four toes, the long flexor alone in the great toe. Proximally each sheath is continuous with the plantar aponeurosis. These sheaths restrain the flexor tendons and increase their efficiency [p. 79]. Cut through one of these sheaths longitudinally to expose the tendons and the synovial sheath.

In the sole the deep fascia is extremely thick in the intermediate region (plantar aponeurosis) but is thin medially and laterally where it covers the abductors of the big and little toes. However, it forms a thick band between the lateral process of the tuber calcanei and the base of the fifth metatarsal. The plantar aponeurosis is separated from the lateral and medial parts by shallow furrows through which the branches of the plantar vessels and nerves enter the skin of the sole. The furrows are formed by intermuscular septa which pass into the sole from the plantar aponeurosis and separate the two abductor muscles from the flexor digitorum brevis [Fig. 189] which lies deep to the plantar aponeurosis.

Plantar aponeurosis

This extremely thick layer of deep fascia is attached posteriorly to the medial process of the calcanean tuber. Anteriorly it increases in width and splits into five slips which are held together by transverse fibres but separate as each passes to one toe. The margins of each slip curve dorsally over the sides of the flexor tendons, and are attached to the plantar ligament of the metatarsophalangeal joint. The intermediate part is attached to the proximal end of the fibrous flexor sheath—the same arrangement as in the hand. Thus each slip of the plantar aponeurosis is firmly bound to the proximal phalanx of a toe by the plantar ligament and the fibrous flexor sheath. So the plantar aponeurosis forms a tie-beam between the ends of the longitudinal arch of the foot. Its attachment to the proximal phalanges results in the slips of plantar aponeurosis being pulled distally when the toes are forcibly extended, e.g. in pushing-off with the foot. This tightens the aponeurosis and pulls the ends of the arch together so that it forms a rigid structure against which the push-off can be effective. Check this in your own foot by passively extending your toes with your hand. The plantar aponeurosis can then be seen and felt as a tight bar which is relaxed when the toes are flexed [Fig. 213].

Dissection

Cut across the plantar aponeurosis 2–3 cm in front of the heel. Split the distal part longitudinally and lift its parts away from the underlying flexor digitorum brevis. As the margins of this muscle are reached, the intermuscular septa will be seen. Divide these and reflect the aponeurosis distally. Avoid injury to the plantar digital vessels and nerves which lie immediately deep to the distal part of the aponeurosis.

Remove the deep fascia from the abductor muscles of the hallux and little toe. Retain the plantar digital nerves already found to these toes.

Structures in the sole of the foot

As the dissection proceeds, these structures will be uncovered in a number of layers. These layers have no significance beyond that of description and are not clearly separated from one another by fascial planes. They represent the order in which the structures are uncovered and the general depth at which they lie.

From superficial to deep, the layers consist of:

1. Abductor hallucis, flexor digitorum brevis, abductor digiti minimi, and the plantar digital vessels and nerves distally.

2. The medial and lateral plantar nerves and vessels.

3. The long flexor tendons—tibialis posterior, flexor hallucis longus, and flexor digitorum longus with the flexor accessorius and lumbrical muscles attached to it.

4. Flexor hallucis brevis, adductor hallucis, and flexor digiti minimi brevis.

5. The deep parts of the lateral plantar artery and nerve and their branches.

6. The bones and ligaments of the foot, the tendon of peroneus longus, the interosseous muscles in which are the perforating branches of the plantar metatarsal arteries and the extensions of tibialis posterior to the tarsal and metatarsal bones.

The student should not attempt to memorize the exact attachments of the small muscles of the foot except in a few cases where these are important and where they will be stressed in the text. It is obvious that the more superficial any particular small muscle is in the sole of the foot, the more likely it is to be long and to be attached to the ends of this arched structure, i.e. from heel to toe. Also that the superficial muscles are more likely to help in the maintenance of the arched structure of the foot than the deeper, shorter muscles which arise further distally.

That the muscles are not used to support the arches in standing is obvious from the absence of electromyographic activity in the leg and foot muscles in this position. However, the muscles are very important in drawing the bones of the arch together when the arch is subjected to powerful forces during activity. Thus they protect the ligaments from the undue stresses to which these ligaments succumb when the muscles are paralysed or weakened.

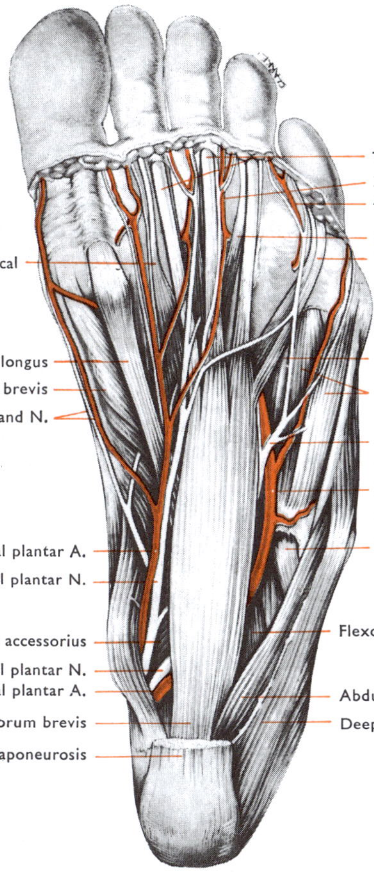

Fig. 189. Superficial dissection of sole of foot. The plantar aponeurosis has been removed. The abductor digiti minimi and the abductor hallucis have been pulled aside.

First layer

Flexor digitorum brevis

It arises from the medial process of the tuber calcanei and the plantar aponeurosis. It divides into four parts which end in slender tendons to the lateral four toes. Each tendon enters the fibrous flexor sheath of the toe and divides into two parts which curve over the sides of the long flexor tendon to the plantar surface of the middle phalanx. **Nerve supply:** medial plantar nerve. **Action:** it flexes the proximal interphalangeal and the metatarso-phalangeal joints of the lateral four toes, and helps to reinforce the longitudinal arch of the foot.

Abductor hallucis

It arises from the flexor retinaculum and the medial process of the tuber calcanei [Fig. 191]. Part of the medial belly of flexor hallucis brevis and the medial part of the expansion formed by extensor hallucis longus pass into the tendon of abductor hallucis and are inserted together on the plantar aspect and adjacent medial surface of the proximal phalanx of the big toe. This plantar position of the insertion of abductor hallucis reduces its efficiency as an abductor of the big toe (see hallux valgus). **Nerve supply:** medial plantar nerve. **Action:** it moves the big toe away from the second toe, i.e. abducts it, at the metatarsophalangeal joint. It is often mainly a flexor of this joint.

Abductor digiti minimi

It passes from both processes of the tuber calcanei [Fig. 191] to the lateral side of the base of the proximal phalanx of the little toe. Part of the muscle is fused with the band of plantar fascia passing from the lateral process of the tuber calcanei to the base of the fifth metatarsal and may be inserted here. **Nerve supply:** lateral plantar nerve. **Action:** it abducts the little toe.

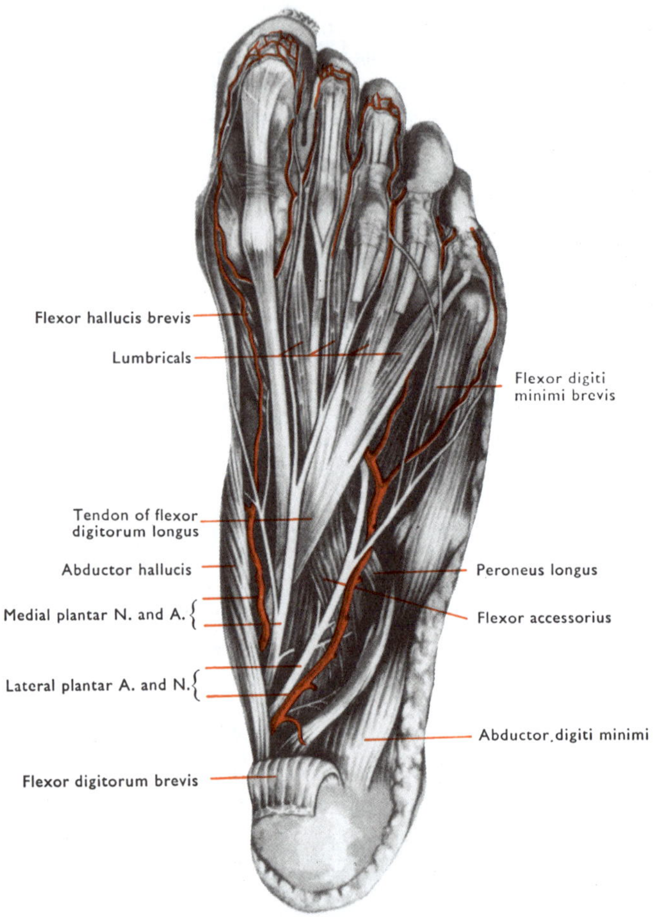

Fig. 190. Dissection of sole of the foot. Most of the flexor digitorum brevis has been removed.

Dissection

Find the proper plantar digital nerves in the toes [Fig. 190] and follow them proximally. Between the toes these nerves unite in pairs to form the common plantar digital nerves. Those from the medial three interdigital spaces can be traced back to the medial plantar nerve, that from the fourth comes from the lateral plantar nerve.

Lift the flexor digitorum brevis and find the nerve entering it from the medial plantar nerve. Cut across the muscle near its middle. Reflect its parts forwards and backwards, avoiding injury to the common plantar digital nerves which pass superficial to its distal part or its tendons [Fig. 189]. Follow at least one of the tendons to its insertion, cutting the fibrous flexor sheath longitudinally to expose it in the toe.

Separate abductor hallucis from the calcaneus. Turn the muscle medially and find the nerve to it from the medial plantar nerve. The greater parts of the medial and lateral plantar arteries and nerves are now exposed. Remove the connective tissue which surrounds the nerves and arteries and follow them distally in the foot. Trace their branches into continuity with (a) the digital branches already exposed

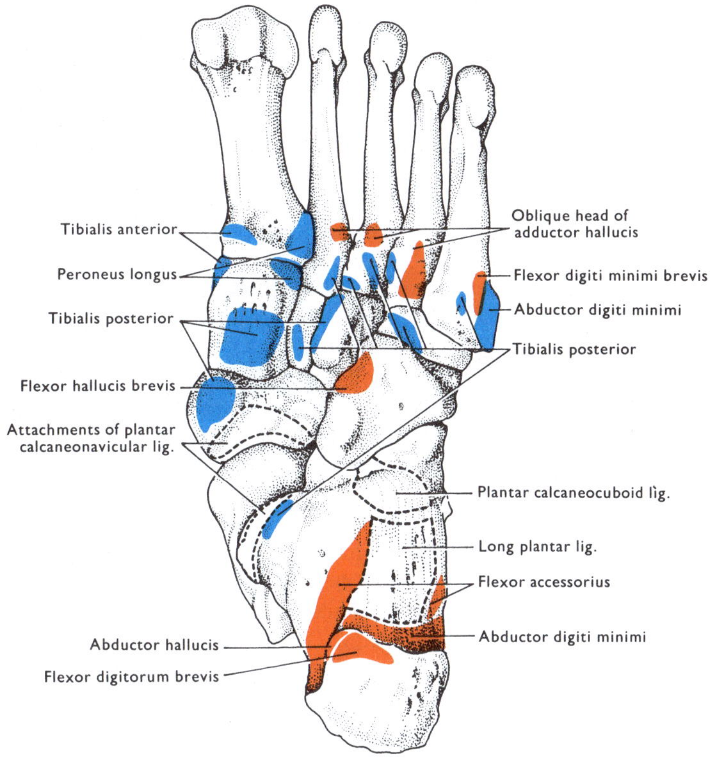

Fig. 191. Muscle attachments to left tarsus and metatarsus (plantar aspect). Interrupted lines show areas of attachment of some ligaments. See Fig. 165.

and (b) the branches to the medial side of the big toe and the lateral side of the little toe. Leave the deep branches of the lateral plantar artery and nerve undissected at present. This dissection exposes the long flexor tendons and the flexor accessorius deep to the vessels and nerves [Fig. 190].

Remove abductor hallucis from the flexor retinaculum. Cut across the retinaculum and follow the plantar nerves and arteries to their origins from the tibial nerve and the posterior tibial artery deep to the flexor retinaculum. Identify and follow the tendon of tibialis posterior to its insertion into the navicular bone. Follow the tendons of flexor digitorum longus and flexor hallucis longus into the sole of the foot. The tendon of flexor hallucis longus may be left in its fibro-osseous tunnel and identified in the foot by pulling on it in the leg. As the tendons are separated in the foot, note the slip from flexor hallucis longus which passes into flexor digitorum longus as they cross each other [Fig. 192] and the insertion of flexor accessorius into the tendon of flexor digitorum longus. Note the branch from the lateral plantar nerve entering flexor accessorius and the origins of the muscle from the calcaneus.

Lift the superficial branch of the lateral plantar nerve and trace its branch into flexor digiti minimi brevis. Do likewise with the medial two digital branches of the medial plantar nerve. The most medial sends a branch to flexor hallucis brevis, the second sends a branch to the first lumbrical [Fig. 189].

Second layer

Plantar nerves

These arise from the **tibial nerve** deep to the flexor retinaculum. They enter the sole of the foot with the corresponding branches of the posterior tibial artery deep to abductor hallucis.

The **medial plantar nerve** gives branches to the abductor hallucis and the flexor digitorum brevis, then runs forwards between them. Here it gives rise to: (1) the **proper plantar digital nerve** to the medial side of the great toe, which also supplies flexor hallucis brevis; (2) cutaneous branches to the medial part of the sole of the foot. Further distally it divides into three **common plantar digital nerves**. These pass superficial to the flexor tendons, to the medial three interdigital clefts where they form the proper plantar nerves of these clefts [Fig. 190]. The distribution in the toes is similar to that of the median nerve in the fingers, that is, to the plantar and terminal parts of the dorsal surfaces of the medial three and a half toes. The medial common plantar digital nerve also supplies the first lumbrical muscle.

The **lateral plantar nerve** passes between flexor digitorum brevis and flexor accessorius, giving branches to the flexor accessorius and the abductor digiti minimi. It then passes forwards, deeply placed between the abductor digiti minimi and the flexor digitorum brevis, and gives cutaneous branches to the lateral part of the sole. It then divides into superficial and deep branches.

The **superficial branch** divides into: (1) the **proper plantar digital nerve** to the lateral side of the little toe; (2) a **common plantar digital nerve** to the fourth interdigital cleft. The first of these also gives branches to the flexor digiti minimi brevis and to the third plantar and fourth dorsal interosseous muscles. The second gives proper plantar digital nerves to each side of the fourth cleft. These are distributed in the same manner as the corresponding branches of the medial plantar nerve. The second also communicates with the most lateral of the common plantar digital branches of the medial plantar nerve. Because of this there is considerable overlap of the territories of the two nerves in the toes, and the area supplied by each may vary.

The **deep branch** supplies the remaining small muscles of the foot by passing medially across the proximal parts of the metatarsals. It will be followed later. The distribution of the lateral plantar nerve in the foot is very similar to that of the ulnar nerve in the hand.

Plantar arteries

The **medial plantar artery** is of variable size. It runs with the medial plantar nerve, supplies the surrounding structures, and gives branches corresponding to those of the nerve. The branches that accompany the common plantar digital nerves are often small or absent. When present, they unite with the corresponding plantar metatarsal arteries. The medial plantar artery ends by anastomosing with the branch of the first plantar metatarsal artery (q.v.) to the medial side of the big toe. Compare Figs. 189 and 190.

The **lateral plantar artery** runs with the lateral plantar nerve. It gives branches to the surrounding skin, muscles, and bones, and forms the plantar arch beside the deep branch of the nerve. The arch sends the proper plantar digital artery to the lateral side of the little toe and then sends a **plantar metatarsal artery** on each intermetatarsal space. Each of these is joined to the corresponding **dorsal metatarsal artery** by a **perforating branch** in the proximal part of the space, and becomes a **common plantar digital artery** after uniting with a digital branch of the medial plantar artery, if present. The common arteries divide into **proper plantar digital arteries** to the adjacent sides of two toes [Fig. 193].

Dissection

Reflect abductor digiti minimi from its origin and expose the lateral head of flexor accessorius. Remove the connective tissue from the long flexor tendons, the flexor accessorius, and the lumbrical muscles. Trace one of the tendons of flexor digitorum longus through a fibrous flexor sheath to its insertion, and at least one of the medial two lumbricals to the proximal phalanx and often to the extensor expansion.

Third layer

This is the layer of the long flexor tendons and associated muscles. The arrangement of the tendons of the long flexors of the toes and of flexor accessorius and the lumbrical muscles is well shown in Fig. 192. Note particularly the pulley-like arrangement of flexor hallucis longus on the plantar surface of the sustentaculum tali, and the slip which it gives to flexor digitorum longus. Also that the long flexor tendons cross each other inferior to the head of the talus.

Flexor accessorius

This muscle arises from both margins of the plantar surface of the calcaneus [Fig. 191]. It is inserted into the tendon of flexor digitorum longus. **Nerve**

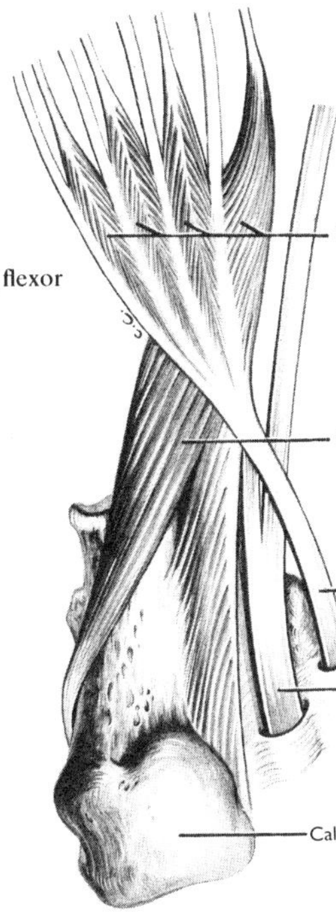

Fig. 192. Layer of long flexor tendons in sole of foot.

supply: lateral plantar nerve. **Action:** it assists in flexing the toes and brings the pull of flexor digitorum longus into line with them.

Lumbrical muscles

These four small muscles which are sometimes reduced to fatty tissue in the elderly arise from the tendons of flexor digitorum longus as shown in Fig. 192. The tendons pass towards the interdigital clefts, and lie with the common plantar digital nerves and vessels between the slips of the plantar aponeurosis which pass to the toes. Here they are inferior to the deep transverse metatarsal ligament and the transverse head of the adductor hallucis [Fig. 193]. One lumbrical tendon enters the medial side of each of the lateral four toes. It then inclines superiorly and is attached to the base of the proximal phalanx and often to the extensor expansion [p. 185]. **Nerve supply:** the first lumbrical by the medial plantar nerve, the other three by the lateral plantar nerve. **Action:** they are weak muscles but they play a part in the flexion of the metatarsophalangeal joints of the lateral four toes and they may also extend their interphalangeal joints. As in the hand, their paralysis prevents the extension of the interphalangeal joints when the metatarso-phalangeal joints are fully extended by the extensor muscles [p. 103]. This leads to a condition known as 'hammer toe' in which the metatarsophalangeal joints of the lateral four toes are fully extended, the proximal interphalangeal joints flexed (flexor digitorum brevis), and the distal interphalangeal joints extended due to pressure on the ground. This makes it difficult to wear any type of shoe with comfort because the acutely angulated toes rub on it.

Flexor tendons in the toes

The arrangement of the tendons and the fibrous flexor sheaths is the same as in the fingers [p. 79]. The only differences are the relative weakness of flexor digitorum brevis and the short, relatively immobile toes.

The **synovial sheaths** are the same in each of the lateral four toes. They begin distal to the attachment of the lumbrical muscles to the flexor digitorum longus tendons, and extend to the base of the distal phalanx where these tendons are inserted. The sheath of the little toe may extend along the lateral side of its tendon to become continuous with the synovial sheath around the main tendon of the flexor digitorum longus. In a similar manner, the sheath of flexor hallucis longus is incomplete where the slip leaves that tendon to join the flexor digitorum longus. Otherwise it usually extends from the lower part of the leg to the insertion of the tendon into the distal phalanx of the great toe.

The tendons within the toes have the same arrangement of **vinculae** as the tendons in the fingers [p. 88].

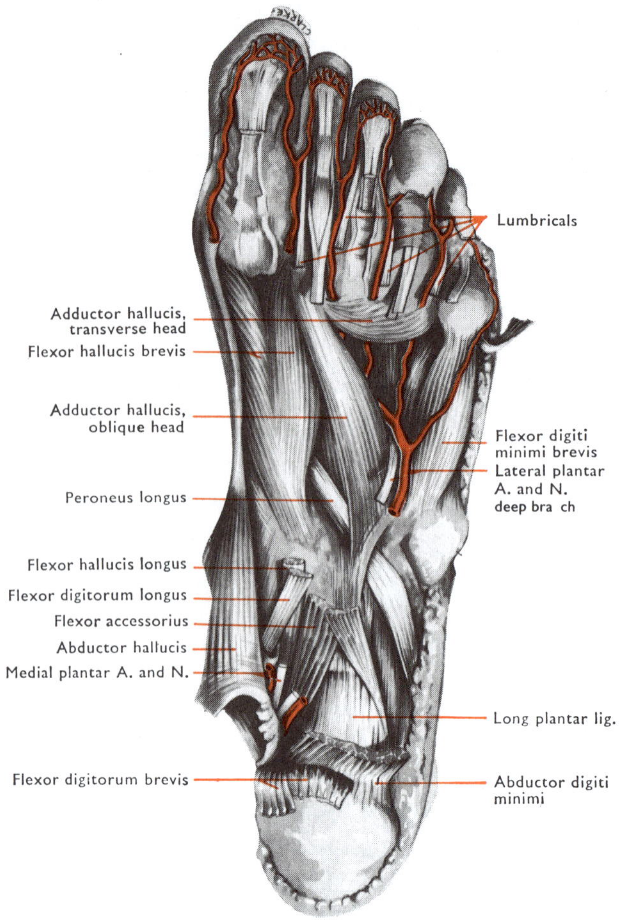

Fig. 193. Deep dissection of sole of foot.

Fourth layer

Dissection

Cut across the flexor accessorius and the tendons of flexor digitorum longus and flexor hallucis longus close to where they unite. Reflect the distal parts of the tendons to uncover the three muscles which form the fourth layer [Fig. 193]. It may be necessary to cut across the medial plantar nerve and reflect it distally to permit sufficient reflexion of the tendons. As the flexor digitorum is turned back, look for the branches of the deep branch of the lateral plantar nerve to the lateral three lumbrical muscles.

Flexor hallucis brevis

This powerful muscle arises from the plantar surface of the cuboid bone [Fig. 191] and the adjoining fascia. It passes anteromedially to the base of the big toe, widening and dividing into two bellies. These are inserted into the medial and lateral margins of the plantar surface of the proximal phalanx of the big toe—the medial with the tendon of abductor hallucis, the lateral with adductor hallucis. Each tendon contains a sesamoid bone [Figs. 214, 215]. **Nerve supply:** medial plantar nerve. **Action:** it flexes the metataraso-phalangeal joint of the big toe, but also tends to produce slight adduction because of its obliquity.

Adductor hallucis

This muscle arises by an oblique head from the fibrous sheath of the tendon of peroneus longus and the bases of the middle three metatarsals. Also by a transverse head from the deep transverse metatarsal and plantar ligaments of the lateral four metatarsophalangeal joints. The fused heads are inserted with the lateral head of flexor hallucis brevis. **Nerve supply:** deep branch of the lateral plantar nerve. **Action:** the oblique head adducts and flexes the metatarsophalangeal joint of the big toe. The transverse head draws the plantar surface of the roots of the toes together and so accentuates the transverse metatarsal arch.

Flexor digiti minimi brevis

It arises from the base of the fifth metatarsal [Fig. 191] and is inserted into the lateral side of the base of the proximal phalanx of the little toe. **Nerve supply:**

superficial branch of the lateral plantar nerve. **Action:** flexion of the metatarsophalangeal joint of the little toe.

Dissection

Define the attachments of these three muscles, but avoid injury to the deep plantar nerve, the plantar arch, and their branches. Detach flexor hallucis brevis and the oblique head of the adductor from their origins. Turn them forwards to expose the nerve and artery. Cut across the abductor hallucis. Turn its distal part forwards with the medial part of the flexor hallucis brevis. Define their common attachment and identify the sesamoid bone in their tendon. Cut this tendon and the bone away from the articular capsule of the metatarsophalangeal joint. Note that the sesamoid bone bears directly on the head of the first metatarsal. Find the nerves to the oblique and transverse heads of the adductor. Then trace the deep branch of the lateral plantar nerve, the plantar arch, and their branches.

Sesamoid bones of the foot

There is a small sesamoid bone in each of the tendons of flexor hallucis brevis. They also extend through the substance of the plantar ligament of the metatarsophalangeal joint of the big toe and articulate directly with the plantar surface of the head of the metatarsal, one on each side. They increase the size of the ball of the big toe and prevent compression devascularization of the tendons of the small muscles which they interrupt and of flexor hallucis longus in the groove between them. Sesamoid bones, or cartilages, are also found in the tendons of peroneus longus and tibialis posterior as they enter the sole, and occasionally in one or more of the other metatarsophalangeal joints.

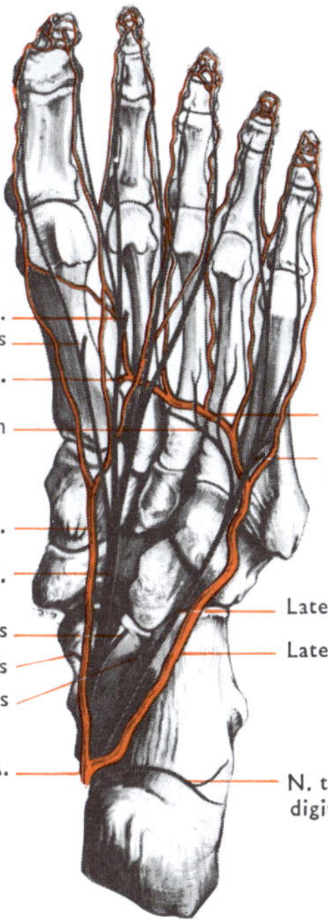

Fig. 194. Arteries and nerves of sole of foot. The plantar nerves and their branches are black.

Fifth layer

Deep branch of the lateral plantar nerve

It arises from the lateral plantar nerve at the base of the fifth metatarsal and crosses the foot on the proximal parts of the metatarsal bones and the interosseous muscles between them. It is deep to the oblique head of adductor hallucis and ends in it. It supplies the adductor hallucis, the lateral three lumbrical muscles, the medial two plantar interossei, and medial three dorsal interossei. It sends twigs to the distal intertarsal, tarsometatarsal, and intermetatarsal joints.

Plantar arch

This continuation of the lateral plantar artery runs with the previous nerve to the proximal end of the first intermetatarsal space. The arch gives a **plantar metatarsal artery** to each of the intermetatarsal spaces. Each of these arteries

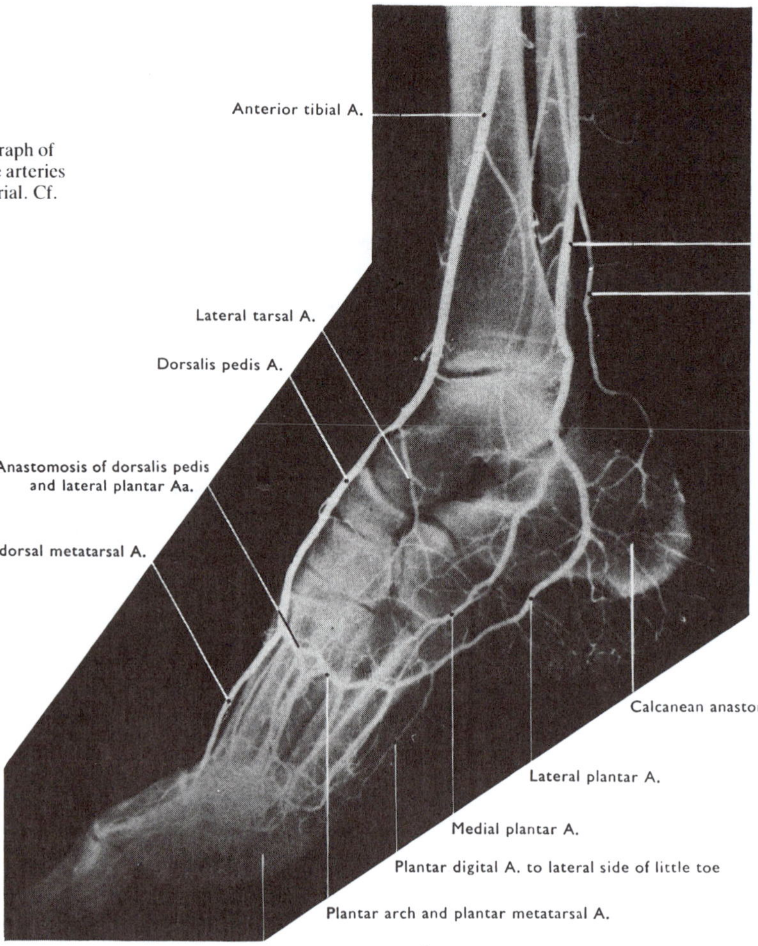

Fig. 195. Lateral radiograph of foot after injection of the arteries with X-ray-opaque material. Cf. Fig. 194.

communicates with the corresponding dorsal metatarsal artery by a **perforating branch** through the proximal (and distal) end of the space. The plantar metatarsal artery may then unite with a branch of the medial plantar artery (medial three spaces) and form a **common plantar digital artery**. In the first space, the perforating branch comes from the arcuate artery (**deep plantar branch**) and is mainly responsible for the formation of the plantar metatarsal artery of that space. Each common plantar digital artery (or plantar metatarsal artery) divides into **proper plantar digital arteries** to the adjacent sides of two toes. That in the first space also gives rise to the proper plantar digital artery to the medial side of the big toe [Fig. 194]. The arch and its branches supply all the surrounding structures, including the bones and joints. The proper digital arteries anastomose with each other and with the dorsal digital arteries in the distal parts of the toes. Thus there is a very free anastomosis between the dorsalis pedis artery and its branches on the one hand and the plantar arteries on the other.

Dissection

Expose the deep transverse metatarsal ligament by detaching the transverse head of the adductor hallucis from its origin and reflecting it medially. Separate a plantar ligament from one of the metatarsophalangeal joints and note its continuity with the deep transverse ligament. Note also the attachment of the fibrous flexor sheath, the plantar aponeurosis, and the extensor expansion to this dense strip of fibrous tissue which forms the anterior surface of the fibrous capsule of each metatarsophalangeal joint.

Cut through the deep transverse ligament on both sides of the middle toe. Find the tendons of the interosseous muscles dorsal to the ligament. Follow them in both directions and separate the interosseous muscles from each other.

It is often helpful to lever the metatarsal bones apart to see the dorsal and plantar interossei clearly even though this tears one of the attachments of the bipennate dorsal interosseous muscle [Fig. 196].

Detach flexor digiti minimi brevis from its origin. Reflect it forwards to expose the interossei in the lateral intermetatarsal space. Pull on the tendon of tibialis posterior. Note its main attachment to the navicular bone and its extensions to other tarsal and metatarsal bones. Pull on the tendon of peroneus longus. Cut through the fibrous bridge (long plantar ligament) which holds it in place on the plantar surface of the cuboid bone. Follow the tendon to its insertion.

Sixth layer

Deep transverse metatarsal ligament

These strong bands unite the plantar ligaments of the metatarsophalangeal joints and so are principally attached through these ligaments to the proximal phalanges. The ligaments help to prevent the bases of the toes spreading and so maintain the transverse metatarsal arch. The interossei enter the toes dorsal to these ligaments; the lumbricals and plantar digital nerves and vessels are on their plantar surfaces.

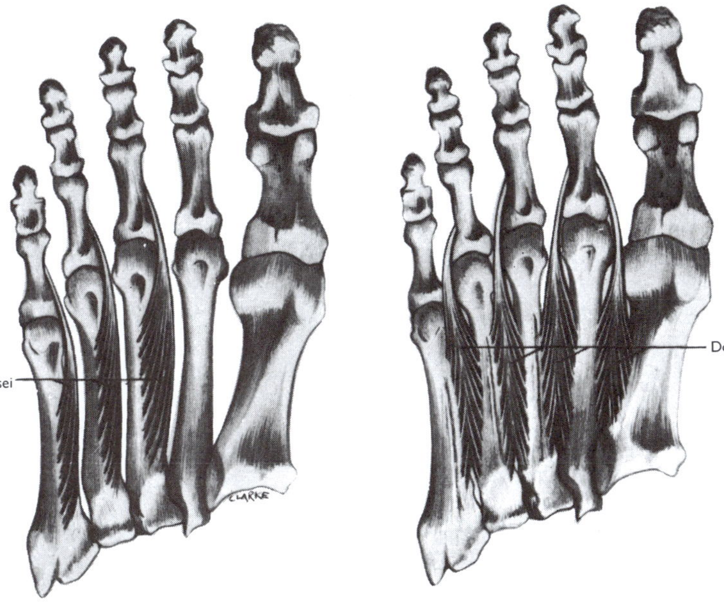

Fig. 196. Interosseous muscles of right foot.

Interossei [Fig. 196]

The general arrangement of these muscles is the same as in the hand, except that the second and not the middle toe has two dorsal interossei. There is a plantar interosseous to each of the lateral three toes and four dorsal interossei to the middle three toes. All the interossei are inserted into the bases of the proximal phalanges with little if any attachment to the extensor expansion. **Nerve supply:** lateral plantar nerve. **Action:** the plantar interossei adduct the lateral three toes to the *axis of the foot,* the line of the second toe, cf. the hand. The dorsal interossei abduct the middle three toes from the axis of the foot. They also flex the metatarsophalangeal joints but usually do not extend the interphalangeal joints.

Tendon of tibialis posterior

This tendon turns over the posterior surface of the medial malleolus (which acts as a pulley for it) and runs forwards beneath the medial part of the plantar calcaneonavicular ligament to the tuberosity of the navicular bone. It also spreads laterally to all the other tarsal bones (except the talus) and to the bases of the middle three metatarsals. The powerful **plantar calcaneonavicular ligament** extends from the sustentaculum tali to the navicular. It supports the head of the talus [Fig. 214] which, transmitting the weight of the body, tends to force its way between the calcaneus and the navicular and stretch the ligament. When tibialis posterior contracts, it pulls the navicular posteriorly and so carries some of the load placed on the ligament. The tendon also has within it a fibrocartilage knob, sometimes ossified to a sesamoid bone, where it lies under and supports the ligament. The extensions of the tendon to the

Fig. 197. Plantar aspect of tarsal and tarsometatarsal joints.

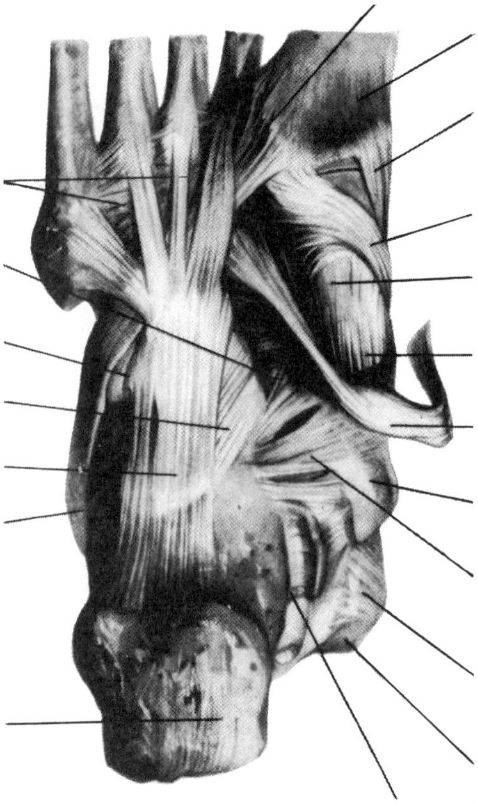

other bones draw the plantar surfaces of the bones together. Thus they strengthen the arches of the foot and protect the various plantar ligaments, e.g. during forced plantar flexion. The extensions to the lateral side of the foot can produce some inversion.

Tendon of peroneus longus

This tendon, containing a sesamoid bone or cartilage, turns over the lateral border of the cuboid bone and then runs anteromedially in the grove on its plantar surface. The **long plantar ligament** [Fig. 197] converts the groove into a tunnel in which the tendon slides in its synovial sheath. The insertion is to the base of the first metatarsal and the adjacent part of the medial cuneiform bone, close to the insertion of tibialis anterior. When peroneus longus contracts, it everts the foot. Tension developed in its tendon in the sole helps to prevent stretching of the ligaments which maintain the transverse arch of the tarsal bones in the same manner as the lateral fibres of the tibialis posterior tendon.

If the proximal end of the first metatarsal is now disarticulated by cutting its ligaments, the communication between the deep plantar branch of the arcuate artery and the plantar arch can be seen.

The joints of the lower limb

The hip joint [see pp. 169–72]

The knee joint

This massive joint carries severe stresses, yet it has a wide range of flexion limited only by contact between the leg and thigh, and a moderate range of rotation when flexed. In all positions of the joint, the femur articulates with the tibia and the patella, and the strength of the joint depends on ligaments and muscles rather than on the close fitting of the bones. Only a relatively small area of each convex femoral condyle articulates with the central area of the corresponding tibial condyle which is slightly concave. The wedge-shaped space left at the periphery of each of these articulations is filled by a C-shaped rim of fibrocartilage (the **meniscus** [Fig. 202]) which extends inwards between the articular surfaces of the bones from the articular capsule. The ends of both fibrocartilages are attached to the median, non-articular, **intercondylar area** of the tibia [Fig. 205]. The synovial cavity extends over the thin, internal edges of the menisci and between them and the articular surfaces of the bones. Thus they are free to slide on these surfaces as far as their attachments to the articular capsule and tibia permit. The menisci deepen the articular surfaces of the tibia and help to spread the synovial fluid between the thrust-bearing surfaces of the femur and tibia.

Ligaments

The **cruciate ligaments** are the most powerful. They pass from the intercondylar area of the tibia to the walls of the intercondylar fossa of the femur, crossing each other on the way. The **tibial** and **fibular collateral ligaments** have been seen already. The **fibrous capsule** is formed by the ligamentum patellae anteriorly, and is strengthened posteriorly by the oblique popliteal ligament—an extension from the tendon of semimembranosus.

Dissection

Remove the structures surrounding the knee joint, but leave the fibrous articular capsule, collateral ligaments, and parts of the muscles or their tendons so that their connections with the ligaments may be seen.

Fig. 198. Fibular collateral ligament of right knee joint.

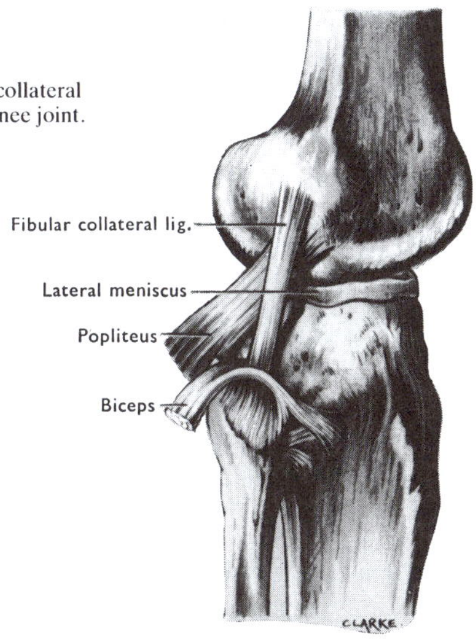

Articular capsule

The fibrous capsule is thin and extensive at the back, but thicker and shorter at the sides. In front it is replaced by the **ligamentum patellae**, the patella, and the tendon of quadriceps—a mechanism which permits the full range of flexion while allowing this part of the membrane to be held taut in any position by the contraction of quadriceps.

Attachments

Posteriorly and at the sides the fibrous capsule is attached close to the articular margins of the tibial and femoral condyles and to the intercondylar line of the femur. Anteriorly, it follows the oblique lines on the tibia downwards to the sides of the tibial tuberosity. Here it blends with the patellar ligament and above that with the sides of the patella and the tendon of quadriceps.

The fibrous capsule is perforated by the tendon of popliteus at the back of the lateral tibial condyle, and by the continuity of the synovial membrane of the joint with the bursa under the medial head of gastrocnemius at the back of the medial femoral condyle.

Fig. 199. Right knee joint from behind.

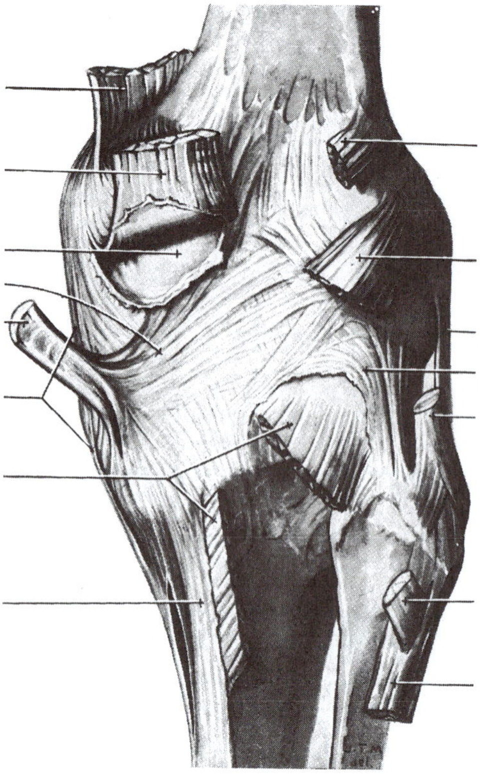

Fibrous structures which strengthen the joint

Ligamentum patellae

This powerful ligament is the continuation of the quadriceps tendon inferior to the patella. It extends from the apex and lower parts of the deep surface of the patella to the smooth upper part of the tibial tuberosity. The upper part of its deep surface is separated from the synovial membrane of the knee joint by the **infrapatellar pad of fat**. The lower part is separated from the upper part of the tibia by the **deep infrapatellar bursa** [Fig. 200].

Fig. 200. Sagittal section of right knee joint to show extension of cavity into suprapatellar bursa. The popliteal vein is not shown.

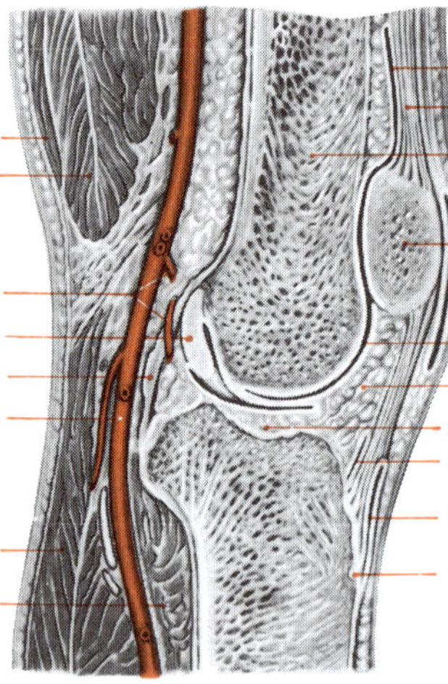

Fibular collateral ligament

This cord-like ligament extends from the lateral epicondyle of the femur to the head of the fibula. Here it pierces the tendon of insertion of biceps femoris. It is separated from the fibrous capsule of the joint, and hence from the **lateral meniscus**, by fatty tissue in which the inferior lateral genicular vessels and nerve run [Fig. 187]. In its turn, the fibrous capsule is separated from the meniscus by the **tendon of popliteus** which is deep to the capsule [Fig. 198].

Tibial collateral ligament

This broad, flat band arises from the medial epicondyle of the femur where it receives fibres from the tendon of adductor magnus. Inferiorly it splits into two layers. The **deep layer** (essentially part of the fibrous capsule) passes to the articular margin of the medial condyle of the tibia and is fused with the

medial meniscus. The **superficial layer**, separated from the medial condyle of the tibia by the inferior medial genicular vessels and nerve and the insertion of semimembranosus, is inserted into the medial surface of the tibia between the medial border and the insertions of sartorius, gracilis, and semitendinosus [Fig. 251].

Oblique popliteal ligament

This is an extension of the semimembranosus tendon. It arises from the tendon close to its insertion, and runs upwards and laterally towards the lateral femoral condyle. It is fused with the fibrous capsule. If the tendon of semimembranosus is pulled on, the ligament becomes obvious.

Patellar retinacula

These are fibrous expansions from vastus medialis and lateralis into the fibrous capsule on the corresponding side of the patellar ligament.

Iliotibial tract

This fuses with the fibrous capsule between the fibular collateral ligament and the ligamentum patellae.

Cruciate ligaments

See below.

Dissection

Cut across the quadriceps tendon immediately proximal to the patella. Carry the ends of this incision downwards to the tibial condyles passing 2–3 cm on either side of the ligamentum patellae. Turn the patella downwards and expose the cavity of the knee joint. Lift the tendon of quadriceps and note that the cavity of the joint extends upwards deep to it to form the suprapatellar bursa. Split the lower part of the quadriceps longitudinally and examine the extent of the bursa. At the upper limit of the bursa, fibres of vastus intermedius are inserted into it (articularis genus muscle). Flex and extend the joint. Note the type of movement which occurs between the tibia and femur. Examine the infrapatellar and alar folds [Fig. 202].

Interior of the knee joint

The cavity of the knee joint may be looked upon as four cavities which have coalesced. (1 and 2) There is one cavity between each femoral and tibial condyle. These are separated posteriorly by a septum of synovial membrane

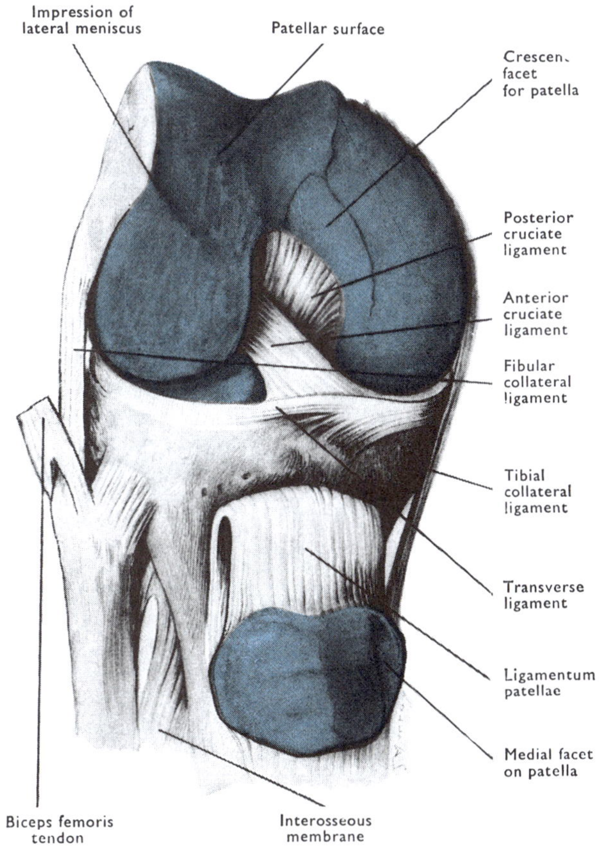

Fig. 201. Dissection of right knee from the front: patella and patellar ligament turned down.

which extends from the intercondylar fossa of the femur to the margins of the intercondylar area of the superior surface of the tibia. The septum covers the front and sides of the cruciate ligaments and its lower part extends forwards as the **infrapatellar fold** of synovial membrane to the posterior surface of the patellar ligament. This fold has a free, crescentic, upper margin over which the two tibiofemoral cavities communicate with each other and with (3) the **patellofemoral cavity** above. The last is continuous superiorly with (4) the **suprapatellar bursa** between quadriceps and the femur, superior to the patella [Fig. 200].

On each side of the infrapatellar fold an **alar fold** extends outwards on to the upper surface of the tibia. The three folds (alar and infrapatellar) cover the **infrapatellar pad of fat** [Fig. 200] and form a soft intracapsular packing between patella, tibia, and femur which can adapt to variations in the shape of the joint space during movement.

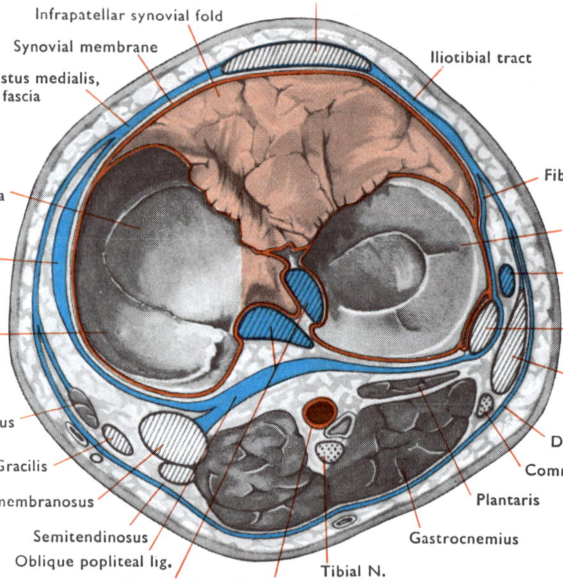

Fig. 202. Transverse section through right knee joint and its surroundings showing synovial membrane (red); fascia and ligaments, blue.
A. Anterior.
P. Posterior.
M. Medial.
L. Lateral.

Synovial membrane

This lines all the structures which form the walls of the cavities of the knee joint, except the articular surfaces of the bones and menisci and the posterior part of the fibrous capsule where the synovial membrane turns forwards from it to enclose the cruciate ligaments [Fig. 202]. It also covers all other non-articular structures within the fibrous capsule, i.e. the infrapatellar pad of fat and the tendon of popliteus. It separates that tendon from the lateral condyle of the femur, posterior to its attachment, and continues with it through the fibrous capsule to separate the tendon from the superior tibiofibular joint. Here it is sometimes continuous with the synovial membrane of that joint.

The **suprapatellar bursa** is a large saccular extension of the joint cavity between the body of the femur and the tendon of quadriceps. It extends a hand-breadth superior to the patella and is almost as wide as this.

Dissection

Remove the infrapatellar synovial fold and pad of fat. Open the deep infrapatellar bursa. Remove the posterior part of the fibrous capsule of the knee joint, and follow the middle genicular artery through it to the cruciate ligaments. Define the posterior parts of these ligaments, and then remove the synovial membrane and connective tissue from their anterior surfaces. Define their attachments to the femur, tibia, and lateral meniscus (meniscofemoral ligaments) [Fig. 204]. Follow the tendon of popliteus and note how it lies between the lateral meniscus and the fibrous capsule of the joint. The fibres of the posterior part of the fibrous capsule which arch over the aperture for the tendon of popliteus are known as the **arcuate ligament**.

If a better view of the cruciate ligaments is required, saw across the

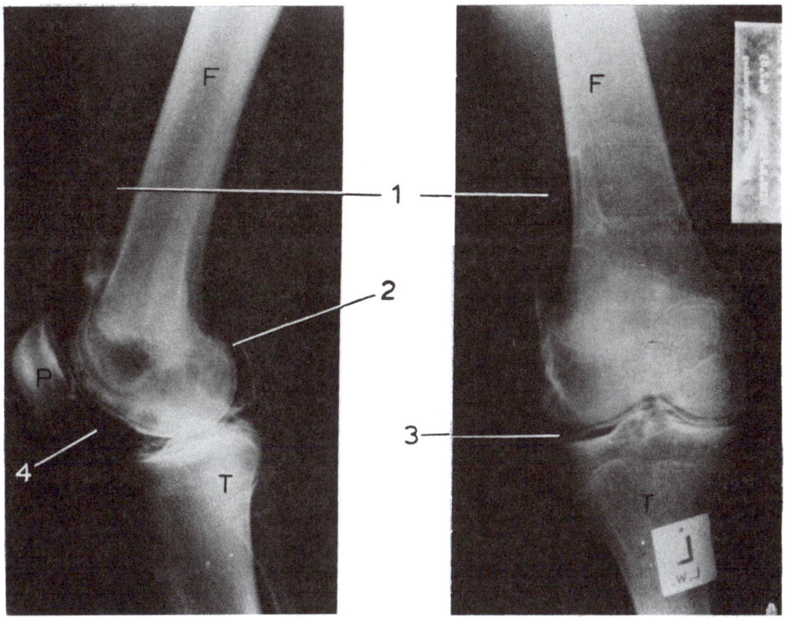

Fig. 203. Double-contrast arthrogram of the knee joint. This is produced by injecting a small amount of X-ray-opaque medium into the cavity of the knee joint, moving the joint to disperse it, and then injecting air to distend the synovial cavity. This leaves a thin film of X-ray-opaque medium (white) on the synovial surfaces which can be identified by contrast with the air (dark) within the cavity.
F, femur; P, patella; T, tibia.
1. Edge of suprapatellar bursa.
2. Posterior recess of synovial cavity behind each condyle.
3. Meniscus with its surfaces covered with X-ray-opaque medium.
4. Infrapatellar synovial fold passing from the posterior surface of the patellar ligament to the intercondylar notch.

femur above the joint, and then divide the distal part of the bone by a sagittal saw cut as far as the intercondylar fossa. Pull the two parts of the femur apart and expose the structures in the fossa.

Cruciate ligaments

These ligaments are so named because they cross each other like the letter X.

The **anterior cruciate ligament** passes upwards and backwards from the anterior part of the intercondylar area of the tibia [Fig. 205] to the posterior part of the medial surface of the lateral condyle of the femur [Fig. 204].

The **posterior cruciate ligament** passes upwards and forwards from the posterior part of the tibial intercondylar area [Figs. 204, 205] to the anterior part of the lateral surface of the medial condyle of the femur. It receives one or more slips from the posterior part of the lateral meniscus (**meniscofemoral ligaments**). The cruciate ligaments hold the femur to the tibia and prevent it sliding forwards (posterior cruciate) or backwards (anterior cruciate) on the flat upper surface of the tibia. The importance of this when the full weight of the body is carried on a flexed knee is obvious. Both ligaments remain

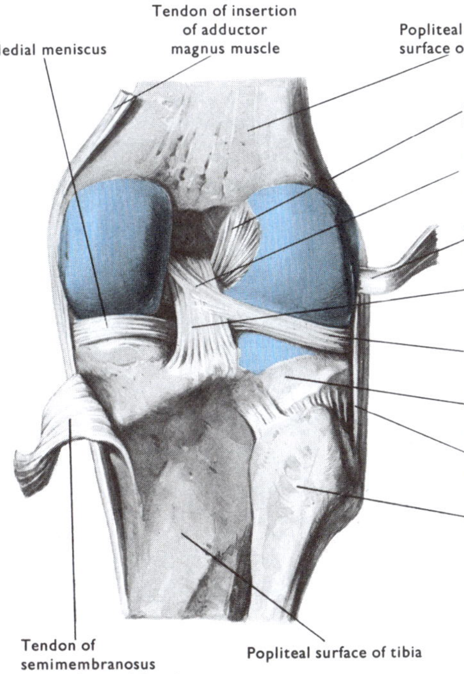

Fig. 204. Right knee joint opened from behind by the removal of posterior part of the articular capsule.

relatively tight throughout the movements of flexion and extension of the knee joint, but do no prevent these movements because of their attachments to the femur close to the axis of the movements. However, the anterior cruciate ligament tightens towards the end of extension and prevents the lateral femoral condyle from sliding backwards on the tibia while the medial condyle continues to do so. This produces *medial rotation of the femur on the tibia* at the end of extension—a process which screws home the joint and 'locks' it in this position.

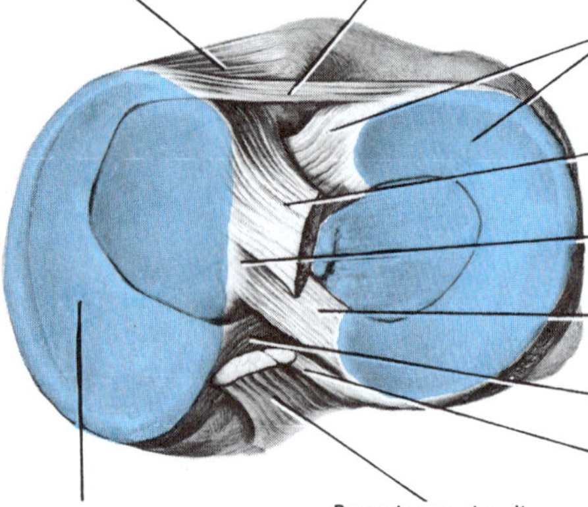

Fig. 205. Upper end of tibia with menisci and attached portions of cruciate ligaments.

Menisci

Each of these C-shaped plates of fibrocartilage lies on the articular surface of a tibial condyle. They are thick at their circumference but thin away to a fine, free, concave edge internally. Both upper and lower surfaces are smooth and articular.

They are mainly attached to the tibia. (1) To the intercondylar area by their fibrous extremities (horns). (2) To the margins of the tibial condyles by their peripheral fusion with the articular capsule of the knee joint. They are not so attached anteriorly, where they are linked to each other by the **transverse ligament of the knee** [Fig. 205], or posterolaterally, where the **tendon of popliteus** intervenes between the lateral meniscus and the capsule. The **lateral meniscus** is nearly circular (in keeping with the more spherical lateral condyle of the femur) so its horns are attached close together near the centre of the intercondylar area. The **medial meniscus** is elongated anteroposteriorly (in keeping with the shape and movements of the medial femoral condyle) so its horns are attached far apart on the anterior and posterior parts of the tibial intercondylar area [Fig. 205]. All these features make the medial meniscus much less free to move on the tibia than the lateral meniscus. This, combined with the greater anteroposterior movement of the medial condyle of the femur and the direct attachments of the lateral meniscus to the femur (anterior and posterior meniscofemoral ligaments) makes it much more likely that the medial meniscus is trapped between the moving surfaces of the tibia and femur. This tends to occur especially in sudden turning movements with the foot fixed on the ground, e.g. in violent changes of direction when running. In such a movement, the medial condyle of the femur pivots around the spherical lateral condyle, and sliding violently backwards or forwards on the tibia while under pressure, may catch the margin of the medial meniscus and tear or avulse it. If such a torn piece of cartilage becomes wedged between the tibia and femur, the joint becomes 'locked' because the ligaments cannot be stretched sufficiently to allow the bones to be forced apart.

Movements of the knee joint [Table 10]

These are mainly flexion and extension. *Flexion* proceeds until the calf and thigh are in contact. *Extension* stops when the thigh and leg are in a straight line. In this position the joint is firmly 'locked'; the anterior cruciate, tibial and fibular collateral ligaments, the oblique popliteal ligament and posterior part of the capsule are all taut, the leg and thigh being converted into a rigid column.

Rotation can also occur at any phase of flexion. It is a natural concomitant

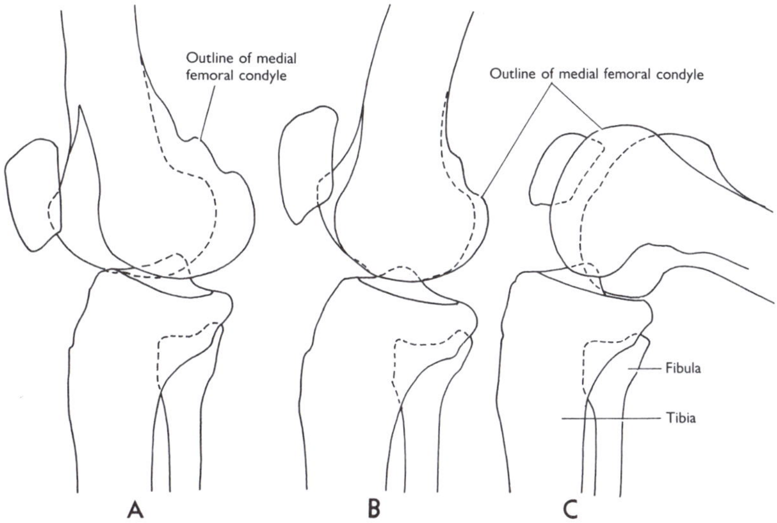

Fig. 206. Tracings of three positions of right knee joint taken from radiographs of three phases of flexion of the knee with the foot firmly fixed on the ground. In this way there is no movement of the tibia and fibula and the full effects of rotation are visible in the femur. The tracings are viewed from the medial side, the parts that are hidden by the more medial structures are shown as broken lines.
A. Position of full extension with the femur fully rotated medially and the knee joint locked.
B. Slight flexion. Note that there has been considerable lateral rotation of the femur, so that the outlines of the condyles are nearly superimposed. This movement occurs at the very outset of flexion.
C. Considerable flexion of the knee with further lateral rotation of the femur on the tibia.

of flexion and extension. Medial rotation of the femur occurs during extension, lateral rotation during flexion [see below and Fig. 206].

In full flexion of the knee, the posterior surfaces of the femoral condyles articulate with the tibia, the patella with the crescentic facet on the medial condyle of the femur [Fig. 201]. As the knee is extended, the femoral condyles roll forwards and slide backwards on the tibial condyles, the points of contact with the tibia moving steadily forwards on the femoral condyles. Because the anteroposterior curvature of the medial femoral condyle becomes flatter anteriorly than the more spherical lateral condyle, the backward translation of the medial condyle increases so that medial rotation of the femur accompanies extension. When the lateral condyle reaches its maximum extension, the groove between its patellar and tibial surfaces [Fig. 201] comes into contact with the lateral meniscus, and the condyle is held forwards by the taut anterior cruciate ligament. The medial condyle continues to slide backwards so that extension is completed by a sudden medial rotation of the femur [Fig. 206A]. This screws the femur home on the tibia, tightens the ligaments, and *'locks' the knee joint*. Flexion is produced by the same movements in the reverse order. It begins with lateral rotation of the femur by **popliteus**. This 'unlocks' the joint and flexion proceeds with lateral rotation of the femur because of the different shapes of the two condyles. Rotation of the flexed joint may be produced independently of flexion and extension by the muscles at the sides of the joint. Biceps femoris is the principal lateral rotator of the tibia; sartorius, gracilis, semitendinosus, and semimembranosus are the main medial rotators of the tibia.

During extension of the joint, the patella rises to progressively higher levels on the patellar surface of the femur. Because the pull of quadriceps on the patella is parallel to the obliquely placed femur, there is a tendency for the patella to deviate laterally as it ascends. This is prevented (a) by the high patellar buttress on the lateral femoral condyle and (b) by the lowest, horizontal fibres of vastus medialis which are inserted into the medial surface of the patella. These two factors help to keep the pull of quadriceps at right angles to the axis of flexion and extension of the knee joint.

Fuller details of the movements of this complex joint should be sought in larger textbooks of anatomy. However, the student should not lose sight of the fact that the knee joint is essentially a hinge. The bolt of the hinge passes through the femoral attachments of the collateral and cruciate ligaments which lie virtually in a straight line. These ligaments suspend the leg after the manner of the ropes of a swing so that rotation is possible when they are relaxed.

Dissection

If it is desired to obtain a clearer view of the proximal surfaces of the tibia and the menisci, cut across the fibular collateral ligament, the remains of the fibrous capsule, and the cruciate ligaments so that the femur may be turned to the medial side.

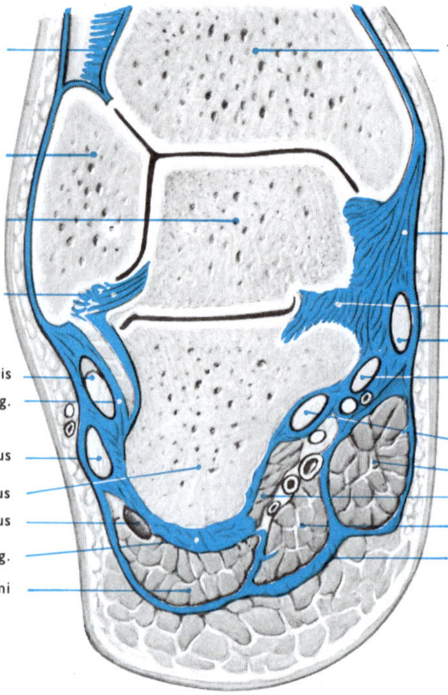

Fig. 207. Oblique coronal section through ankle and subtalar joints.

Ankle joint

This is a hinge joint of great strength. Its stability is ensured: (1) by the powerful ligaments and tendons around it; (2) by the insertion of the trochlea tali into the deep socket between the medial and lateral malleoli. The trochlea bears on the malleoli and on the distal surface of the tibia between them. The socket is not entirely rigid but has some spring because of the flexibility of the body of the fibula. If the talus is forced laterally, the lateral malleolus can move slightly outwards because, acting with the tibiofibular ligaments as a fulcrum, it springs the body of the fibula medially. In extreme cases this may lead to fracture of the fibula in the leg. The socket is deepened posteriorly by the inferior part of the posterior tibiofibular ligament (transverse tibiofibular ligament [Fig. 211]).

Dissection

Remove the remains of the extensor and flexor retinacula. Cut through and displace the tendons which are in contact with the joint, but do not remove them. Define the anterior and posterior parts of the fibrous capsule of the joint. Both are extremely thin and easily

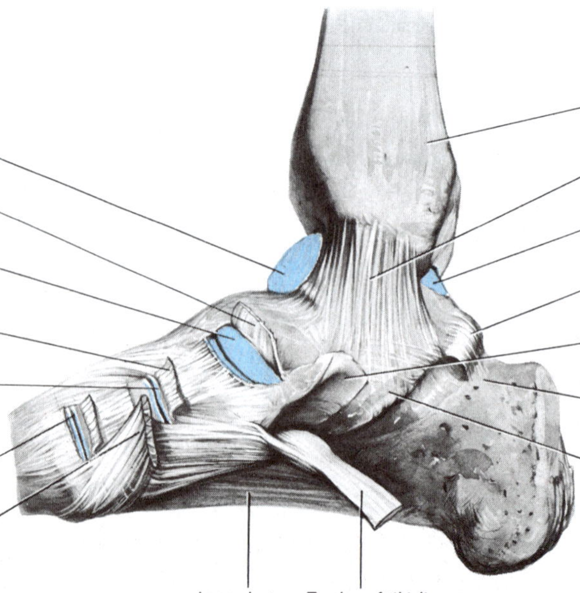

Fig. 208. Ankle joint and tarsal joints from the medial side.

damaged. Now remove these parts of the capsule in order to bring the strong ligaments at the side of the joint more clearly into view. Identify these ligaments and define their attachments [Figs. 208, 209].

Ligaments of the ankle joint

Because this is a hinge joint, the main ligaments are lateral and medial. The anterior parts of the fibrous capsule are thin and consist mainly of transverse fibres. The anterior part extends from the anterior margin of the distal end of the tibia to the superior surface of the neck of the talus. The posterior part passes from the posterior margin of the distal end of the tibia and the posterior tibiofibular ligament to the posterior surface of the body of the talus.

Medial (deltoid) ligament

This very strong ligament radiates from the distal border of the medial malleolus to the medial side of the talus, the sustentaculum tali, the medial edge of the plantar calcaneonavicular (spring) ligament, the navicular bone, and the neck of the talus [Fig. 208]. Thus the medial ligament not only strengthens the ankle joint, but also holds the calcaneus and the navicular against the talus.

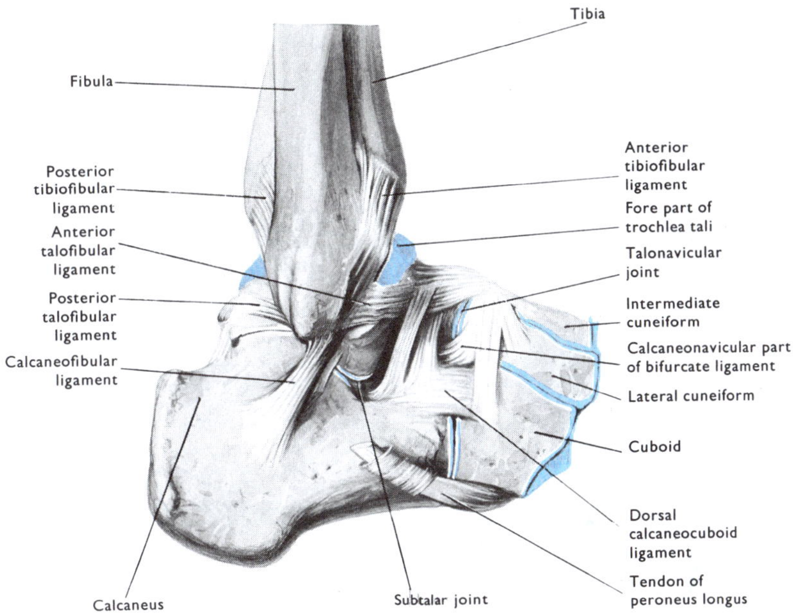

Fig. 209. Ligaments of lateral side of ankle joint and dorsum of tarsus.

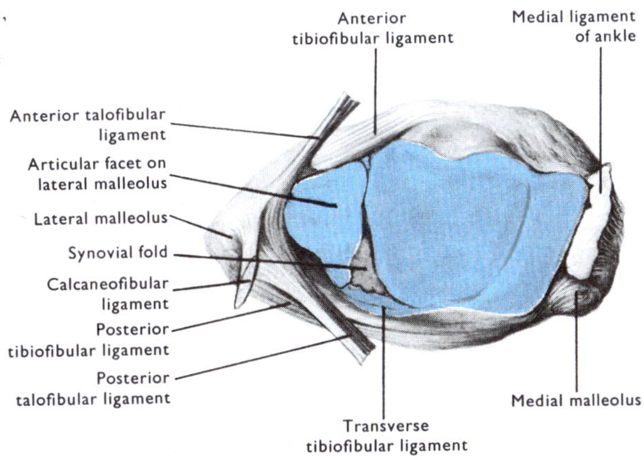

Fig. 210. Surfaces (blue), of tibia, fibula, and transverse tibiofibular ligament which articulate with the talus at the ankle joint.

Lateral ligament

This ligament consists of three bands, of which the anterior and posterior are thickenings of the fibrous capsule. The **anterior talofibular ligament** passes anteromedially from the anterior border of the lateral malleolus to the neck of the talus. The posterior talofibular ligament is much stronger. It runs medially and backwards from the fossa of the lateral malleolus to the **posterior tubercle of the talus** [Figs. 209, 210]. This tubercle of the talus ossifies from a separate centre. It appears, therefore, as a separate bone until it fuses with the rest of the talus. Until it does so, it may be mistaken for a fracture. Rarely it fails to fuse with the remainder of the talus. In this case, it remains in the adult as the **os trigonum**.

The calcaneofibular ligament is a round cord which passes postero-inferiorly from the distal end of the lateral malleolus to the lateral surface of the calcaneus [Figs. 207, 209, 211]. It is separate from the articular capsule of the ankle joint and functions also as a ligament of the talocalcanean joint because it crosses that joint also.

Fig. 211. Ankle joint dissected from behind and part of articular capsule removed.

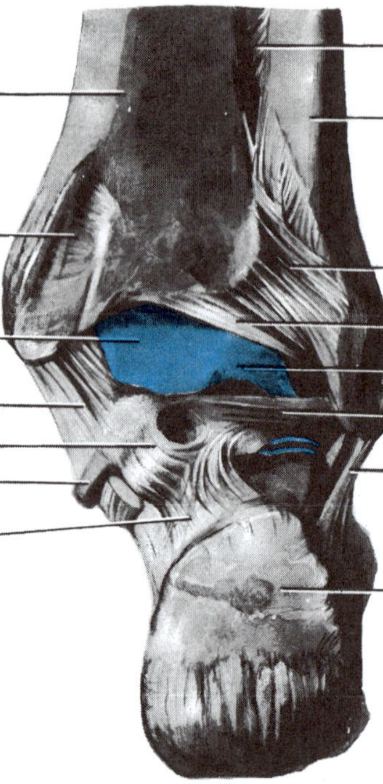

Synovial membrane

It lines the fibrous capsule, but is separated from it by fatty pads which lie deep to the anterior and posterior parts of the capsule. There is a short extension of synovial membrane between the tibia and fibula, inferior to the thickened lower end of the interosseous membrane (interosseous tibiofibular ligament).

All the structures passing into the foot from the leg lie close to the ankle joint, except the tendo calcaneus. Tendons, vessels, and nerves from the anterior compartment lie on the anterior surface; from the posterior compartment they lie on the posteromedial surface; from the lateral compartment (peroneal tendons) they lie on the posterolateral surface.

Movements

The surfaces of the trochlea tali which articulate with the malleoli are wider apart anteriorly, and the socket is also broader in front. Thus the talus fits snugly into the socket when the foot is dorsiflexed. When the foot is plantar flexed, the talus is slightly loose and some slight lateral movement is possible. Hence maximum stability of the ankle is achieved in the standing position. Plantar flexion and dorsiflexion are the only significant movements at the ankle joint.

Tibiofibular joints

The tibia and fibula approach each other at their ends. Superiorly, they articulate by a synovial joint, the proximal tibiofibular joint. Inferiorly, they are bound close together by the thickened lower end of the interosseous membrane (interosseous tibiofibular ligament) and by anterior and posterior tibiofibular ligaments. Here there is no synovial cavity. Elsewhere they are united by the interosseous membrane, except where the anterior tibial vessels pass through it.

Fig. 212. Arthrogram of ankle joint. The synovial cavity has been filled with X-ray-opaque material and a lateral radiograph taken. This outlines the extent of the synovial cavity when distended and passes between the articular surfaces (a) which are not held in apposition when they are not load-bearing and atmospheric pressure cannot act because of the fluid introduced. A thin film of X-ray-opaque material also separates the malleolar articular surfaces from the talus.
a. X-ray-opaque material between the tibia and the trochlea of the talus, the dark line on each side of this is the articular cartilage.
b. Posterior extension of synovial cavity.
c. Margin of lateral malleolus.
ca. Calcaneus.
d. Anterior extension of synovial cavity.
f. Fibula overlapping tibia (the light area immediately below f is due to material entering the recess of the joint cavity between tibia and fibula).
T. tibia.
ta. Neck of talus
The V-shaped white area posterior to the edge of the lateral malleolus is the lowest extent of the joint cavity between the malleolus and the talus.

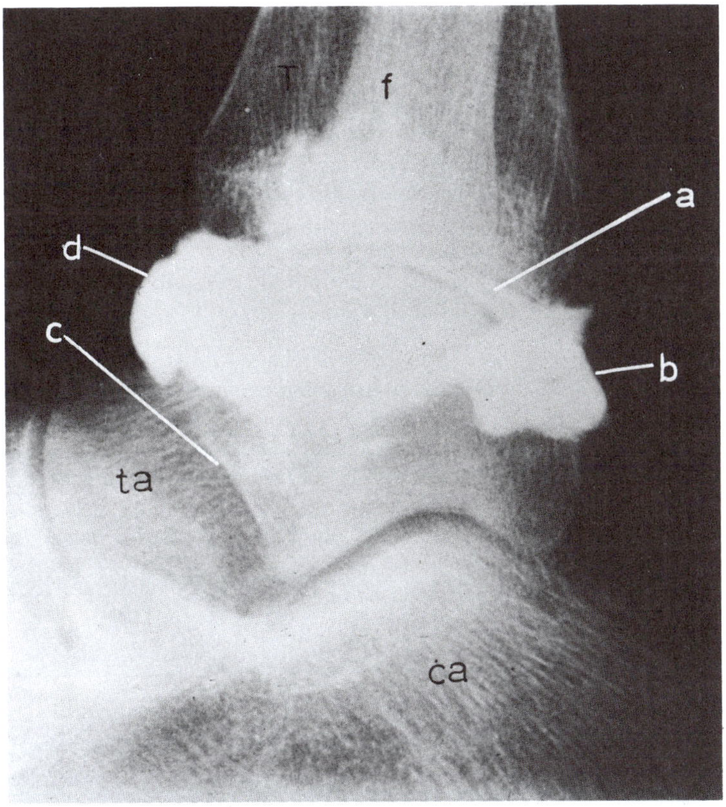

Dissection

Define the anterior and posterior tibiofibular ligaments [Figs. 210, 211]. Strip the muscles from the front of the interosseous membrane and define its attachments. Follow it as far inferiorly as possible. The posterior surface may also be exposed if it is not desired to retain the muscles.

Define the fibrous capsule of the proximal tibiofibular joint. Reflect the tendon of popliteus from its posterior surface. The synovial extension from the knee joint deep to popliteus may be in continuity with the cavity of the proximal tibiofibular joint. Open the joint and confirm its synovial nature.

Interosseous membrane of the leg

This strong membrane stretches between the interosseous borders of the tibia and fibula [Figs. 250, 252]. It is composed of strong fibres which run downwards and laterally from the tibia to the fibula. There is an oval opening in the upper part of the membrane for the passage of the **anterior tibial vessels**, and a small aperture for the **perforating branch of the peroneal artery** a short distance above the ankle joint. Tibialis posterior and flexor hallucis longus arise in part from the back of the membrane; all the muscles of the anterior compartment of the leg have a partial origin from it.

Proximal tibiofibular joint

This joint is between the head of the fibula and the postero-inferior surface of the lateral tibial condyle. The articular capsule is attached near the articular margins. It is strengthened anteriorly and posteriorly by fibres which run downwards and laterally from the tibia to the head of the fibula. The fibular collateral ligament of the knee joint and the tendon of biceps femoris cross the upper lateral surface of the joint. The tendon of popliteus with a synovial extension from the knee joint cross the posteromedial surface of the joint. Here the synovial cavities of the two joints may communicate. **Nerve supply** of the joint is from the nerve to popliteus and the recurrent genicular nerve.

Distal tibiofibular joint [Figs. 207–211]

At this joint the tibia and fibula are firmly bound together mainly by the short but strong **interosseous tibiofibular ligament** which extends from the longitudinal groove on the lateral side of the tibia to the rough medial side of the distal part of the fibula which is fitted into the groove. The lowest part of the groove may be covered with articular cartilage for the upper part of the lateral malleolar facet.

The interosseous ligament is strengthened and hidden by the **anterior** and **posterior tibiofibular ligaments**. These pass upwards and medially from the corresponding surfaces of the lateral malleolus to the distal end of the tibia. They are continuous with the corresponding parts of the fibrous capsule of the ankle joint. The transverse tibiofibular ligament is a strong, yellowish band of fibres which passes from the malleolar fossa of the fibula to the entire length of the inferior margin of the posterior surface of the tibia. This part forms a posterior lip to the socket for the ankle joint [Figs. 210, 211] and articulates with the posterolateral part of the body of the talus.

Movements

Only a small amount of movement of the fibula on the tibia is possible. Slight medial movement of the body of the fibula occurs when the lateral malleolus is forced laterally by the trochlea of the talus. This movement takes place around the powerful tibiofibular ligaments which act as a fulcrum. The resilience of the body of the fibula, acting in the opposite direction, keeps the lateral malleolus pressed against the trochlea of the talus. This increases the stability of the ankle joint and also gives its socket a measure of resilience.

Dissection

The interosseous tibiofibular ligament may be exposed by sawing transversely through the tibia and fibula approximately 5 cm from the distal end of the tibia. Then make a coronal saw cut through the distal parts of both bones approximately at the middle of the tibia. The ligament and any extension of the cavity of the ankle joint between the tibia and fibula are now exposed [Fig. 207].

Joints of the foot

These numerous joints occur between the tarsal, metatarsal, and phalangeal bones. Thus there are: (1) intertarsal joints; (2) tarsometatarsal joints; (3) intermetatarsal joints; (4) metatarsophalangeal joints; (5) interphalangeal joints.

Arches of the foot

The general shape of the articulated tarsal and metatarsal bones of the foot is that of a half dome, concave inferiorly. When the feet are together, the two half domes form a single dome. The rim of each half dome consists of the heel, the lateral border of the foot, and the heads of the metatarsal bones. It is the skin covering these parts of the foot which comes into contact with the ground and forms the *footprint* of a bare foot. It is conventional to describe

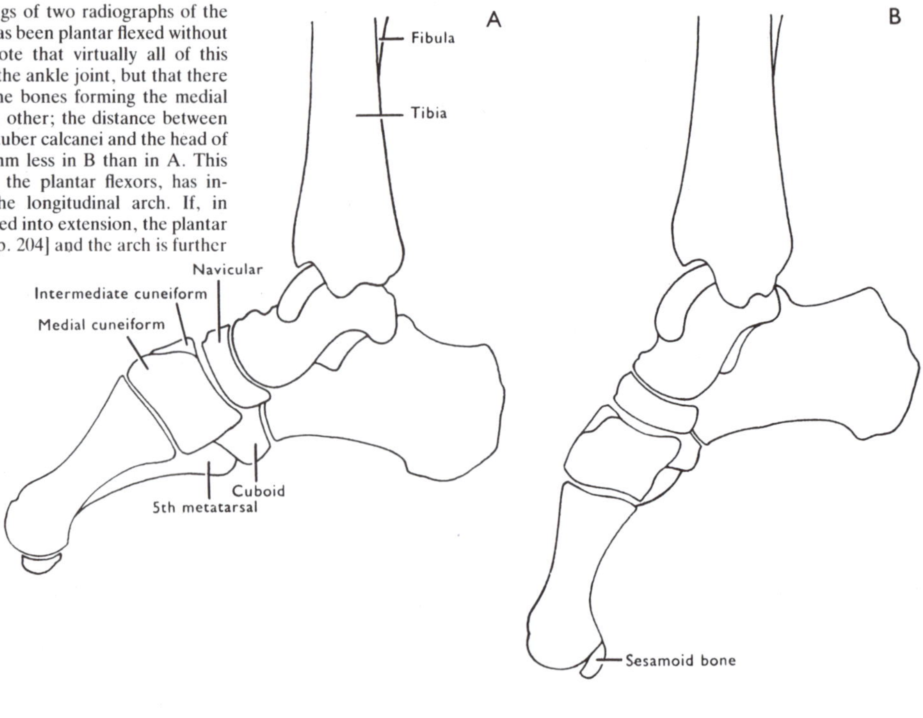

Fig. 213. Outline drawings of two radiographs of the same foot. In B the foot has been plantar flexed without any other movement. Note that virtually all of this movement takes place at the ankle joint, but that there is also slight flexion of the bones forming the medial longitudinal arch on each other; the distance between the medial process of the tuber calcanei and the head of the first metatarsal is 7 mm less in B than in A. This movement, produced by the plantar flexors, has increased the height of the longitudinal arch. If, in addition, the toes are forced into extension, the plantar aponeurosis is tightened [p. 204] and the arch is further heightened.

each foot as having longitudinal and transverse arches, even though the transverse arch is a half arch except at the heads of the metatarsals which form a complete but flat transverse arch.

Longitudinal arch

This bony arch has a greater height and a wider span on the medial than on the lateral side of the foot. On the lateral side it is nearly flat. The talus ('keystone' [Fig. 214]) lies at the summit of the arch. The posterior pillar is the short, thick calcaneus. The longer anterior pillar consists of the remaining tarsal bones and the metatarsals. It is divisible into a medial column (the navicular, cuneiform, and medial three metatarsal bones) and a lateral column (the cuboid and lateral two metatarsal bones).

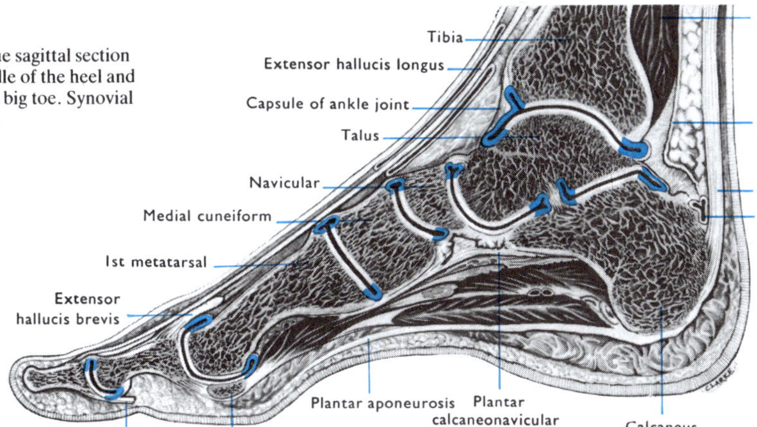

Fig. 214. Oblique sagittal section through the middle of the heel and the middle of the big toe. Synovial membrane, blue.

The talus transmits the weight of the body: (1) posteriorly, to the heel through its subtalar joint with the calcaneus; (2) anteriorly, to the medial column (medial longitudinal arch) through the articulation of the head of the talus with the navicular bone; (3) laterally, the lateral column (lateral longitudinal arch) through both its articulations with the calcaneus.

The **head of the talus** fits into a deep socket between the anterior end of the calcaneus and the navicular, and appears between them on the plantar surface. It is prevented from driving them apart, and so flattening the arch, by the presence of the **plantar calcaneonavicular** ('spring') **ligament** which fills the gap, binds the navicular to the sustentaculum tali (on which the head of the talus also rests), and completes the socket for the head [Figs. 214, 216]. All other ligaments on the plantar surfaces of the bones of the foot (**plantar ligaments**) play a part in maintaining the arches of the foot. They are assisted by the plantar aponeurosis which acts as a 'tie beam' between the ends of the arch. It is capable of being tightened by dorsiflexion of the toes [p. 204]. The fibrous expansions of the insertion of **tibialis posterior** also help to maintain the arches as do the short muscles of the sole and the long muscles through

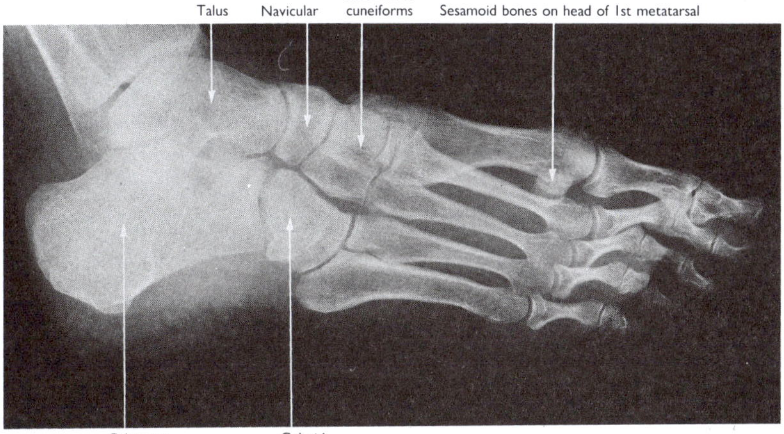

Fig. 215. Oblique radiograph of the left foot. It is only in this view that most of the foot bones are visible separately.

the bracing action of their tendons passing forwards from their pulleys at the ankle. It is not necessary, however, to have contraction of the muscles to maintain the arches when standing, but when the muscles are paralysed or weakened by disuse, the ligaments give way to the stresses applied to them when unprotected by muscular contraction during movement.

Transverse arch of the foot

This arch is seen best in the region of the tarsometatarsal joints. Here the cuneiform bones and the metatarsal bases are wedge-shaped. Their narrow plantar surfaces are held tightly together by plantar and interosseous ligaments and by the tendon of peroneus longus. This arrangement gives the plantar surfaces of these bones a much smaller radius of curvature than their dorsal surfaces, thus forming a well-defined transverse arch.

Dissection

Remove all the muscles and tendons from the tarsal and metatarsal bones. Define the ligaments between the various bones. Note that those on the plantar surfaces are much thicker than those on the dorsal surfaces.

Subtalar joint

This is a cylindrical joint between the concave lower surface of the body of the talus and the convex upper surface of the middle of the calcaneus. These curvatures run transversely and permit the calcaneus to turn around its long axis on the inferior surface of the talus in the movements of inversion and eversion. The fibrous capsule is attached near the margins of the articular surfaces [Fig. 216]. The medial and calcaneofibular ligaments of the ankle joint assist in holding the bones together. The ligament of the neck of the talus (ligamentum cervicis) which passes from it to the calcaneus [Fig. 216] also keeps the bones in contact.

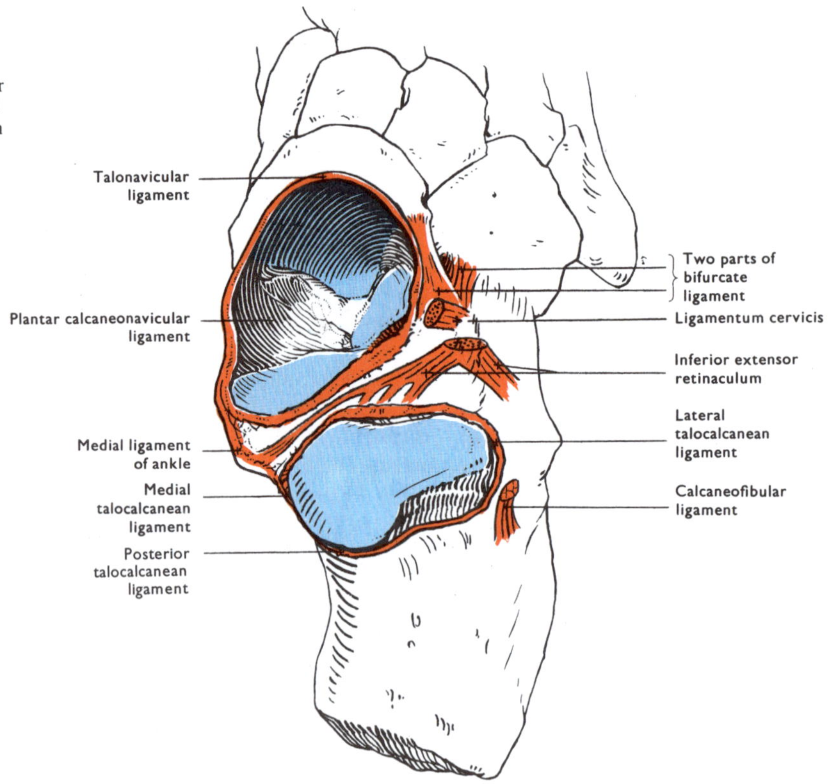

Fig. 216. Ligaments and inferior articular surfaces of subtalar and talocalcaneonavicular joints seen from above after removal of the talus.

Talocalcaneo-navicular joint

This is a complex 'ball-and-socket' type of joint. The ball is the head and adjacent part of the body of the talus. The socket is formed by the proximal surface of the navicular bone, the plantar calcaneonavicular ligament, and the anteromedial part of the calcaneus, including the sustentaculum tali. This joint moves with the subtalar joint in inversion and eversion, so the axis around which these movements take place must also pass through the head of the talus, i.e. upwards, forwards, and medially through the calcaneus and the head of the talus. The talus, locked between the malleoli, remains stationary while the other tarsal bones move on it around this axis. A single fibrous capsule encloses all elements of the talocalcaneonavicular joint [Figs. 166, 216]. It is continuous with the plantar calcaneonavicular ligament, and is strengthened by: (1) medially, the medial ligament of the ankle joint; (2) laterally, the calcaneonavicular ligament [Fig. 209] and ligamentum cervicis; (3) superiorly, the talonavicular ligament; (4) posteriorly, it forms the **interosseous talocalcanean ligament** with the anterior part of the fibrous capsule of the subtalar joint [Fig. 216]. Both these lie in the **sinus tarsi** (the tunnel separating the talus and calcaneus between these two joints) with the stem of the inferior extensor retinaculum arising from the calcaneus between them.

Dissection

Cut across the ligaments which hold the talus to the calcaneus on the lateral, posterior, and anterior surfaces of the two joints. Turn the other tarsal bones away from the talus and examine the articular surfaces of the bones. Alternatively, it is possible to study the surfaces on the articulated bones of a foot, but the involvement of the plantar calcaneonavicular ligament in the joint is not so obvious.

Examine the articular surfaces of the talocalcaneonavicular joint. The head and anterior part of the body of the talus has a minimum of three articular surfaces for this joint. (1) Anteriorly, for the navicular. (2) Postero-inferiorly, for the anterior part of the upper surface of the calcaneus and sustentaculum tali (these two may be separate). (3) Inferomedially, for the plantar calcaneonavicular ligament.

Calcaneonavicular ligaments

The **plantar calcaneonavicular** ('spring') **ligament**, is a thick, triangular sheet which stretches from the sustentaculum tali to the plantar surface of the navicular bone. It fills the angular interval between these bones, and its tough, fibrocartilaginous, upper surface articulates with the head of the talus [Fig. 216]. Medially it is continuous with the fibrous capsule of the talocalcaneonavicular joint and the **medial ligament of the ankle joint**. The tendon of tibialis posterior lies inferior to the ligament and supports it. This plantar calcaneonavicular ligament plays an important part in maintaining the medial longitudinal arch of the foot and in preventing the development of flat-foot.

The anterior part of the superior surface of the calcaneus, lateral to its articulation with the talus, is bound by the **bifurcate ligament** to the lateral surface of the navicular (**calcaneonavicular ligament**) and to the dorsomedial surface of the cuboid (**calcaneocuboid ligament**) [Figs. 209, 216].

Calcaneocuboid joint

This is an oblique, saddle-shaped joint which permits a little rotatory sliding of the cuboid on the distal surface of the calcaneus in a dorsomedial direction. This joint lies almost in the same transverse plane as the **talonavicular joint**. The two constitute the **transverse tarsal joint** though they have separate synovial cavities. The movement of the transverse tarsal joint adds a little to the movements of inversion and eversion (see below).

The calcaneocuboid joint is strengthened by the dorsal calcaneocuboid ligament (see above) but mainly by the **long plantar** and **plantar calcaneocuboid ligaments** on its plantar surface. These ligaments arise from the greater part of the plantar surface of the calcaneus [Fig. 256]. The plantar calcaneocuboid ligament, merely spanning the calcaneocuboid joint, is attached close to it, while the long plantar ligament, passing inferior to the other, arises more proximally and passes distally to both lips of the groove for peroneus longus tendon on the cuboid and to the bases of the middle three or lateral four metatarsals. Both these ligaments are important in maintaining the lateral longitudinal arch of the foot.

Dissection

Define the margins of the long plantar ligament [Fig. 217]. Lift it from the anterior part of the calcaneus by passing a knife between it and

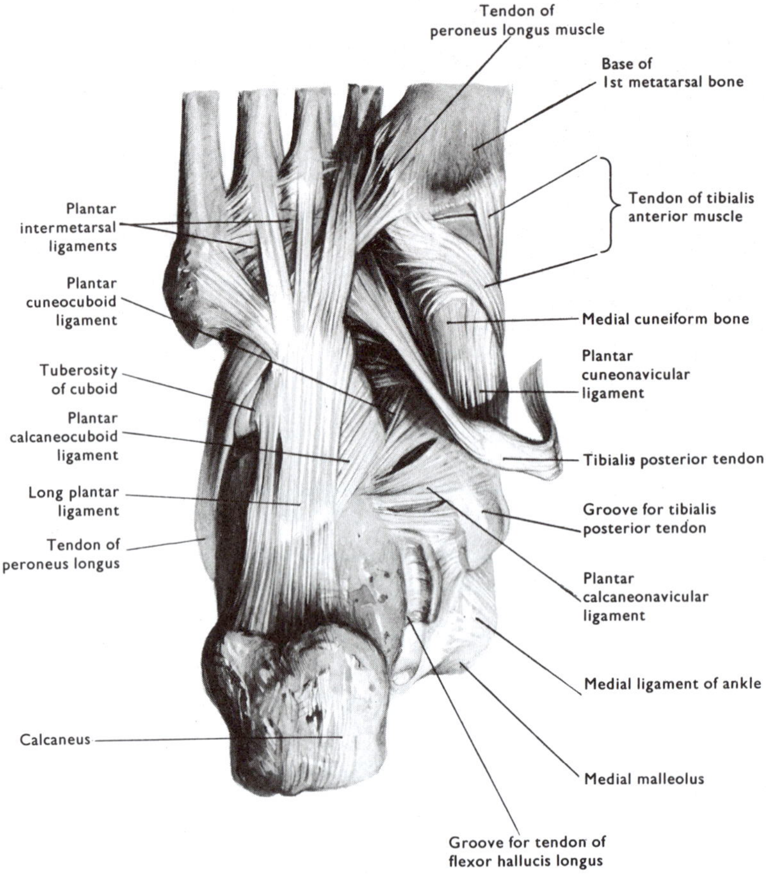

Fig. 217. Plantar aspect of tarsal and tarsometatarsal joints.

the plantar calcaneocuboid ligament which projects beyond its medial edge. Detach the long plantar ligament from the calcaneus to expose the plantar calcaneocuboid ligament.

Cut through the dorsal ligaments of the cuneonavicular, intercuneiform, and cuneocuboid joints. Draw the bones apart to see the articular surfaces and any interosseous ligaments.

Smaller joints of the tarsus

The three cuneiform bones articulate with each other and with the distal surface of the navicular bone by a single joint, and the lateral cuneiform and usually the navicular articulate with the cuboid. The articular surfaces of all these joints are flat, and all have dorsal and plantar ligaments. The intercuneiform, cuneocuboid, and cuboideonavicular joints also have interosseous ligaments. These joints give a certain resilience to the tarsus, but the amount of movement at each is small.

Movements of the intertarsal joints

The joints as a whole increase the resilience of the foot, but the main movements of inversion and eversion occur at the **subtalar** and **talocalcaneonavicular joints** when the rest of the tarsal bones move on the talus. **Inversion** is the movement which raises the medial border of the foot and turns the sole to face medially. **Eversion** is the opposite movement which raises the lateral border of the foot and turns the sole to face inferolaterally. Eversion is more restricted than inversion and both only take place to a small degree at the transverse tarsal joint as can be shown by the virtual disappearance of the movements when the heel is fixed. Inversion and eversion are important movements concerned with adjusting the foot to uneven ground. The student should study the part played by the various leg muscles in the production of these movements [Table 11, p. 237]. The principal evertors are the three peronei; the chief invertors are tibialis anterior and posterior.

Maintenance of the longitudinal arches of the foot. The main ligaments are the plantar calcaneonavicular, the long plantar, the plantar calcaneocuboid, and the plantar aponeurosis. Tibialis anterior raises the medial longitudinal arch. Tibialis posterior has a similar action. It draws the navicular against the head of the talus and tightens the plantar surface of the foot through its widespread insertion into the tarsal and metatarsal bones. The short flexors draw the ends of the longitudinal arches together, and the long flexors of the toes have a similar action as they run horizontally forwards from their pulleys at the ankle.

When the heel is held and the heads of the metatarsals are twisted into the position of eversion, the medial longitudinal arch is exaggerated. The reverse movement produces a marked diminution of the arch so that the foot appears flat. The essential deformity in *'flat-foot'* is an eversion of the heel relative to the anterior part of the foot. This happens when the plantar calcaneonavicular ligament stretches and the sustentaculum tali moves backwards and laterally relative to the navicular bone so that the tuber calcanei swings laterally into an everted position while the remainder of the foot remains stationary. In the reverse deformity of *'club-foot'*, the heel is strongly inverted relative to the forepart of the foot with the consequence that the arch is greatly exaggerated and the plantar calcaneonavicular ligament is short.

Tarsometatarsal joints

Each of the medial three metatarsals articulates with the corresponding cuneiform bone; the lateral two articulate with the cuboid bone [Figs. 254, 255]. There are three separate joint cavities—one for the first metarsal base and one for each of the other two pairs. All these joints have strong plantar and dorsal ligaments.

The joint surfaces of the bases of the middle three metatarsals are flat, but are not in line with each other because the articulation of the third metatarsal is distal to those of the other two. The wedge-shaped bases of all three are firmly fitted together and are set round the lateral cuneiform so that they form a sort of mortise joint with the tarsus. Thus they have only minimal mobility on the tarsus and on each other. The **second metatarsal** is the least mobile. Its base articulates with the short intermediate cuneiform and so is wedged in a socket between the distal parts of the medial and lateral cuneiform bones [Fig. 254]. It articulates with the adjacent parts of the sides of these bones, and is always bound to the medial by a strong **interosseous ligament** and sometimes to the lateral by a weaker ligament. Thus the base of the second metatarsal is so firmly fixed that its thin body is particularly liable to fracture when sudden stresses are applied to the distal part of the foot. The base of the fourth metatarsal (and sometimes the third) is bound to the lateral cuneiform by an interosseous ligament. Thus the middle three metatarsals form a relatively rigid beam in the centre of the distal part of the foot.

The articular surfaces of the bases of the first and fifth metatarsals are slightly curved. Hence they have a greater degree of mobility than the other three, though even this is small because of the strong fibrous capsules.

Intermetatarsal joints

The bases of the lateral four metatarsal bones articulate with one another. They are firmly bound together by plantar, dorsal, and interosseous ligaments.

Dissection

Cut through the dorsal ligaments of the tarsometatarsal and intermetatarsal joints. Force the bones apart to expose the interosseous ligaments and articular surfaces.

Joint cavities of the foot

Six separate joint cavities are present in the foot.

1. The subtalar joint.
2. The talocalcaneonavicular joint.
3. The calcaneocuboid joint.
4. The cuneonavicular joint. This is continuous forwards with the cavities of the intercuneiform and cuneocuboid joints. These are continuous, in their turn, with the cavities of the cuneometatarsal joints at the bases of the second and third metatarsals, and through them with the cavities (intermetatarsal) between the bases of the second, third, and fourth metatarsal bones.

5. The medial cuneometatarsal joint.

6. The cuboideometatarsal joint. This extends into the intermetatarsal joint between the fourth and fifth metatarsal bases.

Dissection

Remove the short muscles of the big toe by detaching them from the sesamoid bones. Note the communication to the tendon of abductor hallucis from the extensor expansion and the attachment of the abductor to the medial sesamoid bone. Identify and cut through the deep transverse metatarsal ligaments on each side of the second toe (if that has not been done already). Trace the tendons of the interosseous muscles of the first two spaces to their insertions and review the course of the lumbrical tendons. Lift the extensor expansions from the dorsal surfaces of the metatarsophalangeal joints of the big and second toes. It forms the fibrous capsule on this aspect of all these joints and is continuous on either side with the thickened lateral part of the capsule—the collateral ligaments. Define these collateral ligaments and then identify the plantar ligament between the long flexor tendon and the joint. Dissect one or more interphalangeal joints in a similar manner. The arrangement of the fibrous capsules is the same as in the metatarsophalangeal joints. However, the collateral ligaments are not loose enough in extension to permit any abduction or adduction at these joints even if the joint surfaces would allow it.

Cut through the medial part of the fibrous capsule on one or more metatarsophalangeal and interphalangeal joints. Separate the bones and examine their articular surfaces.

Metatarsophalangeal joints

In these joints the bases of the phalanges articulate towards the dorsal surfaces of the heads of the metatarsals and move on to these surfaces in extension. In flexion, they move towards the plantar surface of the head, but the range of this movement is much less than in the metacarpophalangeal joints so that the heads of the metatarsals are never uncovered as knuckles, though this can be achieved to some extent by passive flexion of the little toe.

The **fibrous capsule** is attached close to the articular surfaces. It is thickened at the sides to form collateral ligaments and on the plantar surface to form the plantar ligament. The dorsal part is formed by the extensor expansion. A synovial sac extends proximally deep to the extensor expansion and the plantar ligament and is their only attachment to the metatarsal.

Each **collateral ligament** radiates from the pit and tubercle on the side of the head of the metatarsal bone to the side of the plantar ligament and the adjacent part of the side of the base of the proximal phalanx.

The thick fibrous **plantar ligament** is attached firmly to the plantar margin of the base of the proximal phalanx and loosely to the plantar surface of the neck of the metatarsal bone. The plantar ligament separates the long flexor tendon from the joint and the plantar surface of the head of the metatarsal bone. The margins of the plantar ligaments are attached to: (1) the fibrous flexor sheath; (2) slips of the plantar aponeurosis; (3) the deep transverse metatarsal ligament; (4) the collateral ligaments; (5) the margins of the extensor expansions. The plantar ligament of the metatarsophalangeal joint of the big toe contains the sesamoid bones which articulate superiorly with the grooves on the plantar surface of the head of the first metatarsal bone. Some of the other plantar ligaments may occasionally contain minute sesamoid bones.

Articular surfaces

The distal surface of the head of each metatarsal has two continuous articular surfaces with different curvatures. (1) On the dorsal half is a circular, convex surface which fits into the concavity of the base of the proximal phalanx to make a shallow ball-and-socket joint. The more lateral the metatarsal, the more this surface is elongated towards the plantar surface to permit a greater range of flexion. The dorsal position of this articulation is the result of the normal position of extension of the phalanx relative to the metatarsal [Fig. 214]. (2) On the plantar half is a parallel-sided, convex area for articulation with the plantar ligament. In the first metatarsal, this surface is deeply grooved on each side by a sesamoid bone.

Movements

The metatarsophalangeal joints permit flexion, extension, abduction, and adduction. Rotation is prevented by the collateral ligaments. *Flexion* and *extension* are produced by the long and short flexor and extensor muscles. The flexors are assisted by the interossei and the lumbricals. When the joints are flexed, the **plantar ligament** slides proximally towards the neck of the metatarsal—when they are extended, the ligament moves on to the distal surface of the head of the metatarsal. This tightens the plantar aponeurosis and the slips of the extensor expansion which are attached to the plantar ligament and so prevents the distal part of the expansion from acting on the interphalangeal joints in this position of the metatarsophalangeal joints [p. 209]. The lumbricals then become the sole extensors of the interphalangeal joints if they reach the extensor expansion.

Abduction and *adduction* take place from the line of the second toe. These movements are produced by the interossei, by the abductor of the little toe, and by the abductor and adductor of the big toe.

Interphalangeal joints

The joints are similar to those in the hand but have a smaller range of movement or may even be fused (little toe). However, the articular surfaces are sinusoidal. The base of the distal bone has a median sagittal ridge with a parallel groove on each side of it. These fit reciprocally curved surfaces on the distal aspect of the proximal bone. This keys the bones together in such a manner that only flexion and extension are permitted. The single interphalangeal joint of the big toe is much larger than any of the others. It also has a flatter curvature and a smaller range of movement. This is in keeping with the relative rigidity of this joint—a necessary feature in view of the forces which are applied to it.

Movements

At rest, most of the interphalangeal joints are in a position of partial flexion by comparison with the extended position of the metatarsophalangeal joints. They are hinge joints at which only flexion and extension take place. In the big toe, these movements are produced by the long flexor and the long and short extensor muscles; in the other toes, there is the additional action of the short flexor on the proximal interphalangeal joint. The lumbricals extend the interphalangeal joints of the lateral four toes, and become essential for this action when the metatarsophalangeal joints are fully extended. Thus, when the lumbricals are weakened or paralysed, the metatarsophalangeal joints move into a position of full extension while the proximal interphalangeal joints are flexed by the long and short flexor muscles, the distal joint remaining extended because of pressure on the ground. This position of the toes is known as '*hammer toe*'.

Hallux valgus

Several references have already been made to this troublesome deformity which is common in women. It consists of a fixed adduction of the big toe at the metatarsophalangeal joint. This may be so extreme that the toe lies transversely across the other toes. As this occurs, the head of the first metatarsal becomes prominent and tends to rub on the shoe. An adventitous bursa then forms between it and the skin. This tends to become inflamed, swollen, and tender, constituting a 'bunion'. The adduction of the big toe arises because of the obliquity of many of the tendons inserted into it (especially extensor hallucis brevis and longus) and because the attachment of abductor hallucis is more to the plantar than the medial surface of the proximal phalanx—a position which makes it a less efficient abductor. Once the adduction starts, the slip of the extensor expansion to the tendon of the abductor hallucis and the medial part of the fibrous capsule of the joint are further stretched by the increasing obliquity of pull of the extensors and flexors of the big toe. Also the tendon of the abductor and the sesamoid bones slide laterally on the plantar surface of the joint. Thus the condition worsens if the toe is not straightened. As in hammer toe, the presence of the big toe on the plantar surfaces of the other toes forces them dorsally against the shoe. Here they rub with the production of painful corns.

Tables 9–12
The muscles, movements, and nerves of the lower limb

These Tables list the muscles in groups according to the joint or joint complex across which they act. The origin, insertion, and action of each muscle is given first, and then the muscles are grouped according to the actions which they produce on the particular joint or joint complex, and the nerve supply of each muscle is given. This allows an easy assessment of the degree of paralysis of a particular movement following destruction of a particular nerve. In Table 12, the total motor distribution of each nerve in the lower limb is shown, together with the paralysis which results from destruction of that nerve at each level in the limb. The total cutaneous nerve supply of each of these nerves is shown in the corresponding figures.

The limitations of these Tables arise from the fact that they show only the actions which a particular muscle produces when it actively shortens. It should be remembered that muscles are also brought into action (1) to fix one part of the trunk or limb so that another part may have a stable base on which to act, e.g. the contraction of the abductors of the left hip joint to stabilize the pelvis when the right lower limb is raised from the ground; or (2) to control the rate or strength of a movement which is in the direction opposite to that which the muscle would produce if it were shortening, e.g. the contraction of the hamstrings when the hip joint is being flexed in the action of sitting down.

The muscles of the lower limb

In movements of the lower limb it should be remembered that when the foot is on the ground the muscles of that limb are being used in a reversed manner—that is, the trunk and proximal parts of the limb are moving while the distal part is stationary. In the limb which is free to move, the muscles are used in the conventional manner, the origins remaining relatively stationary while the insertions move. Thus in walking, when the right limb is raised from the ground the abductors of the left hip joint act on the pelvis with the hip joint as a fulcrum and support the body weight on the left lower limb by preventing the pelvis from sagging to the right. At the same time, the abductors of the right hip, acting from the pelvis, prevent the right limb from falling against the left. Similarly, the muscles which move the ankle joint act on the tibia and fibula when the foot is on the ground. Items which appear in The Table in brackets are equivocal or depend on the position of the limb.

Table **9**

Muscles acting on hip joint only [Figs. 125, 141, 242, 243, 247, 249]

Muscle	Origin	Insertion	Action
Adductor			
longus	Body of pubis	Femur, linea aspera	Adduction
brevis	Pubis, body and inferior ramus	Femur, linea aspera	Adduction
magnus	Pubis, inferior ramus Ischium, ramus and tuber	Femur, linea aspera, med. supracondylar line, adductor tubercle	Adduction, extension, (med. rotation)
Psoas major	Lumbar vertebrae	Lesser trochanter	Flexion (medial rotation)
Iliacus	Iliac fossa	Line inferior to lesser trochanter	Flexion

Muscle	Origin	Insertion	Action
Pectineus	Pubis, body and superior ramus	Back of lesser trochanter to linea aspera	Adduction, flexion
Gluteus			
minimus	Ilium, between ant. and inf. gluteal lines	Gtr. trochanter, ant. surface	Abduction, med. rotation, fixes pelvis on thigh*
medius	Ilium, between ant. and post. gluteal lines	Gtr. trochanter, lat. surface	Abduction, med. rotation, fixes pelvis on thigh*
maximus, deep ¼	Sacrum, post. surface, sacrotuberous lig.	Femur, gluteal tuberosity	Extension, lat. rotation
Piriformis	Sacrum, pelvic surface, middle 3 parts	Gtr. trochanter	Abduction, lat. rotation
Obturator			
externus	Obturator membrane, ext. surface, margin of obt. foramen	Trochanteric fossa	Lat. rotation (flexion)
internus	Internal surfaces of ilium, pubis, and ischium in lesser pelvis, and obturator membrane	Gtr. trochanter, med. surface	Lat. rotation
Gemelli	Ischium, each side of lesser sciatic notch	With obt. internus	As obturator int.

*This action prevents the pelvis sagging towards the opposite side when the lower limb on that side is raised from the ground.

Muscles acting on hip and knee [Figs. 141, 241, 243, 251, 253]

Muscle	Origin	Insertion	Action
Hamstrings			
Biceps femoris long head	Ischial tuberosity	Head of fibula	Hip, extension Knee, flexion, lat. rotation of leg*
Semimembranosus	Ischial tuberosity	Tibia, med. condyle, post-med. surface	Hip, extension Knee, flexion, med rotation of leg* (Semimembranosus and Semitendinosus)
Semitendinosus	Ischial tuberosity	Tibia, med. surface, upper ¼	
Gracilis	Pubis, body and inf. ramus	Tibia, med. surface, upper ¼	Hip, adduction Knee, flexion, med. rotation of leg*
Sartorius	Ilium, ant. superior spine	Tibia, med. surface, upper ¼	Hip, flexion, lat. rotation Knee flexion, med. rotation of leg*
Tensor fasciae latae	Ilium, crest, ant. ¼	Tibia, lat. condyle, ant. surface via iliotibial tract (Tensor fasciae latae and Gluteus max. superficial ¾)	Hip, flexion, abduction. Stabilizes pelvis on thigh Knee extension
Gluteus max. superficial ¾	Ilium, post. to post. gluteal line. Sacrum, post. aspect Sacrotuberous ligament		Hip, extension, lat. rotation. Stabilizes pelvis on thigh Knee, extension
Rectus femoris	Ilium, ant. inf. spine and area above acetabulum	Patella, thru' quadriceps tendon	Hip, flexion Knee, extension

*When the knee is flexed.

Movements at the hip joint

Movement	Muscles	Nerve supply
Flexion	Iliacus and Psoas major	Lumbar ventral rami
	Rectus femoris	Femoral
	Sartorius	Femoral
	Tensor fasciae latae	Superior gluteal
	(Pectineus	Femoral)
	(Adductors longus and brevis	Obturator)
Extension	Gluteus maximus	Inferior gluteal
	Semimembranosus	Sciatic (tibial part)
	Semitendinosus	Sciatic (tibial part)
	Biceps femoris, long head	Sciatic (tibial part)
	Adductor magnus, ischial part	Sciatic (tibial part)
Adduction	Adductors longus, brevis, and magnus	Obturator
	Gracilis	Obturator
	Pectineus	Femoral
	Quadratus femoris	L. 4, 5 & S. 1 ventral rami

Movement	Muscles	Nerve supply
Abduction	Gluteus medius and minimus	Superior gluteal
	Tensor fasciae latae	Superior gluteal
	Piriformis	L. 5, S. 1 & 2 ventral rami
	(Obturator internus in flexion	L. 5, S. 1 & 2 ventral rami)
Medial rotation	Tensor fasciae latae	Superior gluteal
	Gluteus minimus	Superior gluteal
	Gluteus medius, ant. fibres	Superior gluteal
	(Adductors	Obturator)
	(Iliopsoas	L. 1 & 2 ventral rami)
Lateral rotation	Sartorius	Femoral
	Gluteus maximus	Inferior gluteal
	Obturator internus and gemelli	L. 5, S. 1 & 2 ventral rami
	Obturator externus	Obturator
	Quadratus femoris	L. 4 & 5, S. 1 ventral rami
	Piriformis, in flexion	L. 5, S. 1 & 2 ventral rami

From this table it is obvious that medial rotation and abduction are seriously disturbed by injuries to the superior gluteal nerve. Adduction loses virtually all its power when the obturator nerve is damaged. Extension is most usually produced by the hamstrings, gluteus maximus being used mainly when extra power is required or in extremes of extension when the hamstrings may be actively insufficient to produce the movement.

Table **10**

Muscles acting on knee only [Figs. 247, 249, 251, 253]

Muscle	Origin	Insertion	Action
Vastus			
medialis	Femur, intertrochanteric, aspera, and med. supracondylar lines, tendon of adductor magnus	Patella, superior and med. surfaces, capsule of knee joint	Extension, medial displacement of patella
intermedius	Femur, ant. and lat. surfaces of body	Patella, superior surface, suprapatellar bursa (articularis genus)	Extension, elevates suprapatellar bursa
lateralis	Femur, gtr. trochanter, linea aspera	Patella, superior and lat. surfaces, capsule of knee joint	Extension
Biceps femoris short head	Linea aspera	Head of fibula	Flexion, lat. rotation of leg*
Popliteus	Femur, lat. condyle popliteal groove	Tibia, post. surface prox. to soleal line	Med. rotation of leg or lat. rotation of thigh. Flexion

*When the knee is flexed.

Muscles acting on knee and ankle [Fig. 249]

Muscle	Origin	Insertion	Action
Gastrocnemius	Femur, lat. surface of lat. condyle, post. surface medial condyle	Calcaneus, via tendo calcaneus	Knee, flexion Ankle, plantar flexion
Plantaris	Femur, lat. condyle post. surface	Tendo calcaneus	Acts with gastrocnemius

Movements at the knee joint

Movement	Muscles	Nerve supply
Flexion	Semimembranosus	Sciatic (tibial)
	Semitendinosus	Sciatic (tibial)
	Biceps femoris	
	long head	Sciatic (tibial)
	short head	Sciatic (common peroneal)
	Gracilis	Obturator
	Sartorius	Femoral
	Popliteus	Tibial
	Gastrocnemius	Tibial

Movement	Muscles	Nerve supply
Extension	Vastus medialis	Femoral
	Vastus lateralis	Femoral
	Vastus intermedius	Femoral
	Rectus femoris	Femoral
	Gluteus maximus	Inferior gluteal
	Tensor fasciae latae	Superior gluteal
Lateral rotation of leg*	Biceps femoris	Sciatic (tibial and common peroneal)
	(Gluteus maximus	Inferior gluteal)
	(Tensor fasciae latae	Superior gluteal)
Med. rotation of leg		
knee extended = lat. rotation of thigh	Popliteus	Tibial
knee flexed	Semimembranosus	Sciatic (tibial)
	Semitendinosus	Sciatic (tibial)
	Gracilis	Obturator
	Sartorius	Femoral

*With flexed knee.
It is obvious from this table that flexion of the knee would be seriously disturbed by sciatic nerve destruction, and knee extension by femoral nerve destruction.

Table 11

Muscles acting on the ankle only [Fig. 253]

Muscle	Origin	Insertion	Action
Soleus	Tibia, soleal line, mid. ⅓ med. border Fibula, post. surface upper ⅓	Tendon calcaneus	Plantar flexion

Muscles acting on ankle and tarsal joints [Figs. 174, 251, 253, 256]

Muscle	Origin	Insertion	Action
Peroneus longus	Fibula, lat. surface upper ⅔	Base first metatarsal and med. cuneiform lat. side	Ankle, plantar flx. Tarsal, eversion Maintains transverse arch of foot
brevis	Fibula, lat. surface lower ⅔	5th metatarsal base	Ankle, plantar flx. Tarsal, eversion
Tibialis anterior	Tibia, lat. surface upper ½, interosseous membrane	1st metatarsal base, med. cuneiform inferomedial surface	Ankle, dorsiflexion Tarsal, inversion
posterior	Interosseous membrane upper ½ and adjacent parts of tibia and fibula	Navicular tuberosity Medial cuneiform. All tarsals except talus, 2–4 metatarsal bases	Ankle, plantar flx. Tarsal, maintenance of arches, inversion
Peroneus tertius	Fibula, ant. surface distal ¼	5th metatarsal base	Ankle, dorsiflex. Tarsal, eversion

Muscles acting at ankle, tarsal, and toe joints [Figs. 251, 253]

Muscle	Origin	Insertion	Action
Extensor hallucis longus	Fibula, ant. surface middle two quarters	Hallux, base of distal phalanx	Ankle, dorsiflex. Tarsal, inversion Hallux, extension
Extensor digitorum longus	Fibula, ant. surface upper ¾	Extensor expansion toes 2–5	Ankle, dorsiflex. Toes, extension 2–5 all joints
Flexor hallucis longus	Fibula, post. surface middle two ¼	Hallux, distal phalanx, base	Ankle, plantarflex Hallux, flexion all joints*
Flexor digitorum longus	Tibia, post. surface middle two ¼	Terminal phalanges toes 2–5	Ankle, plantarflex Toes, 2–5 flexion all joints*

*Both these muscles may assist in maintenance of the longitudinal arches of the foot when they are active. However, they are not essential unless the foot is under stress.

Movements at the ankle joint

Movement	Muscles	Nerve supply
Plantar flexion	Gastrocnemius	Tibial
	Soleus	Tibial
	(Plantaris	Tibial)
	Tibialis posterior	Tibial
	Flexor digitorum longus	Tibial
	Flexor hallucis longus	Tibial
	Peroneus longus	Superficial peroneal
	Peroneus brevis	Superficial peroneal
Dorsiflexion	Tibialis anterior	Deep peroneal
	Extensor hallucis longus	Deep peroneal
	Extensor digitorum longus	Deep peroneal
	Peroneus tertius	Deep peroneal

Movements at tarsal joints, particularly talocalcaneonavicular joint

Inversion	Tibialis anterior	Deep peroneal
	Extensor hallucis longus	Deep peroneal
	Tibialis posterior	Tibial
Eversion	Peroneus longus	Superficial peroneal
	Peroneus brevis	Superficial peroneal
	Extensor digitorum longus (lateral)	Deep peroneal
	Peroneus tertius	Deep peroneal

From the last two tables it is obvious that dorsiflexion is abolished (foot-drop) and inversion seriously impaired if the deep peroneal nerve or the common peroneal nerve from which it arises is destroyed. In addition, when the common peroneal nerve is destroyed the superficial peroneal nerve is also put out of action and eversion is lost.

When the tibial nerve is destroyed superior to the origin of the branches to gastrocnemius, plantar flexion is seriously impaired leaving insufficient strength (peronei only) to rise on the toes or push off in walking.

Muscles acting on tarsal joints and toes [Figs. 191, 256]

Muscle	Origin	Insertion	Action
Extensor digitorum brevis	Calcaneus, superior surface, ant. part	Hallux, prox. phalanx Toes 2–4, ext. expansion	Hallux, MP extension Toes 2–4, extension all joints
Flexor digitorum brevis	Tuber calcanei, medial process	Toes 2–5, middle phalanges	Tarsus, support* Toes 2–5, MP & PIP flexion
Flexor accessorius	Calcaneus, plantar aspect medial and lateral	Tendon of flexor digitorum longus	Straightens pull of flx. digitm. longus
Abductor hallucis	Tuber calcanei medial process and flexor retinaculum	Hallux. prox. phalanx, medial side, med sesamoid	Tarsus, support* Hallux, MP abduction or flexion
Abductor digiti minimi	Tuber calcanei, both processes	Toe, 5, prox. phalanx, lat. side. Base of 5th metatarsal	Toe 5, MP abduction Metatarsal 5 abduction

*Support in this case means that the pull of these muscles may assist in the maintenance of the longitudinal arches of the foot when the muscles are contracting.

Muscles acting on toes only [Figs. 192, 193, 196]

Interossei dorsal	Adjacent sides of two metatarsals	Prox. phalanx, lat. side toes 2–4 and med. side toe 2	Toes 2–4 abduction at MP from line of toe 2
plantar	Metatarsals 3–5, medial side	Toes 3–5, prox. phalanx medial side of base	Toes 3–5, adduct to line of toe 2
Lumbricals	Tendons flexor digitorum longus	Toes 2–5, extensor expansion	Toes 2–5, MP flexion, IP extension
Flexor hallucis brevis	Cuboid, plantar surface, medial side	Hallux, prox. phalanx, med. and lat. sides of base	Hallux, MP flexion
Adductor hallucis	Metatarsals 2–4, bases Plantar ligs., MP 2–4	Hallux, prox. phalanx, lat. side of base	Hallux, MP adduction. Approximates prox. phalanges of toes and accentuates anterior transverse arch
Flexor digiti minimi brevis	Metatarsal 5, base	Toe 5, prox. phalanx, lat. side of base	Toe 5, MP flexion

IP = interphalangeal joints

Movements of toes

Movement	Muscles	Nerve supply
Flexion		
All joints	Flexor hallucis longus	Tibial
	Flexor digitorum longus	Tibial
	Flexor accessorius	Lateral plantar
MP & PIP (2–5)	Flexor digitorum brevis	Medial plantar
MP only	Flexor hallucis brevis	Medial plantar
	Flexor digiti minimi brevis	Lateral plantar
Toes 2–5	Lumbricals	Medial plantar, toe 2 Lateral plantar, toes 3–5
Toes 2–5	Interossei	Lateral plantar
Extension all joints	Extensor digitorum longus*	Deep peroneal
Toes 2–4	Extensor digitorum brevis*	Deep peroneal
Hallux	Extensor hallucis longus	Deep peroneal
MP only	Extensor hallucis brevis	Deep peroneal
IP only toes 2–5	Lumbricals (see below)	Lateral plantar, toes 3–5 Medial plantar, toe 2

*Full extension of MP prevents these muscles from extending IP joints which are then only extended by the lumbricals. If the lumbricals are weak, paralaysed, or fail to reach extensor expansion 'hammer toes' result.

Movement	Muscles	Nerve supply
Abduction at MP from line of toe 2		
Toe 1	Abductor hallucis*	Medial plantar
Toes 2–4	Dorsal interossei	Lateral plantar
Toe 5	Abductor digiti minimi	Lateral plantar
Adduction at MP to line of toe 2		
Toe 1	Adductor hallucis	Lateral plantar
Toes 3–5	Plantar interossei	Lateral plantar
Toe 2	Dorsal interossei when toe 2 already abducted by other dorsal interosseous	Lateral plantar

*This muscle is often inserted with the flexor hallucis brevis through the medial sesamoid to the plantar aspect of the proximal phalanx so that it acts as a flexor rather than an abductor. Thus it may fail to prevent the tendency of the adductor hallucis and the oblique tendons of extensor hallucis brevis and longus to cause the proximal phalanx of the great toe to deviate laterally. This condition, known as hallux valgus, exposes the medial side of the head of the metatarsal of the great toe to rubbing on the shoe. A bursa tends to form between it and the skin and this becoming inflamed and swollen forms a bunion.

Table **12**

Nerves of the lower limb motor distribution

In the following tables are shown the positions in the limb where the various muscles are innervated, the muscles, and the effects of paralysis of these muscles following injury to the nerves or their major branches. Where a nerve innervates muscles in more than one segment of the limb (thigh, leg, foot) the effects of injury to the nerve depend on the level of injury. Thus when the sciatic nerve is destroyed in the popliteal fossa, the hamstring muscles supplied by it in the thigh are not paralysed though those in the leg and foot area. Since, for example, leg and foot muscles may act together on the same joints, the degree of paralysis of some movements is increased the more proximal the destruction of the nerve. The more proximal destruction also adds paralysis or weakness of further movements because other muscles are paralysed. In those cases where a number of muscles assist in an action and some innervated by nerves other than those which are destroyed, the muscles which are still active are shown in brackets after the statement of the effect of the muscle paralysis. In some cases it is difficult to demonstrate any disability as a result of the paralysis of a single muscle within a group producing a particular movement. In this case, no statement of the effects of paralysis is given.

Abbreviations.

The toes are numbered 1–5 from the medial side. 1 is the big toe, 5 the little toe. MP = metatarsophalangeal joint. IP = interphalangeal joints. PIP = proximal interphalangeal joint(s). DIP = distal interphalangeal joint(s).

Femoral nerve [For cutaneous supply, see Fig. 218]

Situation of muscle innervation	Muscles	Effects of paralysis by nerve destruction
Abdomen	Psoas (part) and Iliacus (part)	Weakened hip flexion (sartorius, rectus femoris, tensor fasciae latae)
Thigh	Pectineus Sartorius Rectus femoris	Weakened hip flexion (iliopsoas)
	Vastus medialis Vastus intermedius Vastus lateralis	Virtual loss of knee extension (Gluteus maximus and tensor fasciae latae through iliotibial tract)

Obturator nerve [For cutaneous supply, see Fig. 218]

Situation of muscle innervation	Muscles	Effects of paralysis by nerve destruction
Thigh	Obturator externus Adductor longus Adductor brevis Adductor magnus (adductor part) Gracilis	Loss of adduction at hip joint Consequent instability in standing and walking (pectineus, quadratus femoris)

Superior gluteal nerve

Situation of muscle innervation	Muscles	Effects of paralysis by nerve destruction
Gluteal region	Gluteus medius Gluteus minimus Tensor fasciae latae	Loss of abduction at hip joint. In walking, the body is flexed to the paralysed side so as to bring the centre of gravity over the supporting limb while the opposite limb is raised from the ground

Inferior gluteal nerve

Situation of muscle innervation	Muscles	Effects of paralysis by nerve destruction
Gluteal region	Gluteus maximus	Loss of power in extension of the hip joint (hamstrings). Some antero-posterior instability of pelvis in standing

Sciatic nerve [For cutaneous supply, see Fig. 218]

Situation of muscle innervation	Muscles	Effects of paralysis by nerve destruction
Thigh	Adductor magnus (hamstring part) Semitendinosus Semimembranosus Biceps femoris (long head) (short head)	Weakened hip extension (gluteus maximus) Severe weakness of knee flexion (sartorius and gracilis) Weakened rotation of leg on thigh, esp. lat. rotation (iliotibial tract)

Common peroneal nerve [For cutaneous supply, see Fig. 218]

Deep peroneal nerve

Situation of muscle innervation	Muscles	Effects of paralysis by nerve destruction
Leg	Tibialis anterior Extensor hallucis longus Extensor digitorum longus Peroneus tertius	Weakened inversion Loss of IP extension to toe 1* *Loss of dorsiflexion of ankle joint* (foot-drop) Weak extra toes 2–4 none in 5 Weakened eversion
Foot	Extensor digitorum brevis	Weakened extension of MP toe 1*. If paralysed with extensor digitorum longus and hallucis longus, there is loss of extension of all joints to toe 1* and loss of MP extension of the other toes (lumbricals)

Superficial peroneal nerve

Situation of muscle innervation	Muscles	Effects of paralysis by nerve destruction
Leg	Peroneus longus Peroneus brevis	Weakened eversion (peroneus tertius, extensor digitorum lateral part)

Tibial nerve [For cutaneous supply, see Fig. 218]

Situation of muscle innervation	Muscles	Effects of paralysis by nerve destruction
Popliteal fossa	Popliteus	Slight weakening of knee flexion (hamstrings, sartorius, gracilis)
Leg	Gastrocnemius Soleus Tibialis posterior Flexor hallucis longus Flexor digitorum longus	*Marked weakness of plantar flexion at ankle joint* (peroneus long, and brev.) Weak MP and loss of IP flexion toe 1 Weak MP & IP and loss of DIP flexion toes 2–5*

Situation of muscle innervation	Muscles	Effects of paralysis by nerve destruction
Foot		
Medial plantar nerve	Abductor hallucis	Loss of abduction toe 1* (if present previously)
	Flexor hallucis brevis	With longus, loss of flexion all joints toe 1*. Without longus, slight weakness MP flexion toe 1*
	Flexor digitorum brevis	With longus, loss of flexion all joints toe 2; weak MP flexion toes 3 & 4 (lumbricals, interossei)
Lateral plantar nerve	Medial lumbrical Lumbricals, lateral 3	Loss of IP extension toes 2–5* when MP fully extended—'hammer toes'
	Flexor digiti minimi brevis	With flexor digitm. longus, loss of flexion all joints toe 5*
	Abductor digiti minimi	No abduction of little toe
	Adductor hallucis	Loss of adduction toe 1*
	Plantar interossei	Loss of adduction toes 3–5 *
	Dorsal interossei	Loss of abduction toes 2–4
	Flexor accessorius	

*Toe 1 = big toe; toe 5 = little toe.

Nerves of the lower limb: cutaneous distribution

[Figs. 218, 219]

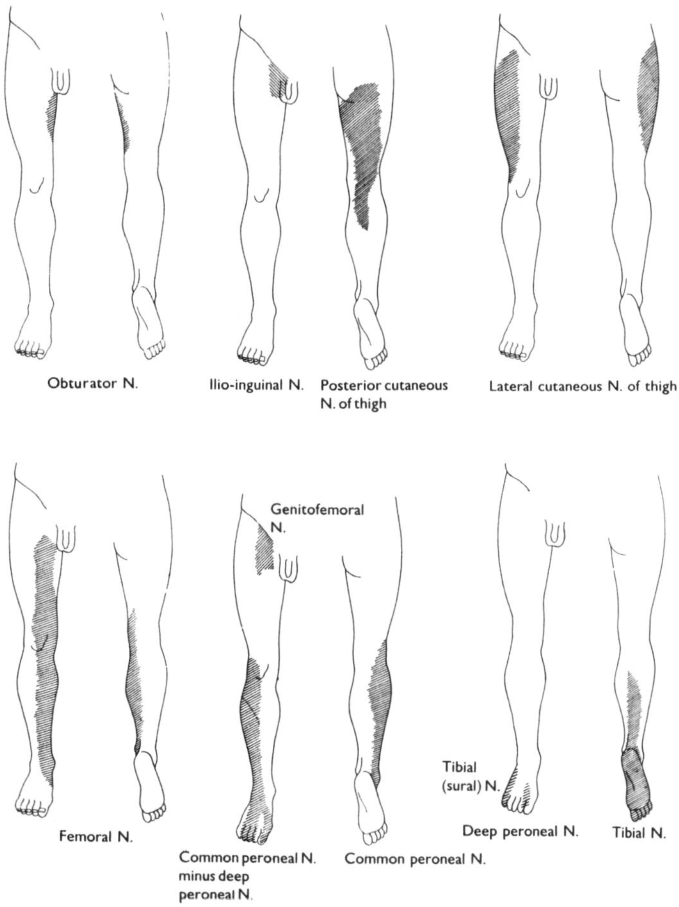

Fig. 218. Diagrams of the approximate cutaneous distribution of various nerves in the lower limb. The areas shown are only approximate because nerves supplying adjacent territories of skin overlap to a considerable degree.

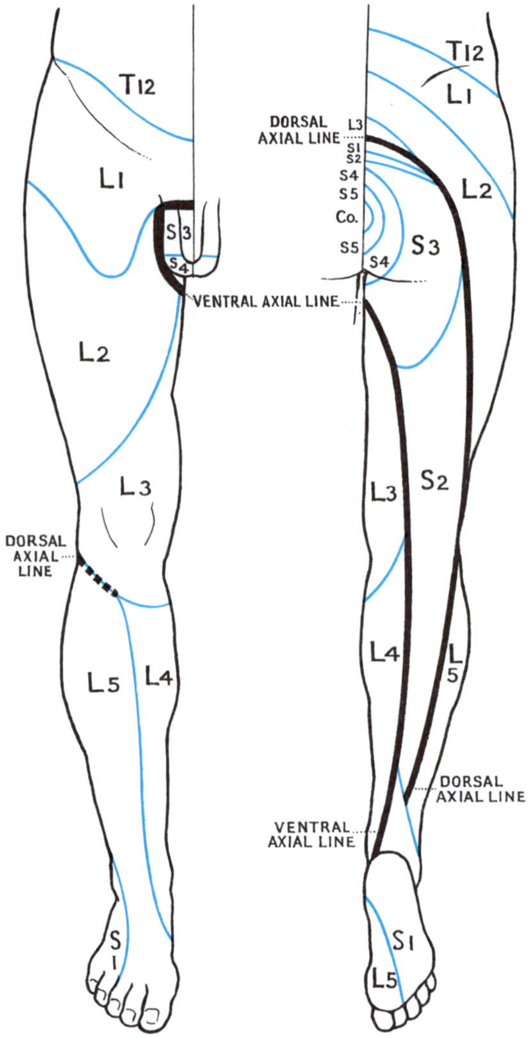

Fig. 219. Dermatomes of lower limb, showing the segmental cutaneous distribution of spinal nerves (T.12, L.1–5, S.1–5, Co.) on A, the front and B, the back of the limb and lower part of trunk. (After Head, 1893, and Foerster, 1933.)

The bones of the upper and lower limbs

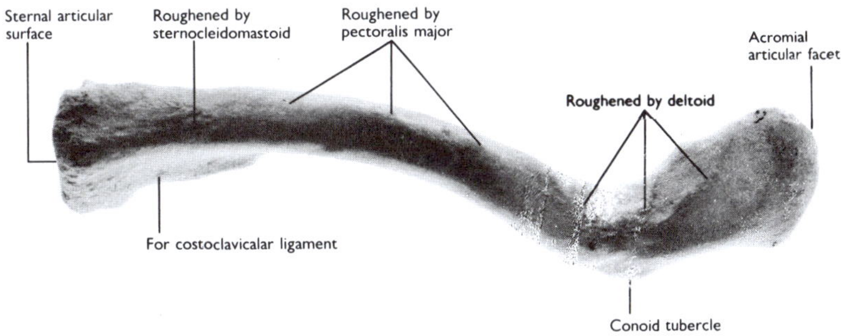

Fig. 220. Right clavicle (superior surface).

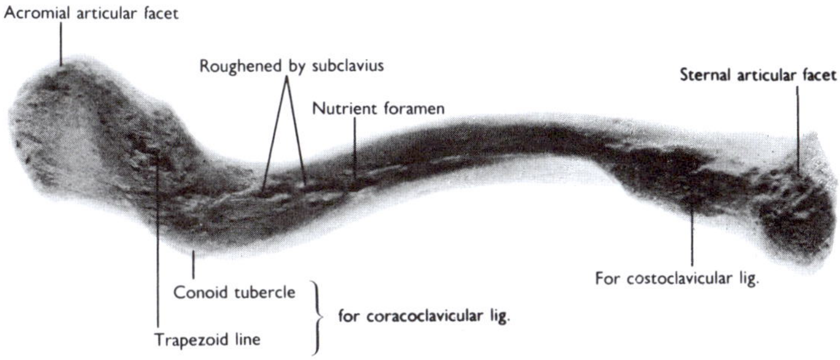

Fig. 221. Right clavicle (inferior surface).

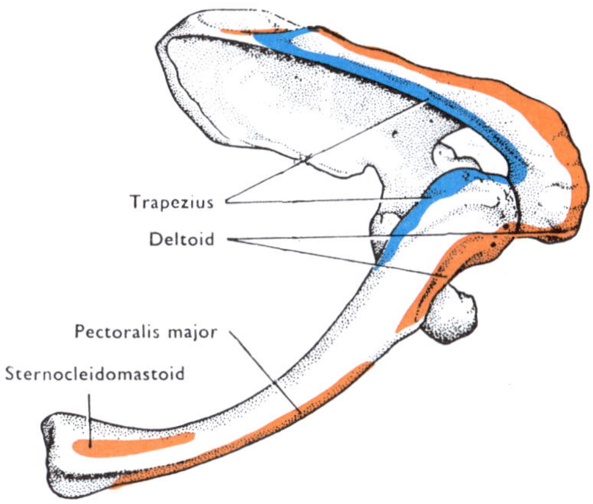

Fig. 222. Shoulder girdle from above showing muscle attachments.

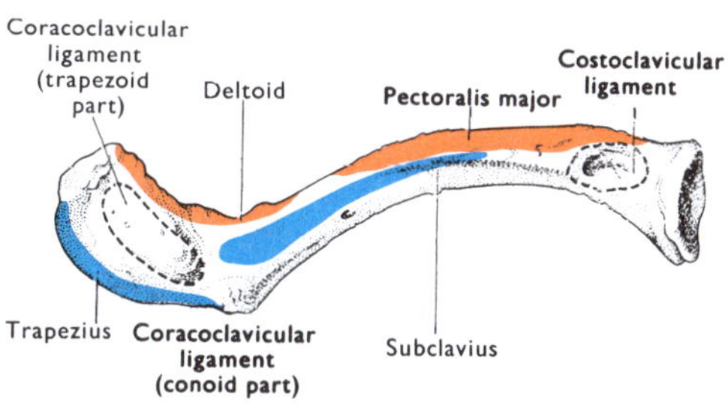

Fig. 223. Muscle attachments of inferior surface of right clavicle.

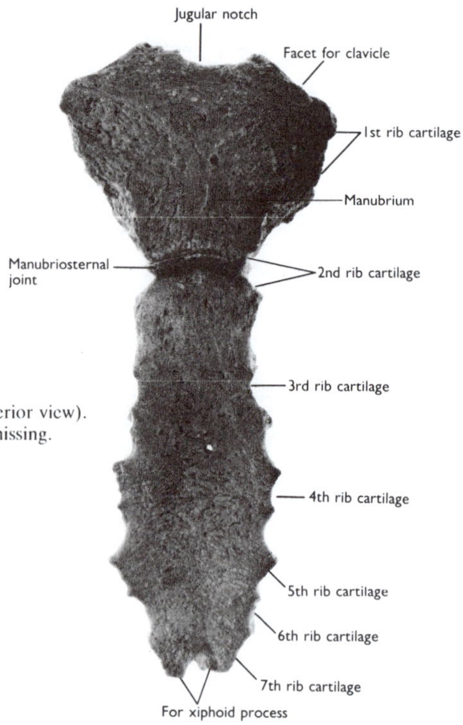

Fig. 224. Sternum (anterior view). The xiphoid process is missing.

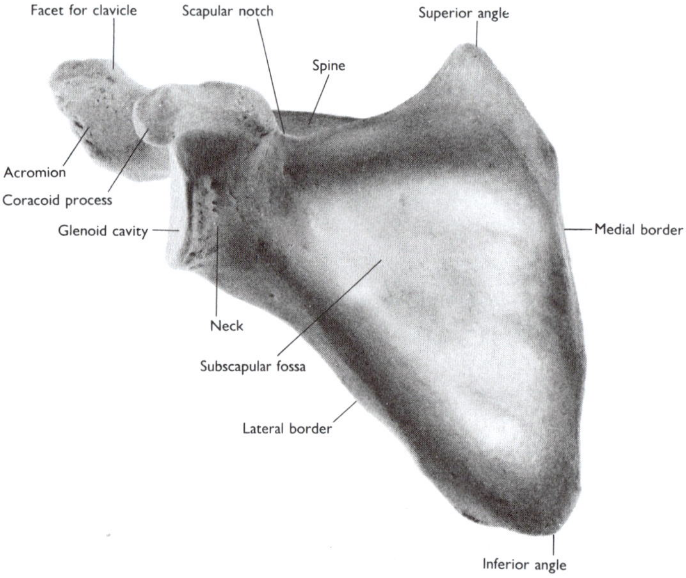

Fig. 225. Right scapula (costal aspect).

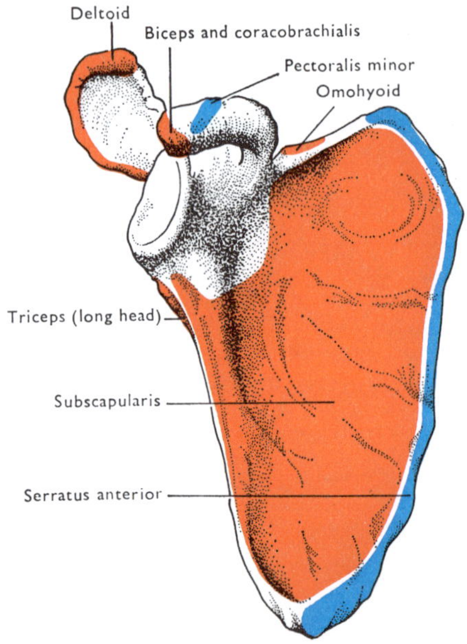

Fig. 226. Muscle attachments to costal surface of right scapula.

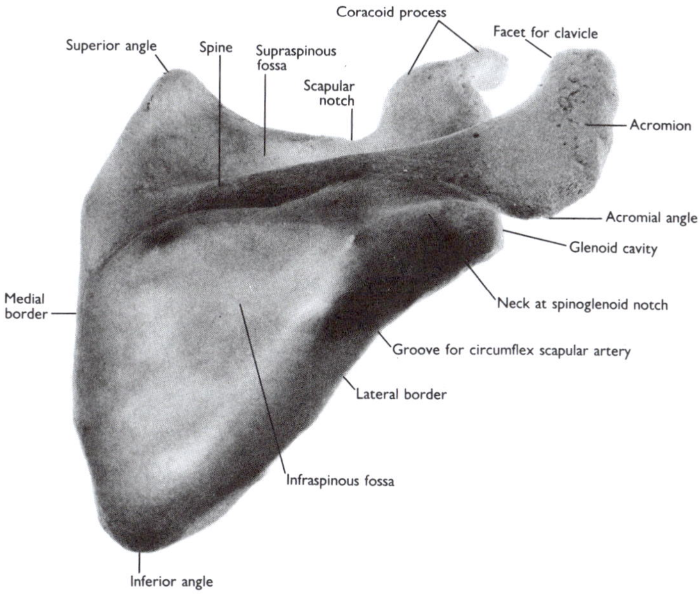

Fig. 227. Dorsal surface of right scapula.

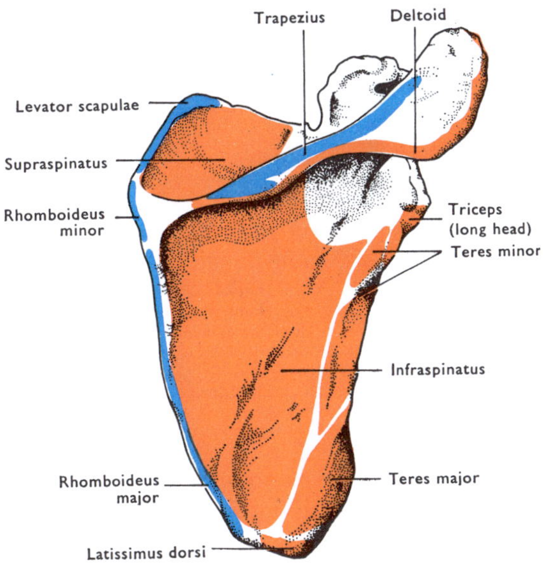

Fig. 228. Muscle attachments to dorsal surface of right scapula.

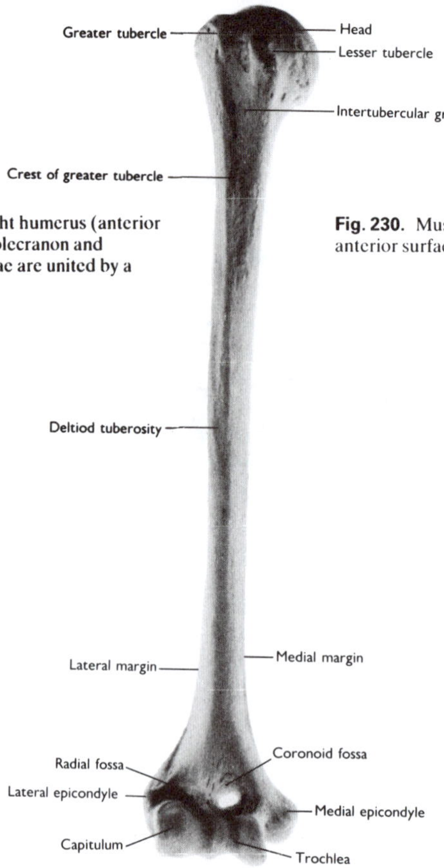

Fig. 229. Right humerus (anterior aspect). The olecranon and coronoid fossae are united by a foramen.

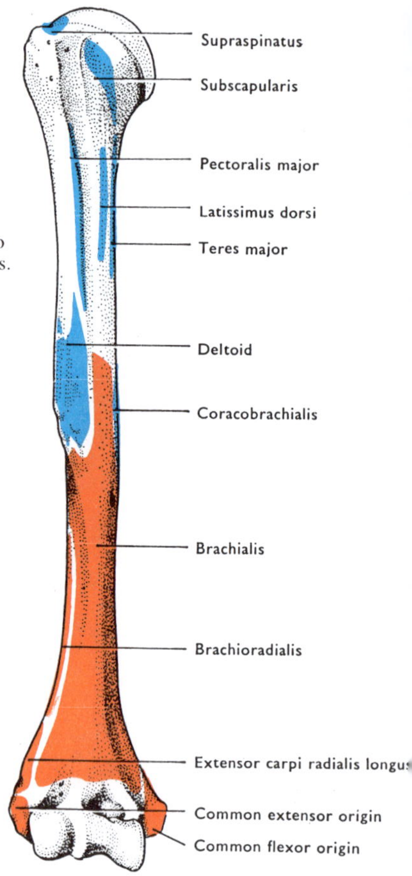

Fig. 230. Muscle attachments to anterior surface of right humerus.

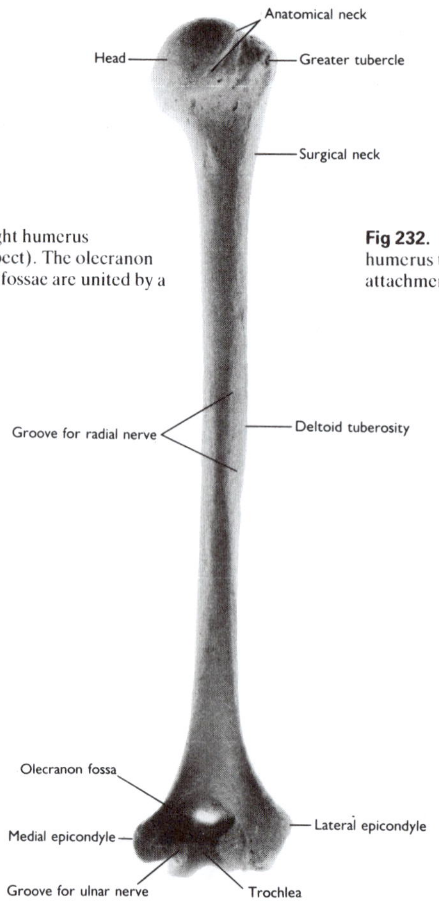

Fig. 231. Right humerus (posterior aspect). The olecranon and coronoid fossae are united by a foramen.

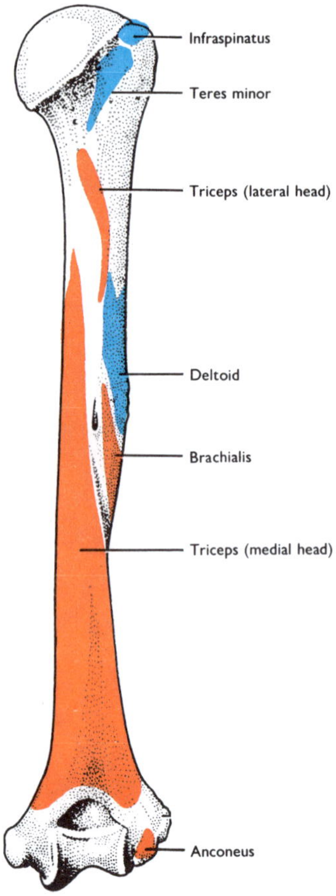

Fig 232. Posterior aspect of humerus to show muscle attachments.

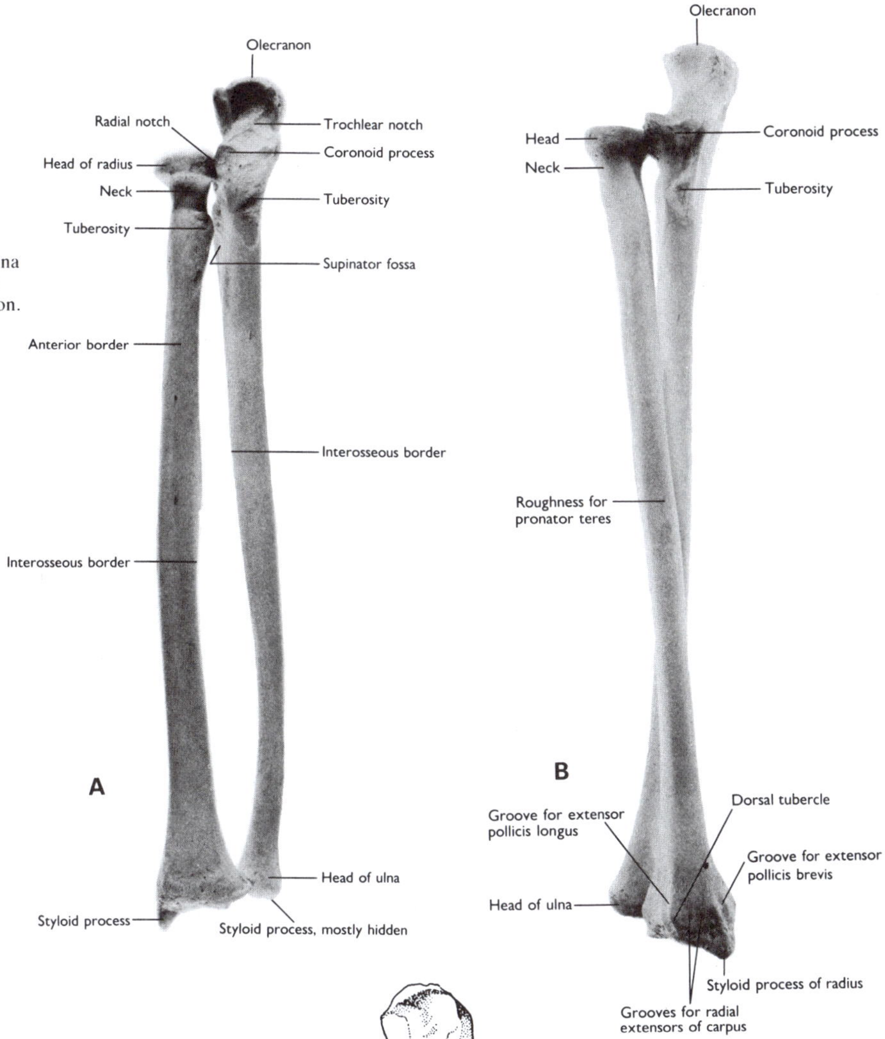

Fig. 233. Right radius and ulna (anterior aspect). (A) Supine position. (B) Pronated position.

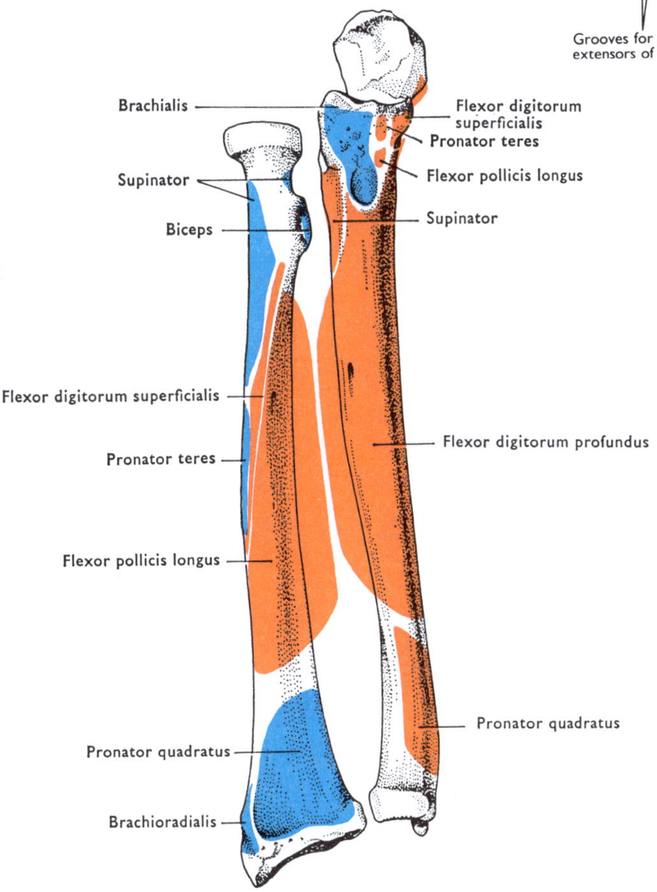

Fig. 234. Muscle attachments to anterior surface of right radius and ulna.

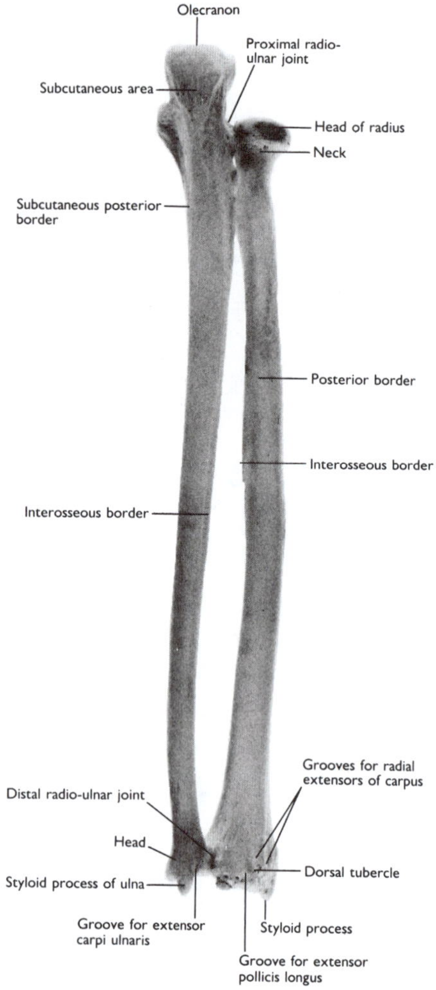

Fig. 235. Right radius and ulna (posterior surface).

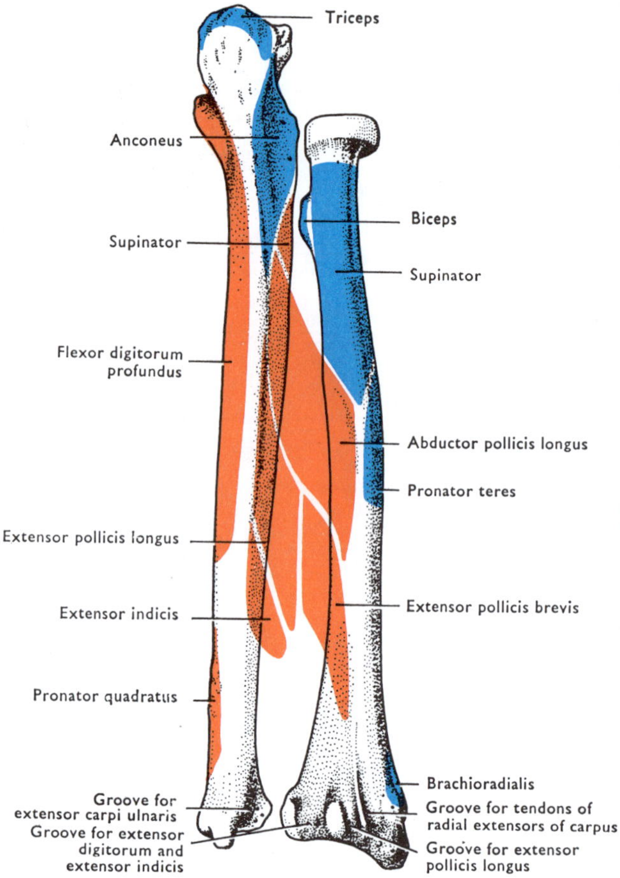

Fig. 236. Muscle attachments to posterior surface of right radius and ulna. The attachment of flexor carpi ulnaris to the posterior border of the ulna is not shown.

Fig. 237. Palmar aspect of bones of right hand.

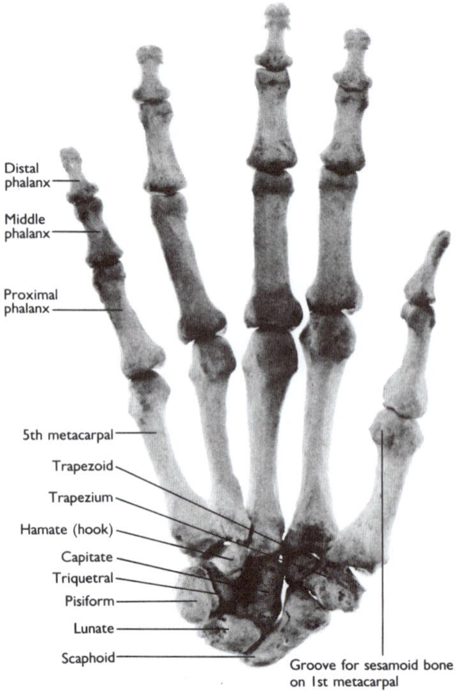

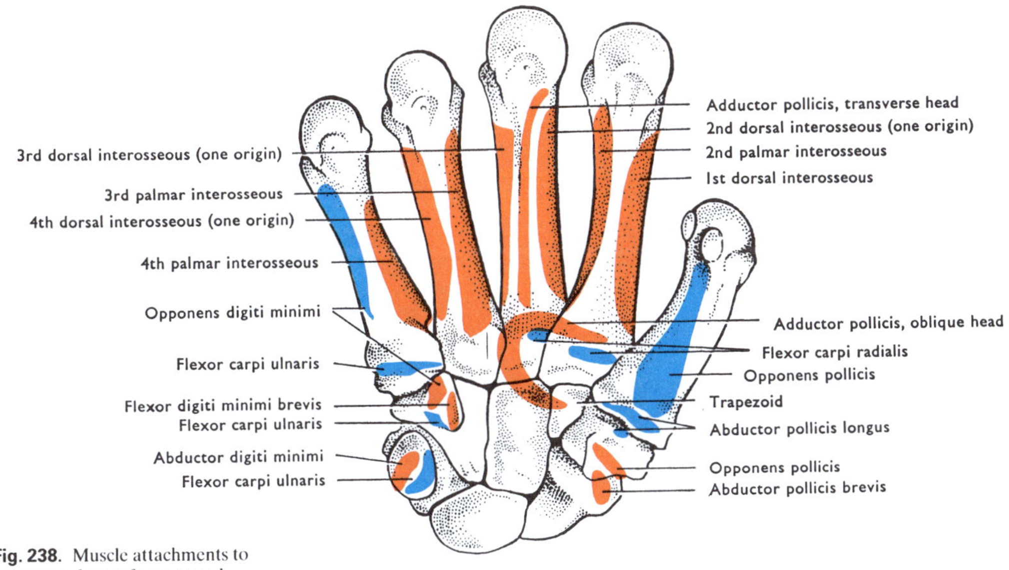

Fig. 238. Muscle attachments to palmar surfaces of carpus and metacarpus.

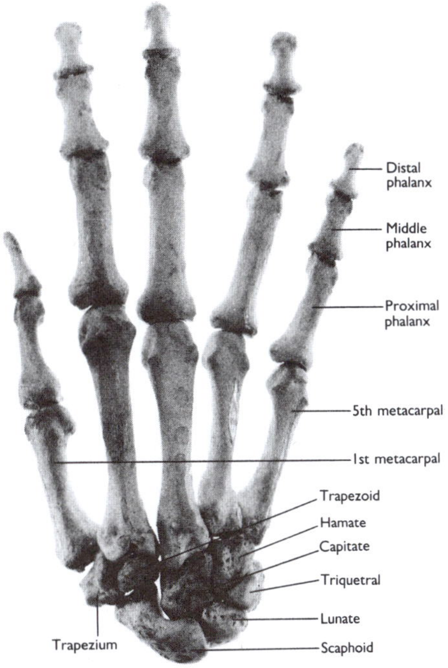

Fig. 239. Dorsal aspect of bones of right hand.

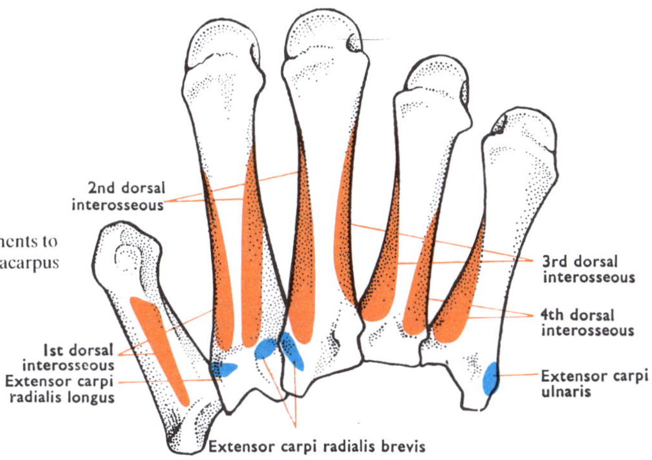

Fig. 240. Muscle attachments to dorsal aspect of right metacarpus

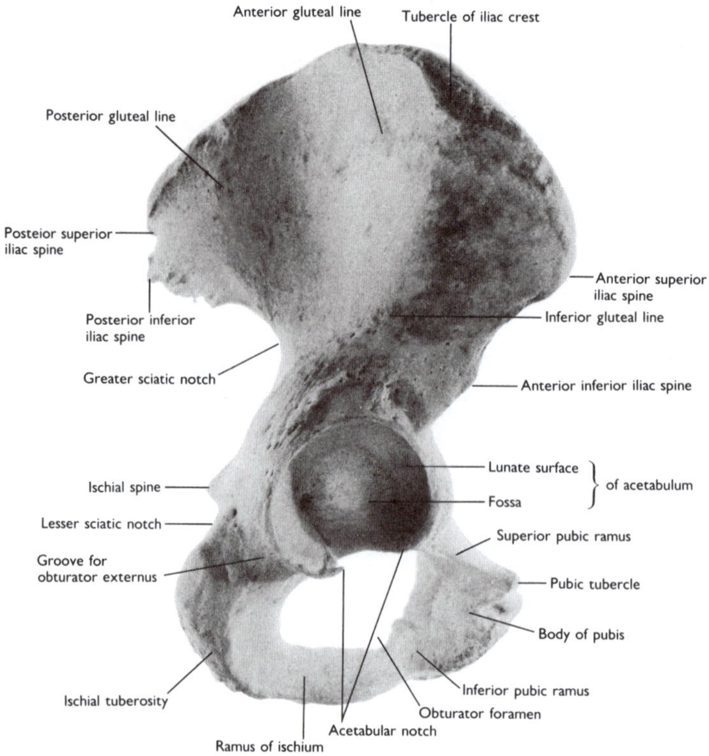

Fig. 241. Right hip bone seen from the lateral side.

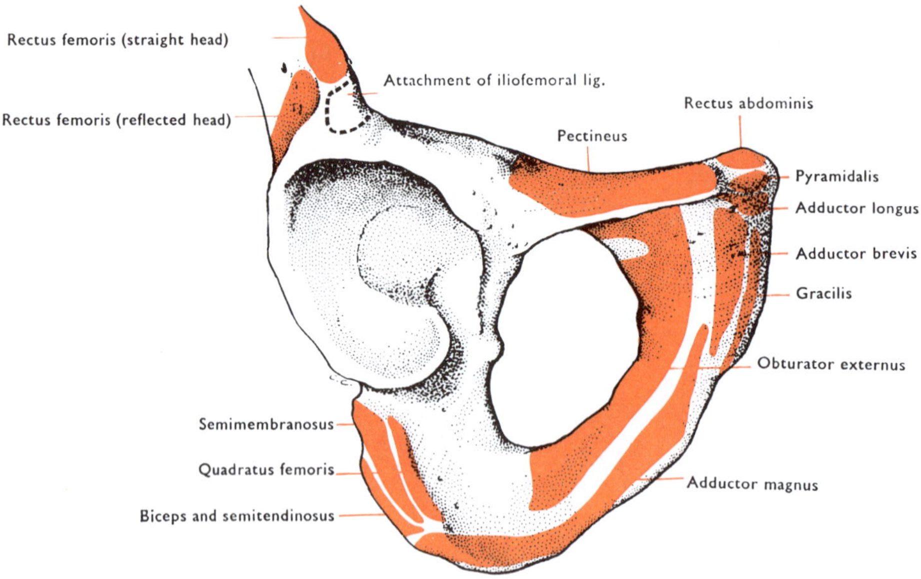

Fig. 242. Muscle attachments to outer surface of right pubis and ischium. The actual origin of the pectineus is not so extensive as shown; it arises from the upper part of the pectineal surface of the pubis and overlies the remainder.

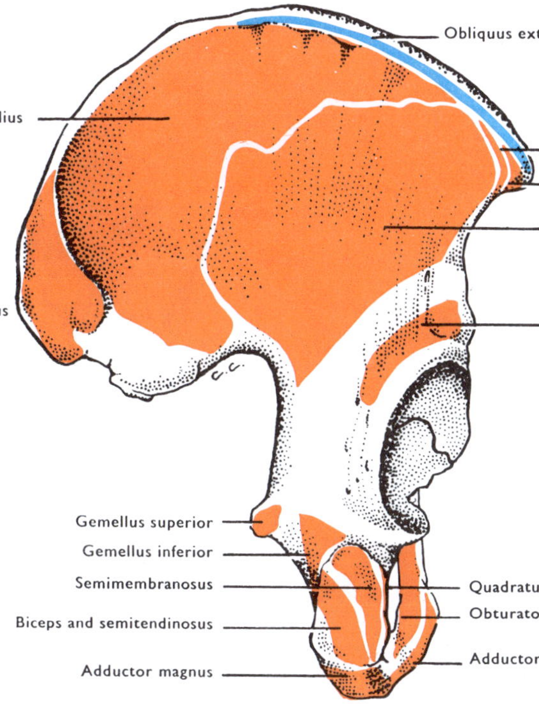

Fig. 243. Muscle attachments to outer surface of right hip bone.

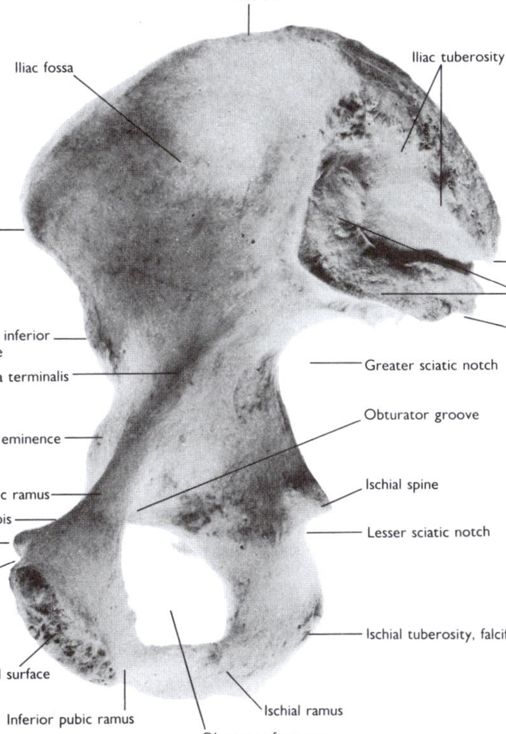

Fig. 244. Right hip bone seen from the medial side.

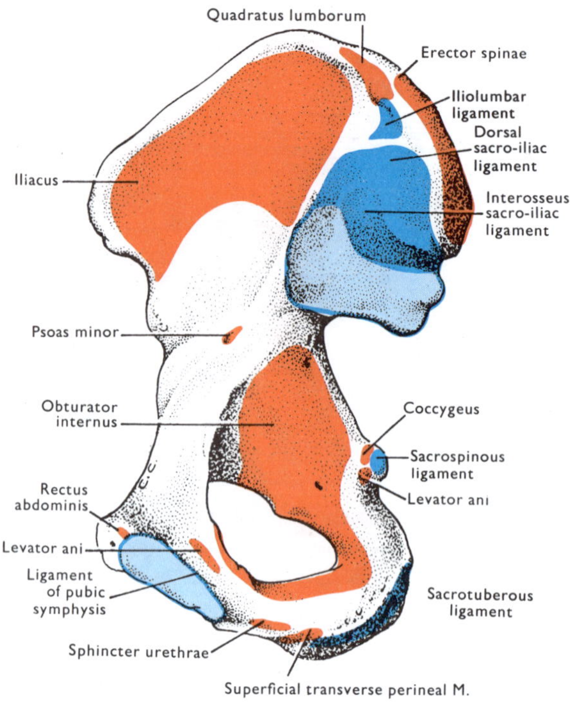

Fig. 245. The medial aspect of the right hip bone. Muscle attachments, red; ligamentous attachment and cartilage, blue.

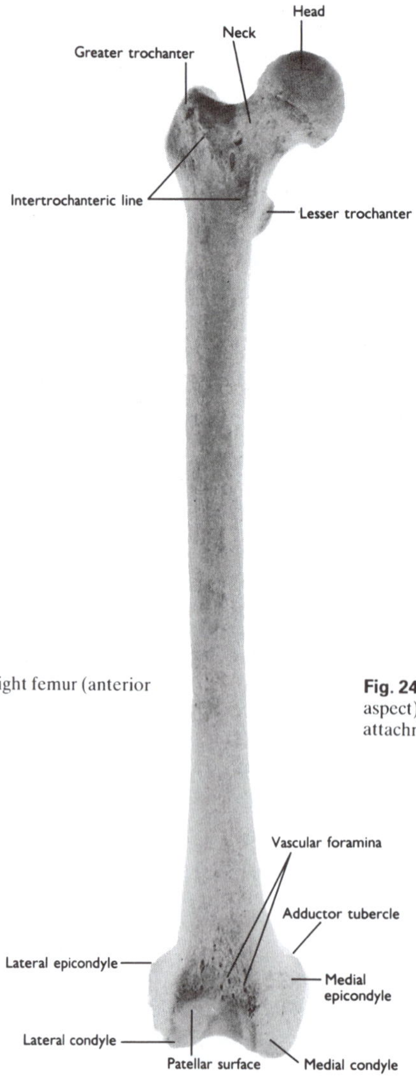

Fig. 246. Right femur (anterior aspect).

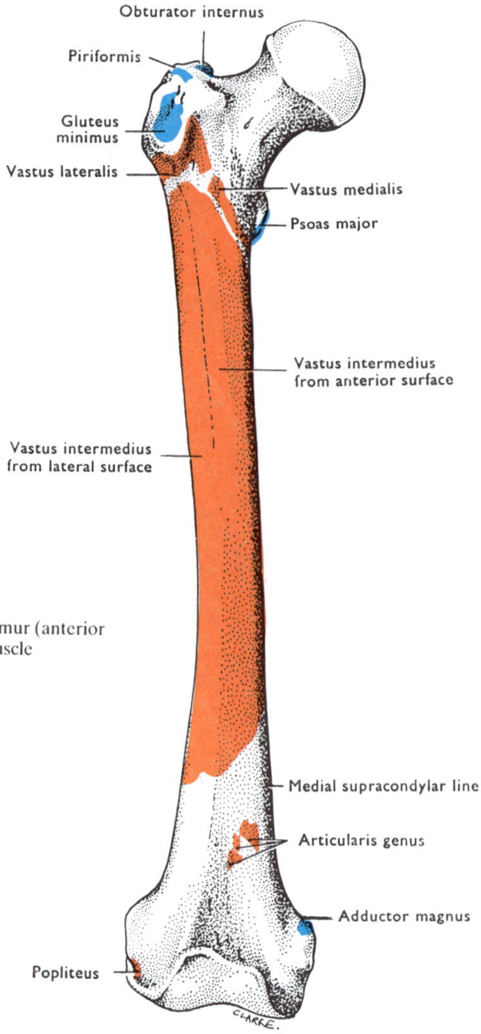

Fig. 247. Right femur (anterior aspect) to show muscle attachments.

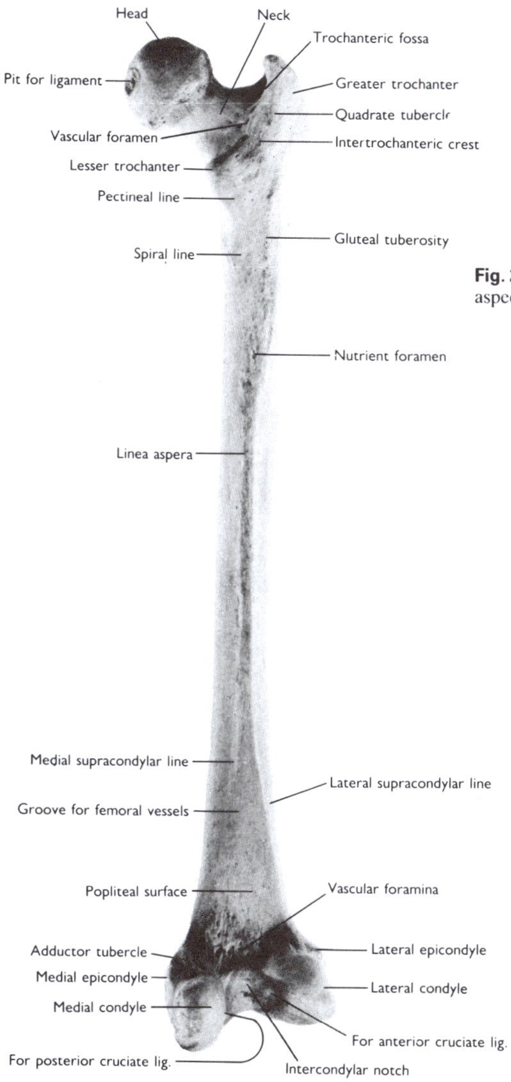

Fig. 248. Right femur (posterior aspect).

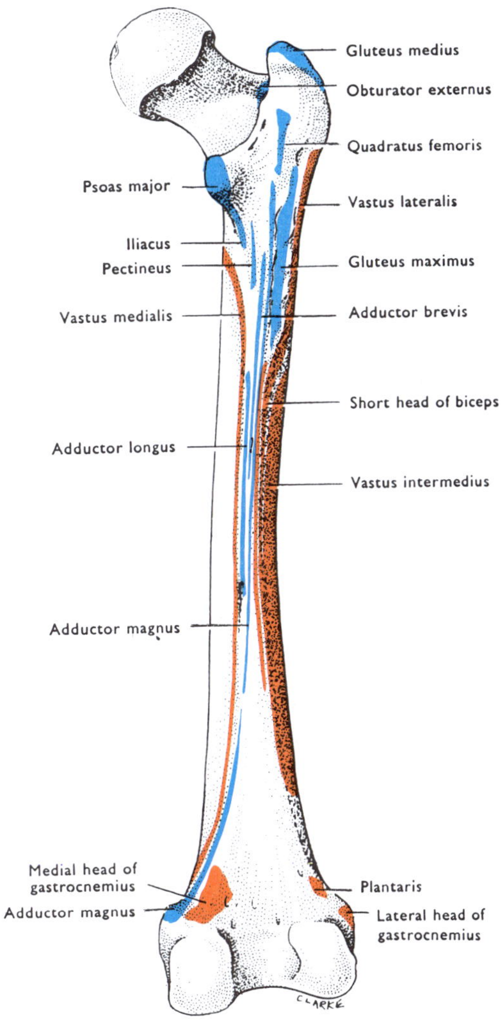

Fig. 249. Right femur (posterior aspect) to show muscle attachments.

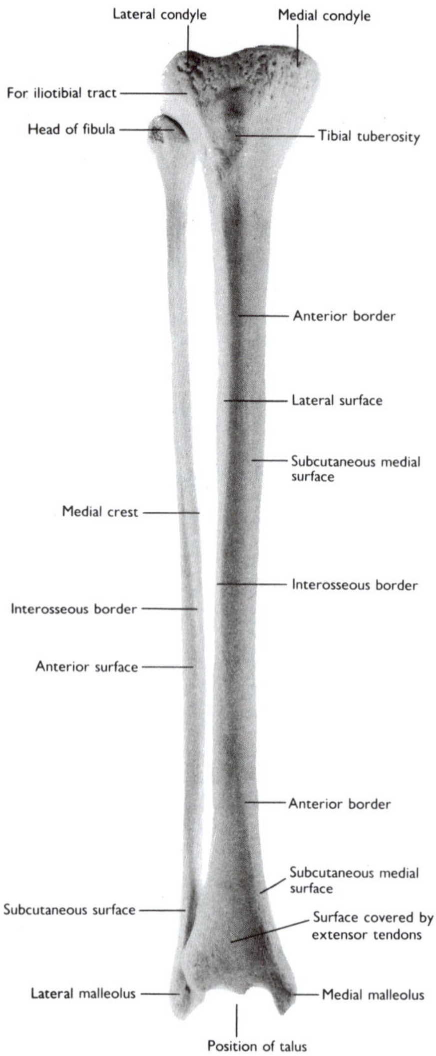

Fig. 250. Right tibia and fibula (anterior aspect).

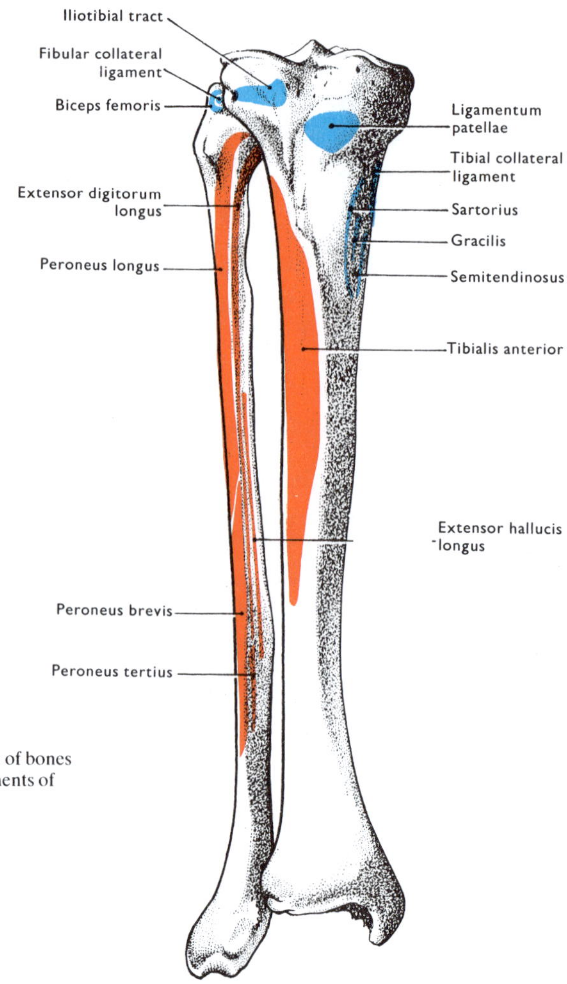

Fig. 251. Anterior aspect of bones of the leg to show attachments of muscles.

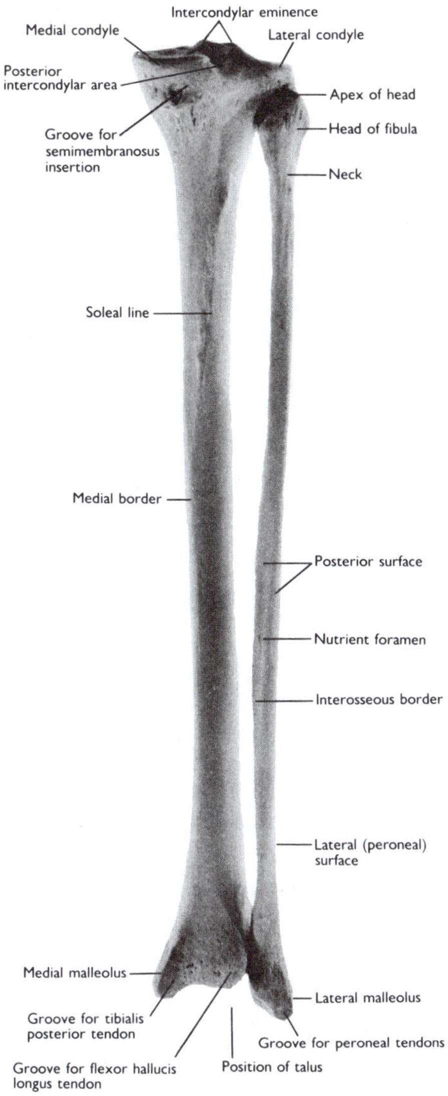

Fig. 252. Right tibia and fibula (posterior aspect).

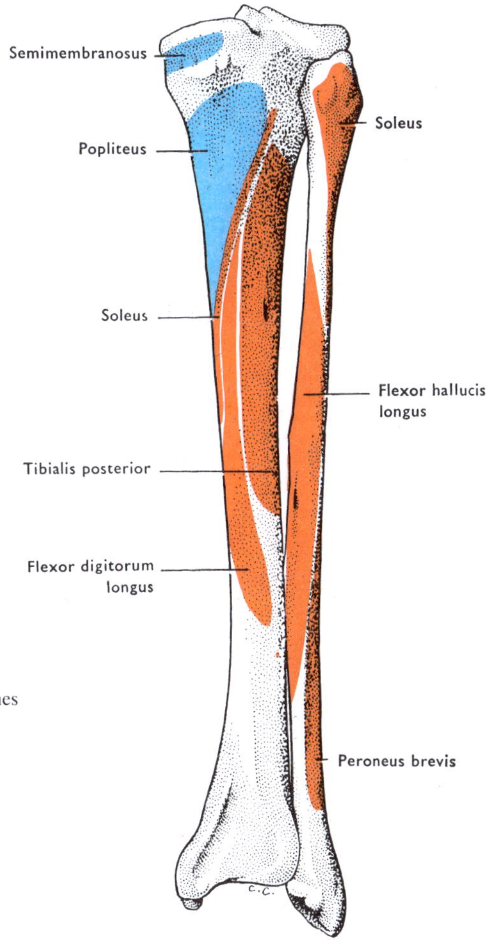

Fig. 253. Posterior aspect of bones of leg to show attachments of muscles.

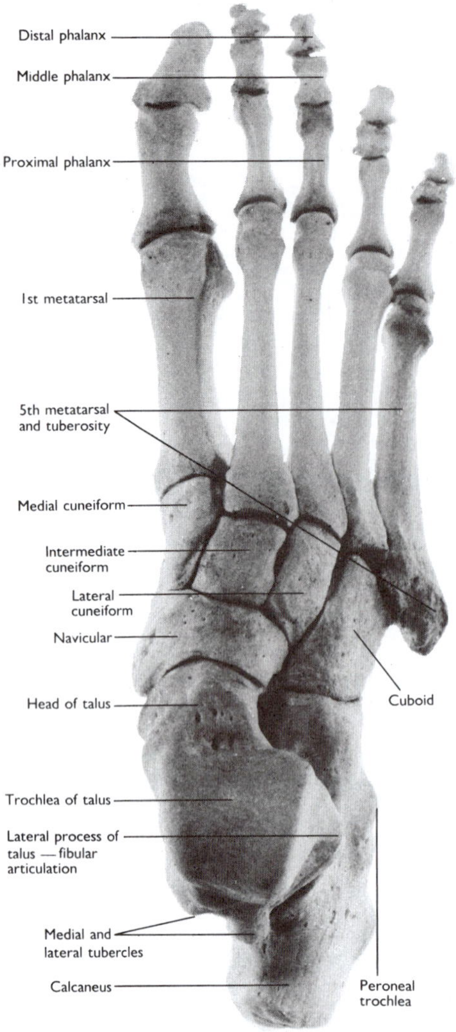

Fig. 254. Superior or dorsal surface of bones of right foot.

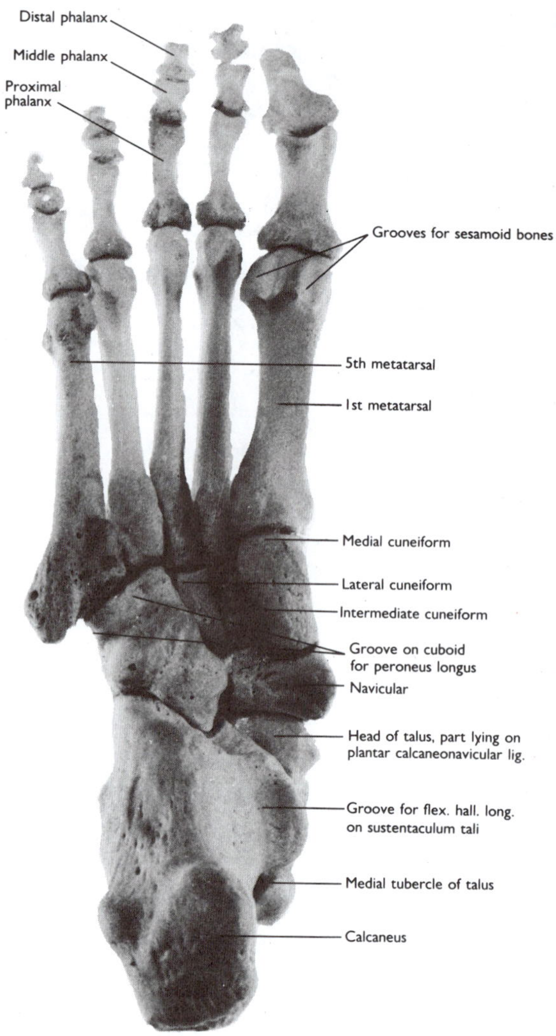

Fig. 255. Inferior or plantar surface of bones of right foot.

Fig. 256. Muscle attachments to left tarsus and metatarsus (plantar aspect).

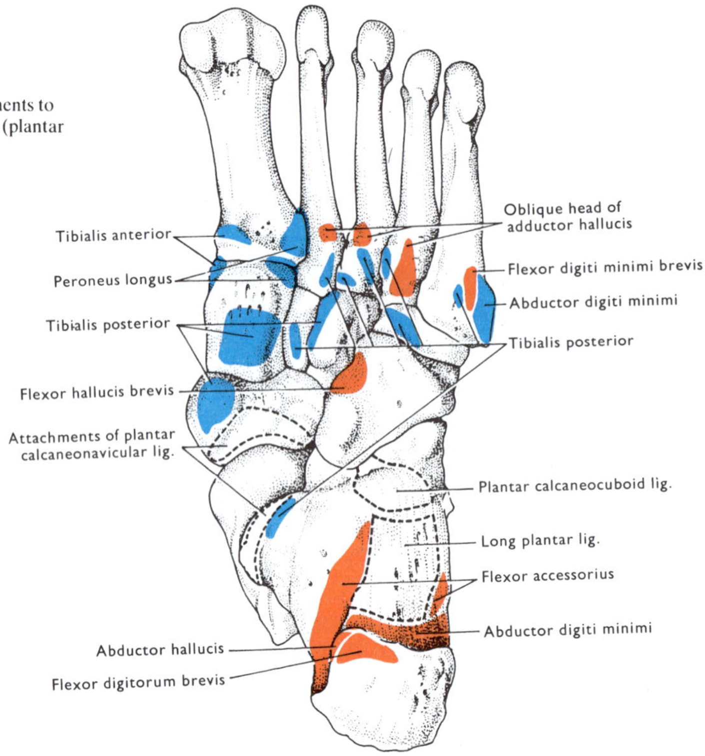

Index

This index contains references to the tables which have been introduced at the end of each of the sections, upper limb and lower limb. These tables give (1) the attachments, actions, and nerve supply of the various muscles of the limb grouped in relation to the joints which they move and the movements which they produce, and (2) the motor distribution of the main nerves of the limb and the paralyses which result from injuries to these nerves. Such page references appear in the index with an asterisk (e.g. Joints, shoulder, movements 116*). Page references are also given to illustrations (e.g. Phalanges, of fingers 20, 44, 113†). These entries are marked by a dagger. References to the main entries are in **bold** type.